LISTENING
TO YOUR
HORMONES

LISTENING
TO YOUR
HORMONES

GILLIAN FORD

PRIMA PUBLISHING

Library of Congress Cataloging-in-Publication Data

Ford, Gillian.
    Listening to your hormones: from PMS to menopause, every woman's complete guide / Gillian Ford.
       p.   cm.
    Includes bibliographical references and index.
    ISBN 0-7615-1002-8 (pbk.)
    1. Endocrine gynecology—Popular works.   2. Psychoneuroendocrinology—Popular works.   3. Hormone therapy—Popular works.   I. Title.
RG159.F67   1995
618.1—dc20   95-23405
                                                                          CIP

    98 99 00 DD 10 9 8 7 6 5 4
Printed in the United States of America

Those wishing to contact the author may call (916) 772-1681.

How to Order:
Single copies may be ordered from Prima Publishing, P.O. Box 1260BK, Rocklin, CA 95677; telephone (916) 632-4400. Quantity discounts are also available. On your letterhead, include information concerning the intended use of the books and the number of books you wish to purchase.

CONTENTS

ACKNOWLEDGMENTS

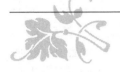

I would like to thank Marian Fritz, Katie Lynch, and Sandra Reeves for their invaluable help with my manuscript and for their friendship and support.

Special thanks to my husband, Dr. Desmond Ford, who has been consistently supportive of my venture to help women. An evangelist and teacher, he believes that mine is a real ministry—helping women with problems that can ruin their lives physically, emotionally, and spiritually.

I would like to pay tribute to Katharina Dalton, M.D., with whom I have corresponded since 1974. Her work spanning over 50 years is still considered controversial by many doctors, but thousands of women in Europe and the U.S. bless her name. Natural progesterone didn't help my PMS, but I have seen many women who found it a long-term cure. I know a number of doctors who have used progesterone on their patients with great success by following Dr. Dalton's directions.

Special personal thanks to psychologist Dr. Judith Bardwick (now an industrial consultant in San Diego, California). She wrote a classic book in 1970, called *The Psychology of Women*. In recommending estrogen for depression, it certainly saved my life. The seeds of many of the ideas on which I built my subsequent work were in her chapter on the physiology of women. Without her book, I couldn't have written mine. Dr. Bardwick was 25 years ahead of her time in pointing out the link between hormones and psychological states, and the beneficial effects of estrogen on the mind. She also risked the disapproval of her peers and met a great deal of opposition in taking her stand.

I would also like to thank John Studd, M.D., a research physician in Britain, who is vehemently opposed to the use of natural progesterone for PMS, but is nonetheless a strong voice supporting the use of estrogen for depression. He was introduced to estrogen implant surgery by Robert Greenblatt, M.D., a wonderful pioneer in hormone work, with a charismatic personality. Dr. Studd trained, among thousands of others, my friend Gordon Campbell, M.D., an OB/GYN (specialist in obstetrics and gynecology) in Australia. Gordon gave me my first estrogen implant—oh, instant bliss!

I would also like to thank the doctors with whom I have worked more closely on a practical level. First, Dr. Myrtle Caton, a board-certified internist, who took an interest in my problems and came with me to hear Dr. Katharina Dalton speak in San Francisco in 1982. This meeting inspired Myrtle to specialize in treating PMS and postpartum depression. She sent me to train as a PMS counselor at PMS Action in Wisconsin that same year, and together we set out to help women with hormonal problems. And we did! Through the years, even when sickness forced her to close her practice, she remained a pivotal support for me and my work.

I would also like to thank Lee Vliet, M.D., whose acquaintance I made at the North American Menopause Society Conference in 1982. She gave an excellent presentation there on estrogen and depression. I thought it was the highlight of the meetings, and realized that I had found a soul mate. We made contact and have since worked together on several projects. Lee is a national pioneer in women's health issues and an expert in hormone replacement therapy (HRT). She is the author of *Screaming to be Heard* (see Foreword), and we look forward to future collaboration in writing projects.

Thanks to Richard Wilkinson, M.D., for his generous help. He virtually dictated the chapter on multiple chemical sensitivities (MCS) to me. I saw the need for this chapter because I have been contacted by many women with MCS and chronic fatigue syndrome, complicated by hormonal swings. I asked Rick to help me with it since this was his expertise. Also, a presentation by Rick on testosterone replacement for men was the foundation and backbone of my chapters on androgens.

Thanks to Dr. Norman Beals, Jr., a retired physician. His father, Norman Beals, Sr., M.D., was a hormone expert before him. Together, they worked for 60 years to help women with severe hormonal problems. Norman's father was a close friend of Robert Greenblatt, M.D., and Norman cherishes the memories of his time as an intern working closely with Dr. Greenblatt. His tremendous influence is still felt among his students today (Don Gambrell, M.D., Penny Wise Budoff, M.D., and Lila Nachtigall, M.D., among many others). Dr. Beals has read my manuscript many times and provided invaluable advice, especially on the testosterone chapters.

Thanks to Philip Warner, M.D., Kathryn Morris, M.D., Denise Mark, M.D., also good friends, who read parts of the manuscript and generously contributed quotes and information.

I have also particularly appreciated working in association with Drs. Mike Jones, Philip Weaver, Byron Lake and his wife Neva Monigatti-Lake, Susan Shapiro, Linda Foshagen, Zane Kime, Gio Morino, Glenn Enochian, and Louis Hertz. I have worked with many physicians, but I owe the ones I have mentioned a special debt.

FOREWORD

Courage, persistence, intuition, inquisitiveness, and ability to listen to women's experiences—these are the qualities which Gillian Ford brings to her work as a PMS and menopause educator, counselor, and writer. As a physician and a women's health advocate for my entire medical career, I have found Gillian to be a valuable colleague in advancing the awareness of these hormonal connections in a variety of clinical problems women experience. I have recommended her previous books to my patients, who have been grateful for the "black and white" validation of their questions and observations.

Women do have a remarkable ability to be in tune with their bodies and to observe connections that physicians and health professionals simply must begin taking more seriously. Gill has been one of the few voices speaking out for women with hormonal components to their health problems, and has, for many years, been a tireless advocate for these issues to be more effectively addressed by the medical community.

The remarkable aspect of working with Gillian Ford is that she is a self-taught layperson. Her unique perspective as a woman who has herself suffered with unrecognized hormonally triggered health problems has added to the passion and compassion with which she speaks on these subjects. It is impressive to find that the scope of her knowledge and understanding of complex hormonal relationships exceeds that of the majority of physicians—even those who specialize in endocrinology. She has painstakingly researched the available medical information to provide women with a synthesis of what is known about these crucial links. I have not found a *medical* textbook which addresses these issues in such a comprehensive manner.

Women who have had difficulties with PMS, postpartum depression, autoimmune disorders, thyroid problems, multiple chemical sensitivities, candida, and many other similar health concerns will find that Gillian provides insights into possible hormonal links which many of us have suspected but which traditional research has overlooked. She and

I have each addressed these connections in our respective books, although from slightly different perspectives. You will find some areas in which we each have a unique point of view, yet our overall explanations and philosophies are quite similar.

Although she and I did not meet in person until 1992—and prior to that we had been working on opposite coasts—she and I have had parallel tracks with our career interests in the important neuroendocrine phenomena women experience. Over the years, both of us have encountered lack of interest or concern about these problems by physicians and researchers. It has been rewarding, personally and professionally, for us now to be collaborating to bring this information to a broader audience and to improve the delivery of healthcare for women of all ages. The current surge of interest in menopause has facilitated increased attention being paid to women's long-standing observations that the brain and the body are affected by hormonal shifts. *Listening to Your Hormones* has updated and expanded references and is a reflection of this expanding field of research and clinical attention to the nuances of hormonal factors.

I encourage women of all ages to read *Listening to Your Hormones*. Then pass it on to your physicians, your daughters, and your friends. It may save you many dollars in fruitless therapies which are not directed to the underlying hormonal needs, and it certainly will help you find innovative ways of improving your *quality* of life. If you are a woman who has ever experienced the agony of premenstrual or postpartum suicidal thoughts, the important connections Gillian Ford has made in this book may even save your life.

—Elizabeth Lee Vliet, M.D., May 1995, Tucson, Arizona

Author, *Screaming to Be Heard: Hormonal Connections Women Suspect . . . and Doctors Ignore* (New York: M. Evans, 1995).

Founder, HER Place: The Women's Center for Health Enhancement and Renewal, Inc., at All Saints Center for Women's Health Fort Worth, Texas, and Tucson, Arizona.

Clinical Associate Professor, Department of Family and Community Medicine, University of Arizona College of Medicine.

INTRODUCTION

Many women know instinctively that they have hormonal problems, because they "listen" to their hormones. I find that women are very intuitive, and most of them know exactly what is happening to their bodies. They know that their problem is hormonal. But when they go to find help, too often the doctor doesn't listen and tells them that their instincts are all wrong.

This book is all about hormones. Why are they important? Is it safe to take hormones? Can hormone therapy help you? What happens when hormone replacement doesn't work properly? Which types of hormone replacement are most natural? How do you know what you need? What are the best ways to take hormones?

First of all, you need to know that hormones have very important functions in your body. The hormones that are needed to create new life—estrogen, progesterone, thyroid, and testosterone—are also extremely important for maintaining your own health. This is why, when women's estrogen and progesterone levels drop, they risk increased heart disease, gradual deterioration of the skeleton, and, potentially, similar degeneration in every part of their body.

HORMONES AFFECT MOODS

The same principle also applies to one's emotional life. Estrogen, in particular, acts in women as a mood elevator and is responsible for a feeling of well-being and joyfulness. Natural progesterone (so called to distinguish it from synthetic progestins) and thyroid also contribute to emotional health. When one or more of these hormones recede (this can happen when women are quite young), women may feel dreadful and experience all sorts of physical and emotional symptoms. Too often, the roles of these hormones are belittled, overlooked, or ignored. Many women spend years trudging from doctor to doctor to find help for what could often be simply resolved with the right hormone replacement therapy (HRT).

Other authors have written about premenstrual syndrome (PMS), menopause, postpartum depression, and low thyroid problems (hypothyroidism) as isolated disorders. But I find that these problems often occur together. As a result, I decided to write this book showing these links.

MY OWN STORY

I also wanted to write this book because of my own experience with severe PMS and hypothyroidism in my teens and twenties, my entry into premature menopause at age 37, my hysterectomy in late 1995, and the experiences I have had over the past 14 years as a PMS and menopause counselor. I would like to explain the circumstances in some detail to show how difficult my problems were, and how hard it was to find any help.

My Mother and Sister

I inherited problems with PMS; my mother and sister both had severe PMS. My mother had terrible monthly migraines, and, long after menopause, still gets them cyclically. Because she had a hysterectomy in her early forties and because she smoked for 60 years, my mother, who is now 85, has osteoporosis.

My only sister had severe PMS and says there were times when she was afraid to go out in the car because she was tempted to kill herself. She once broke an entire set of china throwing it at the dining room wall. She and I have lived in different countries since our twenties and saw little of each other until recent years. Her husband told me that each month he had to beg her not to kill herself. She and I went through essentially the same problems with PMS and major depression. She has also had a hysterectomy.

Both my mother and my sister had goiters and had surgery on their thyroid glands, though neither of them was given thyroid medication.

Going Through Puberty

I started having PMS at age 13 when I started menstruating. But even as a child, I was moody and experienced a lot of fatigue. The first symptom I recall began at age 11, when I went with my family on vacation. Traveling around the beautiful Devon countryside in England by car, I slept in the back almost the whole three weeks. I was like a bear in hibernation, difficult to wake up when they stopped to see something. As soon as they would let me, I would instantly fall asleep again. It could have been mononucleosis, but there were no viral symptoms—just the exhaustion. Or perhaps it was the imminent onset of menstruation or borderline hypothyroidism that began the fatigue that plagued me much of my adult life.

Sleeping Through My Teens

In my teens, I could easily sleep until noon. I struggled through the afternoon, feeling as though I could sink through the floor with fatigue. I was a night person and felt very energetic around 8:00 at night, but the next morning I woke up feeling as though I had a hangover. I also felt the cold deep in my bones. I was unable to sleep at night unless I had a hot-water bottle or an electric blanket. Without one or the other, I would wake up in the night shivering. I had dry skin that chafed easily, and my eyelashes frequently fell out. I had these symptoms of low thyroid all my life, though my tests were always normal until it was discovered in my mid-forties that I had thyroiditis.

From the time I started my periods, they were extremely regular—25 days each month for 13 years until age 26, when they became irregular because of stress. I never missed one period until they stopped in my forties. My periods were light to moderate, and I had occasional minor cramping. My problems with PMS started at puberty and lasted, at the beginning, about four days a month. Four days may seem short, but while it lasted the sudden drop in mood was intense and frightening. I felt as though my emotions fell off a cliff, and the suddenness and violence of the change frightened me. I first went to a physician for PMT (premenstrual tension, as it was called then) in 1961. I was 17 and living in New Zealand at the time. The doctor gave me Valium, but I decided not to take it because I didn't like the idea of being tranquilized.

Going to College and Getting Married

I went to a private college for five years, from age 21 to 26. I was responsible for my own financial support the whole time. I remember my constant struggle with chronic fatigue while there. The last two years of my stay were especially difficult, because I was an assistant dean of women and had to stay up late to lock the doors. I found it hard to stay awake late (even though, for much of the rest of my life, I have had most of my energy at night).

I met my future husband, Des, while at college. He was my religion teacher, and I became his secretary for a year. He was married to a wonderful woman, Gwen, who was dying from breast and bone cancer. About a year and a half before her death, Gwen and Des discussed the possibility of his getting to know me better, if I was interested, with a view to marrying me later. This may seem strange, but it's not unusual for dying women to let their husbands know they want them to remarry, partly to provide for their children. Gwen was a very sane, unselfish person, and it was in character that she would initiate this.

Gwen felt that, because Des was a public figure, we would not have a chance to get to know each other after her death. She also wanted him to marry as soon as possible because there were three children and one was only three years old at the time. So, Gwen, Des, and I spent many hours together. Gwen was in a wheelchair, and we covered hundreds of miles on pleasant walks.

It must have been a very hard situation for Gwen to be so sick and to know that her life would shortly end and another would take her place. But you would never have known it. She treated me like a beloved sister. During her last three years, she weighed only 60 pounds. Her patience and humor lasted right to the end when, after years of dreadful suffering, she died radiantly.

Gwen's passing was a terrible loss, particularly for her two older children. She was a mature Christian, able to look beyond her present problems, but the children took her death very hard. It seemed so unjust to them because Gwen was a loving, kind, patient, and guileless person, with no enemies. She wouldn't hurt a fly, and yet she suffered terribly.

Gwen died in April of 1970, and I graduated from college in November of that year. A month before my graduation, Des received a request to go to Manchester University in England to complete a second Ph.D. I told my parents that I was getting married, and then worked on completing my exams. I had taken all my major subjects in my last two years and was practice-teaching that last year. We had to get passports and make all the other arrangements necessary for such a trip, and I had to graduate. I married at 7:00 A.M. on the morning I graduated, and Des and I went away for a few days' honeymoon. A week later, Des's youngest child returned home after living with friends for a year, and that night we all left for England.

The Birth Control Pill and How It Made Me Worse

I tell you all of this so you can understand that I was under a lot of stress. In the months before I married, the stress affected my periods. They suddenly became irregular—nothing drastic: 23 days, 21 days, and 19 days. But I had been as regular as clockwork (25-day cycles) for 13 years, and I thought there was something wrong. I didn't realize that the stress of my circumstances was causing the changes. I also didn't know that most women's periods weren't as regular as mine. Had I known, I wouldn't have worried about this slight irregularity. But because I didn't know, when I went to my doctor for a premarital checkup, I told her about the irregularity and she suggested that I go on the birth control pill.

Before I married, I did have a couple of premenstrual upsets, but Des attributed my emotionality to the stress I was under. There is no doubt that birth control pills made me much worse. During our trip to England, Des and I had our first real argument. The following day, I started my period. This cycle of argument and resolution was the pattern for the following years. I stayed on the birth control pill for about three months. Then, because I realized that it was making me continually depressed, I went off the pill and all hell seemed to break loose. My cycles changed completely and, from then on, they were rarely 28 days, and usually well over 30 days, apart. I started having problems for at least two-and-a-half weeks during the second half of the cycle, and sometimes for as long as a month.

How My Symptoms Changed

I found that my symptoms started, like clockwork, every twelfth day of the cycle. Beginning in puberty, I had always known when I ovulated because I had pain on the right side of my navel each twelfth day of the cycle. This timing of ovulation remained the same after I went off the birth control pill, even if I didn't bleed until the thirty-ninth day. Once I ovulated, I began my symptoms, and they would worsen until I began my period. The longer the cycle was, the longer my symptoms lasted, and the more intense they became. But as soon as I began to bleed, the symptoms completely disappeared as though a veil had been lifted, and I felt perfectly normal for 12 days.

Some women have worse PMS every second or third cycle, depending on which side they ovulate. My symptoms were always bad, though worse during longer cycles. The pattern of symptoms was predictable. On day 12, I would feel a sudden change, as though someone had thrown a switch in my body, and I began to feel the symptoms come on. First, I became extremely irritable. Within a day or two, I became exhausted. Then I went into a gradually deepening depression and withdrew into sullen silences, punctuated by sudden uncontrollable outbursts of anger. I could never tell when these were going to happen, and ended up retreating into my bedroom for hours and days at a time. I would shut myself away from my family because I felt violent, and I was afraid of what I might do or say. I became very volatile and angry. My skin, which had always been very clear, became riddled with acne after being on birth control pills. Just before my period, I felt emotionally as though I was about to fall off a cliff, and I became extremely suicidal. I also started to have severe cramps for the first three days of my period. I'd had minor cramps before, but nothing like this. Nothing seemed to take the pain away.

But every month, as soon as I began to bleed and cramp, I felt instant emotional relief. Then I had 11 good days (apart from the three days of cramps). I felt my normal, happy self at that time. Looking back, I feel that something "broke down" in me, because of taking birth control pills, which has never been permanently resolved. I take hormones, and they make a tremendous difference, but, if I go off them I quickly regress emotionally and physically. At this time, I was on a vegetarian diet and running several miles a day. I was doing everything I knew to be right, but nothing helped.

Every Month Was Hell

Going through this experience each month was like living on an unpredictable seesaw. My husband, with typical male logic, said to me, "Why can't you decide in the good part of the month how you will behave in the bad part?" I told him that if I always felt like I did in the good 11 days, I would have no conception of what the other part was like. I felt as though I was in a watertight compartment during the bad days, unable to imagine that I ever had any good days. It was like finding myself in the path of a huge tidal wave, or a battalion of marines; I was defenseless, totally unable to respond normally or to pull myself out of the depression.

My husband thought my behavior was a reflection of my personality—that I had hidden this side of my nature prior to marriage and was now revealing it. As for me, I didn't really know what was happening, and I was terribly confused. Inside I felt like a trapped animal, and the thought that this was going to keep coming back filled me with panic. I couldn't control my feelings or my behavior, and I felt terrified and guilty.

How PMS Undermined My Self-Worth

It's very difficult to explain what PMS is like to someone who doesn't have it, but it is devastating to one's feelings of self-worth. You constantly ask yourself, "Who am I? Am I the nice person who emerges at the onset of my period for 11 or 12 days, or am I the cyclical bitch?" When you take a vote on yourself and the bad days drastically outweigh the good, it is very difficult to believe that you have much value. This experience in my mid-to-late twenties was very different from the one I had at age 17, when the PMT lasted only four days each cycle. In my twenties, the problems lasted so long in the cycle (up to 27 days before my period), that I could hardly think of it as premenstrual.

I started to question my marriage. I had thought that God had led me into marriage, and that I had done the right thing taking on the family, and suddenly it seemed like a disaster. I felt terrible that I was making everyone miserable when inside I wanted to be part of their healing. I did recognize that it had something to do with my menstrual cycle, but when I started visiting doctors, none of them believed that the problem was hormonal. All I knew was that it occurred between ovulation and menstruation, and I realized that the birth control pill was a large factor in my change of personality.

Searching for Causes of Pain

While we were in England, from 1970 to 1972, I began trying to get medical help. I had a recurrent pain mid-cycle on my right side. It was only mittelschmerz (pain at ovulation), as I found out later, but at the time I thought it might indicate a problem that could be the cause of my PMS. I kept going to doctors looking for the source of the pain. Maybe it had something to do with my emotional problems.

A couple of doctors thought that I might have appendicitis, and I went into the hospital to be checked, but that diagnosis was ruled out. The surgeon sent me to a psychiatrist who told me that there was nothing wrong with me, and that I needed to learn to like myself. Later I had surgery, supposedly for polycystic ovaries. Doctors I visited later challenged this diagnosis. They said that I didn't have the symptoms of polycystic ovaries; I was extremely thin, had periods every month, and had no male hair pattern on my body. The surgery, supposedly a wedge resection for one of my ovaries, didn't help my PMS symptoms at all; they returned immediately to my great disappointment. Twelve years later, I had triple surgery for massive adhesions—a result of the surgery in 1970 which, I feel on looking back, was totally unnecessary. Another 13 years later, I had an even more extensive surgery for adhesions at the time of my hysterectomy and oophoroectomy. Adhesions, unfortunately, tend to reform.

Given Heavy Medication

After we returned from England to Australia, I continued trying to find relief during the years from 1972 to 1977. We moved to the United States in 1977, and I continued my search here, alternating mainly among internists, gynecologists, and psychiatrists. Since I came from a family with a history of depression, it was probably understandable that much of the treatment I received grew out of the assumption that I had biologically based depression. I was also told that I was manic-depressive.

My second encounter with a psychiatrist was in Australia when we returned from England in 1972. This psychiatrist,

Dr. P., told me that I was transferring anger from my father to my husband. He put me in a private mental facility for a month to stabilize me on Parstellin, which was a combination of an antidepressant (which carries certain food restrictions) and a major tranquilizer. The medication seemed to help during the first cycle, but not afterward. Still, I continued taking it for about eight months. Then, by accident, I ate the wrong food (a raw fava bean out of my garden), and had an immediate and violent heart reaction. My blood pressure fluctuated wildly—first soaring high, then low—and I felt like I was dying. At that time, I was grateful for this adverse reaction. I thought it was God's way of taking me away from all my troubles. But I didn't die. I just had to go cold turkey off the Parstellin, which made me feel even worse.

Subsequently, I went on a series of medications—Valium, Librium, Tofranil (imipramine hydrochloride), Norpramin (desipramine hydrochloride), Pamelor (nortriptyline hydrochloride), and Elavil (amitriptyline hydrochloride). None of this medication helped my depression. In fact, some of it made me worse—more nervous, more anxious, more phobic. I often woke up in the night terrified. During those years in Australia, when I was on medication and my depression would get out of control, a local doctor friend would occasionally put me in a private hospital overnight. These were the most difficult years of my life.

No One Called It PMS

I found that the majority of doctors I visited weren't really listening as I recited what was happening to me. They never recognized that there was a hormonal connection. I was told by one psychiatrist (I visited six through the years) that my problems were continual, not cyclical as I thought. He said my problems were connected to the stresses of early childhood and the circumstances of my marriage, and that I was being stubborn and not facing facts. I would go home and think about what he said, but I knew it wasn't correct. Whenever I asked questions or didn't agree with the doctors' conclusions, I was told that I was being stubborn.

Over the years, I have learned that PMS is a disease that drops between the cracks that separate medical specialties. Most doctors would treat the individual symptoms—headaches, depression, skin problems, heart arrhythmias, seizures, bronchial problems, etc.—and miss the common thread: the hormonal imbalance. A family physician might send a woman with PMS to an OB/GYN. He might put her on the pill, (which landed me in trouble in the first place), give her a tranquilizer, or (as in my case) look for something that needs surgery. Frequently, women treated for the individual symptoms of PMS become treatment failures because the basic problem is hormonal.

If a woman mentioned that she was suicidal, as I was for years, the OB/GYN (trained mainly in surgery and obstetrics) might take fright and send her to either a psychologist or a psychiatrist. The psychologist would want to know about her early childhood, and the psychiatrist would treat her with psychotropic drugs. I have rarely met a psychiatrist who will acknowledge that there is such a thing as hormonal depression. It has always seemed to me that PMS is an endocrine problem, and that endocrinologists are the logical physicians to treat it. But in fact they generally don't, because they are so blood-test oriented, and very little that is abnormal shows up in the hormones of a young woman with PMS.

The First Gleams of Light

I was living in Australia in 1974 when I received my first gleam of hope in the form of three books that I read within months of each other.

The first book was called *The Pill on Trial*, written by Paul Vaughan, a medical journalist for the British Medical Association, and published by Penguin in 1970. Vaughan wrote a section on women who became temporarily psychotic because of their extreme sensitivity to the synthetic progestin in birth control pills.

Shortly after reading this, I mentioned it to a friend who was a physiology teacher, and told her I that knew my problems had something to do with my periods. She lent me *The Menstrual Cycle*, by Katherina Dalton, M.D. My friend used the book as a textfor teaching about the process of menstruation. But it was really a book about PMS, and it described my problem exactly. When I read the case histories in that book, it was like reading about myself. At last, my problem had a name: premenstrual syndrome. I now knew that many other women had been through the same experience.

Within weeks, another science teacher at the college where my husband taught referred me to *The Psychology of Women*, which had just come into the college library. It was a book on women's sexuality, written by Dr. Judith Bardwick, an American psychologist. Dr. Bardwick's book was not about PMS, but it contained a chapter on women's physiology which explained how the menstrual cycle worked and the role of the birth control pill in producing depression. She showed, using research evidence, that a woman's mood is universally at its highest just before ovulation when the estrogen is high and progesterone is absent, and lowest premenstrually when both estrogen and progesterone are low. These books confirmed my instinctive belief that my problem was basically hormonal and connected with taking birth control pills—even though the differences of opinion about estrogen and progesterone were initially confusing.

Back in the seventies, trying to find information about hormonal problems was extremely difficult. I remain very grateful to these and other authors who wrote about these subjects even though they were sometimes ridiculed for doing so. I had been telling physicians for years that this problem must have something to do with my menstrual periods because it was so cyclical, but they always tried to convince me otherwise: "You just think you're all right half the month, but actually you are continually depressed. You just won't face up to the facts."

The Same Problem in My Teens, but Getting Worse

As I have already mentioned, I had known at the age of 17 that I had PMT. It was the same problem but only lasted four days. After using the birth control pill, it just lengthened and worsened over the years. I had trouble recognizing that what I was experiencing in my late twenties was essentially the same problem I had had at age 17, because it lasted so long each cycle. Doctors generally say that PMS cannot last any longer than two weeks because there is a timed connection between ovulation and menstruation; the average is 14 days, but it can, they say, range from 10 days to 16 days. I always started symptoms at the same time each month: on the twelfth day. But my cycle varied a lot and could be 34 to 39 days long. I would have PMS for almost a month *after* ovulation until my period began. Then I had 11 or 12 symptom-free days *before* ovulation. Even though some doctors felt that I could not have PMS because my symptoms lasted too long each cycle, I have met other women who had symptoms that lasted longer than normal.

Searching for Treatment

Still living in Australia in 1974, I set about trying to find Dr. Dalton's recommended treatment: natural progesterone. This therapy was not available in Australia in 1974, and this remains true today. Another friend, a social worker, recommended that I see Dr. M., a psychiatrist who was familiar with Dr. Katherina Dalton's material on hormonal problems. While Dr. M. had good intentions, he inadvertently made things worse for me.

Not knowing the difference between natural progesterone and synthetic progestins, he arranged for me to be given Depo-Provera. I was given a 100-milligram (mg) injection and told to take 10 mg of oral progesterone per day for 20 days and then wait to bleed. I found out, like many women with PMS, that I was extremely sensitive to synthetic progestins. Provera sent my emotions spiraling rapidly downhill within hours of the injection. At the end of the month, I was crying uncontrollably. When I went back to Dr. M., he sent me to an endocrinology hospital in Sydney. They told me that we were on the right track, but it was the wrong hormone. They put me on another synthetic progestin, norethisterone, at a dosage of 10 mg a day.

I couldn't understand why I was feeling worse on the hormones, but was sure that they were making me more depressed. I decided to go home to my parents in New Zealand, and while there I saw yet another psychiatrist, Dr. S., who told me that my childhood and marriage were full of reasons why I should be depressed. At the time, I didn't understand why I was feeling worse and worse on the synthetic progestins, and I was terribly disappointed after feeling such hope. But, fortunately, I had written to Dr. Dalton, who kindly wrote and told me that I was on the wrong medication and that synthetic progestins were not the same as natural progesterone. In fact, she told me, synthetic progestins lowered the levels of progesterone in the body and often made symptoms worsen. She told me that it was the synthetic progestin in the birth control pills I had taken at the time of my marriage that had exacerbated my PMS in the first place. This made sense to me.

When I returned to Australia, I was still feeling suicidal. My psychiatrist, Dr. M., arranged to have 400-mg progesterone suppositories made especially for me. They did stop me from feeling suicidal, though I had been given so much synthetic progestin that I now was having bleeding problems. I bled for 50 days continuously, stopped for a week, and then started again. At about this time, I read an article on Provera injections. In Australia, they were giving them to female inpatients in mental facilities, as a convenient contraceptive, because their sex lives were so difficult to control. A 100-mg shot, I read, would make a woman infertile for three months. I had taken a lot more than that. The article also said that women could have bleeding irregularities for up to six months after having a single shot. Note that Depo-Provera injections were approved by the FDA for use as birth control in 1992.

Diagnosed as Manic-Depressive

I had been on progesterone only for three weeks when Dr. M. received a report from the psychiatrist I had seen in New Zealand. As a result, Dr. M. said that I did not have hormonal problems—I was manic-depressive. He said that they were going to take me off all hormones, and arranged to send me to a gynecologist to help regulate my periods. Then I was to go on lithium.

I told him that I had already been on lithium, and that it hadn't helped. Dr. M. said that when I was on it before, I did not have regular blood tests for lithium levels. He had me speak to his superior at the hospital, supposedly a world authority on bipolar disorders, who said that I was indeed manic-depressive; the pattern was not classical, but occurred on a monthly basis instead. When I told Dr. M. that I was sure I had PMS, he told me that I was stubborn, refusing to face the truth about my background and the circumstances of my marriage.

I went, that day, to see the gynecologist Dr. M. had recommended. He wanted to take me off all hormones and let nature regulate my periods. I told him that I had finally found out what was wrong with me and had just found the proper hormonal help, and now they were going to whisk me off before I had time to see if it helped. I asked him if he had ever been depressed.

"No," he replied, "I have a very even personality."

"Well," I told him, "I have been terribly depressed for a long time. I was desperate when I came to see Dr. M., and he has made me much worse. You may both be responsible for my death if you take me off progesterone and I don't get some help."

I went home that evening feeling very desperate, and cried myself to sleep.

Back On Track

Amazingly, the next day I was handed one of the key books I mentioned earlier, *The Psychology of Women*, written by Dr. Judith Bardwick. At the time, she was a teacher at Michigan State University. Dr. Bardwick had been researching the subject of women's psychology and found that the most popular theory at the time was Freud's penis envy. The reason we get depressed is that we are jealous of men for having a penis!

Dr. Bardwick thought this was ridiculous and wrote her book in 1968 as an attempt to rethink the subject. Though based on limited research, much of the material stemmed from her remarkable intuition. She was 25 years ahead of her time in making the connections she made between women's hormonal changes and moods.

The book was largely about women's sexuality, but there was an excellent chapter on the physiology of women and its impact on a woman's emotions. In this chapter, Dr. Bardwick described how different kinds of contraceptive pill—the combination and the sequential—with their different proportions of estrogen and progestin caused different and predictable patterns of depression. I had been on both kinds of pill. The portrayal of the differences in their effects on depression matched my experience exactly.

The combination pill, said Dr. Bardwick, contained both synthetic estrogen and progestins taken every day, though in different proportions—more estrogen and less progestin at the beginning of the cycle, more progestin and less estrogen in the last half. Women on the combination pill who became depressed experienced depression every day.

The sequential pill, no longer on the market, contained high levels of estrogen in the first part of the cycle, and progestins during the last part of the cycle. Women on the sequential pill who became depressed experienced typical PMS; they would feel fine while on the estrogen and depressed while on the progestin.

Bardwick had also done research on women's moods in relation to their normal menstrual cycles. She claimed that women universally felt at their best before ovulation, when estrogen is at its highest. Then premenstrually, when estrogen levels were lower, women experienced their lowest mood and were more negative; had low self-esteem and more nightmares; recalled bloody, violent episodes in their lives; and coped less well emotionally. Dr. Bardwick blamed PMS on a lack of estrogen. This was the opposite of Dr. Katherina Dalton's original theory that PMS is caused by a lack of progesterone and an excess of estrogen.

Estrogen Helped Me Dramatically

I had tried progesterone, and it helped only marginally (though admittedly the form I took it in was not the best). When I read Dr. Bardwick's book, it gave me another great ray of hope. Here was a logical expression of my problem and a possible solution. Armed with Judith Bardwick's book, at age 29, I headed for my local physician in Australia and begged him for estrogen. Dr. E. was manic-depressive himself, and later sadly committed suicide. He was a very kind man. I remember his visiting my son night after night when he had a bad case of measles. Dr. E.'s own horrific depression made him very sympathetic, and he was wonderfully sensitive to my problems.

I asked him if I could try estrogen, and showed him Dr. Bardwick's book. I told him that the book suggested that estrogen was what I needed. Most physicians would have said, "No," because I was only 29 at the time, had periods every month, and showed no obvious symptoms of estrogen deficiency such as hot flashes and drying of the vagina.

He responded, "Why not? It can't hurt you." He gave me a prescription, and I went on estrogen that day. It was a fairly high dose and it was synthetic estrogen, but it worked like a miracle. I had a dramatic response to taking estrogen and literally felt better overnight. After I had gone off the birth control pill, I had acne for several years and began having severe menstrual cramps. My hair was lank. I lost weight and looked emaciated. As soon as I went on estrogen, my physical and emotional state changed for the good overnight. My skin immediately began to clear up, and I never returned to having the acne problem I'd had for the previous four years. My cramps went away. Most important of all, the depression lifted like a veil. In my case, I found that estrogen was far more helpful than progesterone, though for years I have taken both in all sorts of forms.

That wasn't the end of my troubles, however. I was supposed to be on both estrogen and progesterone to avoid endometrial cancer. I couldn't get natural progesterone in Australia and found that taking any synthetic progestin, even in small doses, made me feel suicidal within a short time of taking it. I also found out a year or two later that I was taking too much estrogen. It gave me a strange feeling as though my head was expanding. About that time, I found a woman family doctor in Sydney whose husband was a university medical professor specializing in hormonal therapy. She formulated a pill that was tailor-made for me. But I found that even the low doses of synthetic progestin she prescribed made me depressed and suicidal.

In subsequent years, doctors repeatedly tried to take me off estrogen because they were afraid of cancer. But, over a period of more than 20 years, I have always had the same positive reaction to estrogen that I had back then. And I am in deep trouble if I go off it.

I have been in contact with Dr. Katherina Dalton ever since those days. I decided to also write to Dr. Judith Bardwick some time ago to thank her for saving my life 20 years ago. *The Psychology of Women* was a landmark book, way ahead of its time. When she replied to my letter, Dr. Bardwick said that her colleagues at Michigan State University thought her crazy to write the book at the time but tolerated her. Her subsequent efforts to help women with hormonal problems were bitterly attacked by feminists who thought that any admission that women had hormonal problems would set their cause back many years. This was unfortunate, because Dr. Bardwick was right on the mark. This attack against her is typical of the attitude of women who don't have hormonal problems, and one of the reasons why there has been little progress 20 years after Dr. Bardwick wrote her book.

Reading Dalton's and Bardwick's books, with their opposite conclusions, so closely together in time left me with an open mind. I realized, even then, that some women responded to different hormones. In many cases of classical PMS, women respond well to natural progesterone alone. I was unusual.

A Change In Estrogen Made Me Depressed

In 1977, my husband and I came to the U.S. to work, and I switched estrogens at that time. I had heard about Premarin from an American friend while in Australia. Because it was from a natural source (pregnant mare's urine), I thought it would be better. I never did quite as well emotionally on Premarin but did not make the connection until much later. When I was counseling some years back, a woman said to me, "I've been on all sorts of estrogen, but whenever they put me on Premarin, I get depressed." Something clicked in my mind, and I realized that I had had the same experience. I started asking women about this afterward, and found that some women with hormonal sensitivities do feel more depressed on Premarin.

A doctor explained to me that it was the "horse factor." He said that Premarin contains about 60 different estrogenic compounds, including equilin equine sulfate. Some of these estrogenic factors will not function well in human cell receptors, and some women get side effects from taking Premarin, including depression. I have found that many women feel fine on Premarin and should stay on it. It has been on the market for over 40 years and is a trusted product. But if a woman finds that she has side effects from Premarin, she should simply switch to another type of estrogen.

Off Estrogen and Back On Progesterone

In 1979, when I had been in the U.S. for two years, I developed endometrial hyperplasia because I had taken high doses of synthetic estrogen in Australia for several years and had only taken progesterone intermittently. I had cryosurgery on my cervix, and then I was fine. My doctor told me to go off estrogen and never to go back on it. In the seventies, there was a cancer scare about estrogen that has since subsided in informed circles.

Around that time, my husband and I went to live in Washington, D.C., for a year. While there, I suffered severely from estrogen deficiency. I can remember feeling as though I had concrete in my legs, and it was very difficult to climb stairs. I was also extremely anxious. Photos showed me biting my lip, because I couldn't stop it from trembling while being photographed. Starting when I went off estrogen, I had a few rough years with a return of my PMS symptoms.

Back in California two years later, I was spending part of each month in bed withdrawing from family and visitors. I thought I could never go back on estrogen, so I found a volume of *Books in Print* at a library and ordered Katherina Dalton's latest books on PMS. At about the same time, I read an article about PMS in *Family Circle* magazine and made contact with PMS Action in Wisconsin. I got on their mailing list and soon received a notice that Dr. Dalton was going to speak at Stanford University in a few weeks. It was amazing providence, because Dr. Dalton didn't speak on this side of the country again for another 10 years. I went to hear her with Dr. Myrtle Caton, a friend who was a board-certified internist. She knew my problems and was interested in the therapy. By another amazing bit of providence, my husband and I were both invited to Europe and would be in London the following week. That was the only time I have been invited to go with my husband on a trip to Europe!

When Myrtle and I arrived to hear Dr. Dalton, there were probably over a thousand people there. She was about to go up onto the platform. I went up and told her that I was coming to England the next week. Could I see her? She said she was booked for four months ahead. I was discouraged, but my husband was determined, and he went and visited her in London. She gave him a prescription for progesterone for me, which Dr. Caton was to monitor.

In September, 1982, Myrtle sent me to PMS Action where I trained as a PMS educator/counselor and began working with her in her medical practice in Northern California. We cooperated in helping women; I did the preliminary workup and education, and Myrtle did the physical exam and prescribed the medication. Unfortunately, after we had worked together for a couple of years, she became seriously ill with a collagen disease and had to relinquish her practice. Then I had to branch out and find other physicians in the area who were willing to treat PMS.

The physicians I have worked with have been open, interested, and genuinely concerned. Most of them weren't initially well informed on the subject. They all told me that they weren't taught about these hormonal problems in medical school. I lent them the books I'd read, and together we built up information and experience—here a little, there a little— over the years. I found that what had helped me to feel better helped a lot of other women with similar problems. I had a premenopausal pap smear at age 37 and went into menopause in my early forties—probably because of the wedge resection done at age 26. A significant amount of each ovary is removed during this surgery. At that point, I started to read more about menopause and began helping older women as well.

Problems with Adhesions

At the end of 1983, when I was 39, I was having a lot of premenstrual cramps which lasted from ovulation until the end of my period. Progesterone was only minimally helping me at that time. My gynecologist, Dr. Jones, could feel what he believed was either an ovarian cyst or a uterine fibroid. It was located higher up in my abdomen than would normally be expected. An ultrasound confirmed the presence of a mass which could have been a fibroid or an ovarian cyst. We decided on surgery. I hoped that I could have a hysterectomy and no longer have my nightmare periods, even though I knew that this is not necessarily a cure for PMS and that sometimes women became even worse afterwards.

During surgery, Dr. Jones found that I had massive adhesions (internal organs adhering to each other) resulting from the surgery I had in 1970. They extended from my navel to my pubic bone and were throughout my abdomen. My right ovary was pulled upward in my abdomen, and my bowel and omentum were wrapped around it.

After surgery I had a bladder infection, and I was put on sulfa and sent home. The infection worsened, and at 2:00 in the morning I had to go to the emergency room where a nurse drew off 1,400 cubic centimeters (cc) of urine. Two days later, I went back into the hospital; large amounts of urine (1,200 and 800 cc) were removed by catheter over the next couple of days. When the infection didn't improve with intravenous penicillin, an abdominal catheter was inserted into my bladder under anesthetic. When I came out of the anesthetic, a nurse put saline solution into the catheter to test it. I nearly jumped off the bed from pain. I was given iodine via the catheter so that X-rays could be taken. This, too, was excruciatingly painful. I returned to surgery to be patched up—the third surgery in 10 days. The surgeon was worried that he had penetrated my bowel, but fortunately he hadn't. Because of the adhesions, and due to the fact that my bladder was distorted from urine retention, the holes in the catheter that should have been inside my bladder were instead somewhere in my abdominal cavity. If this hadn't been fixed, I could not have urinated. The surgeon stretched the ureter and patched me up, and after that I was all right for a while.

Back On Estrogen

A couple of months after the surgery, I hit a real low, physically and emotionally, with my hormonal problems. I was almost back to the state I had been in during the earlier years in Australia. I knew I had to get help, or I would be in dire trouble. I couldn't live feeling the way I was.

Through the detective work of a fellow sufferer and friend who had called around nationally to find a hormone expert for her own problems, I went to Dr. B. in Los Angeles. I stayed there for a month while he tried to get me stabilized on medication. He gave me shots three times a week with a combination of estrogen, natural progesterone, and occasionally a little testosterone. He also put me on thyroid therapy. I started on 0.1 mg of Synthroid. At the end of a month, I felt no better, so Dr. B. raised the Synthroid dosage. Within a couple of days I felt completely normal.

From then on, I did a lot better, but unfortunately I developed side effects from the Synthroid. For a while, I was unable to take even tiny doses occasionally without getting a severe pain in the back of my head. I tried changing the type and dose of thyroid medication several times with no success. My body gradually adjusted to thyroid medication, and this no longer seems to be a problem; I still take thyroid medication.

Several years later, I had contact with Dr. C., an Australian OB/GYN who specializes in menopausal problems. He was interested in progesterone therapy and came to the U.S. with his wife to visit me and attend a lecture by Dr. Dalton. We all traveled to Texas to hear Dr. Dalton speak. But when Dr. C. and his wife returned to Australia, they found that they could not import progesterone, as it was not approved for use there except under research conditions.

Dr. C. read about the work of Dr. John Studd in London—a former student of Dr. Robert Greenblatt from Atlanta, Georgia. Before his recent death, Dr. Greenblatt was a specialist in hormone therapy and had developed the use of the estrogen pellet implant. Dr. Studd was now using it at St. Thomas' Hospital in London as a treatment for PMS, because the pellets give a continuous output of estrogen and stop ovulation. Dr. Studd believed that you couldn't have PMS if you didn't ovulate. (In a recent conversation, he agreed that it is the positive antidepressant effect of estrogen on the brain that is responsible for the improvement.)

Dr. Studd is vehemently opposed to the use of natural progesterone for PMS, which I think is an unfortunate position to take. Both estrogen and progesterone help different women.

Estrogen and Testosterone Implants   On a visit to Australia about five years ago, Dr. C. gave me my first estrogen implant, a minor operation requiring only a local anesthetic. He made a small incision and implanted the tiny pellet of estradiol (100 mg), into the fatty tissue of my abdomen (it can also be put in the buttocks). This first implant lasted me only about three months. More recent ones last four to five months. For many women, implants last six to twelve months. Now I have my implants done in the U.S. by Dr. Phillip Warner. He uses three 25-mg estradiol pellets and a 75-mg testosterone pellet. Several small pellets are actually better for absorption than one large one, because they have more surface area. Dr. Warner has special permission from the FDA to implant pellets. Approval from the FDA for a gel pellet is expected within a few years.

As with the transdermal patch, which delivers estrogen through the skin, the estrogen in the pellet goes directly into the bloodstream and straight to the estrogen receptors in the brain. I find that taking estrogen via the implant is much better for me than using any other form. I always feel wonderful within a couple of hours of having the surgery.

Though reading my history may make it sound as if I had one long, protracted battle, there were years when I did fairly well. But the estrogen implant helped me more than anything else, and I have felt a lot better in every way since I went on it.

SOME THINGS I LEARNED
FROM MY OWN EXPERIENCE

Through this experience, I learned a lot of things about life spiritually and emotionally, but my concern here is what I learned about hormones:

- Hormonal problems are real medical problems which should be taken seriously. Diet and exercise alone won't cure severe cases.
- Some women with PMS receive tremendous benefit from taking progesterone, and others don't. The ones who respond to progesterone are often classic in their symptoms and patterns.
- Estrogen will help some women with PMS—particularly women whose symptoms occur after the end of their period, a time when estrogen levels normally rise. Estrogen particularly helps women with severe depression and nontypical PMS.
- Estrogen and progesterone work together, and some women find benefit from both. There is probably a good case for prescribing both hormones for some women with PMS.
- Many women with PMS come from families where there is a common incidence of thyroid problems—more often hypothyroid than hyperthyroid.
- Women with depression may have chronic depression or hormonal depression or both. These two categories of depression are quite different and respond to different treatments. Most of the books I have read on menopause say

that depression at that time comes from sleep disturbances. I don't believe this is true. I think depression is a bona fide symptom on its own.

MY PRESENT PROTOCOL

My present protocol, which works very well, is that I have an estrogen implant every four to five months. I also take oral Estrace (estradiol) daily after I have been on the implant for three months, as it begins to run out.

Taking the oral estrogen without the implant would give me a measure of relief from physical symptoms, but it doesn't work nearly as well as the implant. If I use estrogen injections, they only last about five days (they are generally given once a month). I have tried to use the patch more than once, but, like many women, I get severe skin reactions to the gel in the patch. I develop lumps the size of a baseball under the bandage. I can tolerate the new Climara patch much better.

The implant works amazingly well for me within a couple of hours of surgery. Both physical and emotional symptoms disappear, and a feeling of well-being dominates. I get maximum benefits around the middle of the life of the pellets. The implant wears off just as quickly as it takes effect. If I don't overexercise (I mainly walk for exercise now), it lasts for four months. If I go to aerobics three or four times a week, it runs out very rapidly. So exercise "uses it up."

The day the implant runs out, I feel an immediate change and begin to have joint pains, headaches, abdominal pains, and stomach aches. These gradually worsen, and I begin to sink back into the emotional fog that I used to experience years ago. But all these symptoms disappear immediately when I get a new implant, and I feel a tremendous calm come over me.

Estrogen is the main hormone that helps me. It completely lifts my depression, my anxiety, and the suicidal feelings I experienced after I went off the birth control pill. Without estrogen, I get migraine headaches, severe joint pains, and abdominal pain from my adhesions. When the estrogen kicks in, all my aches and pains disappear.

Until my hysterectomy I took progesterone from time to time to counter the effect of the estrogen on the lining of my uterus and on my breasts. This used to bring on a menstrual period until I was truly through menopause. I never felt well while on it, but it was nothing like I used to experience in my late twenties. I found progesterone helpful for some symptoms such as joint pains.

I have also taken 0.1 mg of Synthroid and 5 micrograms (mcg) of Cytomel at times, but my need for thyroid medication varies. I can take it for months at a time, and then not be able to take it for months because of its side effects. I now take Westhroid, which is an animal thyroid like Armour, and I find I do better on this.

As I look back over the years, I am grateful for the people who have spent much of their lives devoted to solving hormonal problems. I feel that without the information I gleaned from them, I would never have found help, and I really think that I would have taken my own life. As it is, I don't get depressed or suicidal, and I am profoundly grateful for this. It is this gratitude that fuels my own desire to help other women suffering with these problems, and I know these women exist everywhere.

I always marvel at the profound effect estrogen has on me—not only physically but emotionally. If I am careless about taking estrogen, I go through a death-and-resurrection experience; and this keeps me sympathetic toward the women I work with. I genuinely know how they feel.

Estrogen is responsible for a sense of joy and well-being in women. Earlier in the book, I mentioned that studies show that women *universally* feel better just before they ovulate, whether they have hormonal problems or not. That is the time of the month when estrogen is high. I know, from repeated experience over the years, the amazing effect that estrogen has on my mind. Estrogen increases blood flow to the brain and raises endorphin levels in the brain, and there is no doubt that estrogen alters my brain chemistry in some marvelous way. Still, fine-tuning my hormones is a process that requires continual adjustment.

I have included this section because I know there are other women like me who have real difficulties balancing their hormones. I should mention that some other women have the opposite effect and become irritable on estrogen—which shows the necessity of looking at the individual response during treatment. Treatment with natural progesterone is similar. Some women respond dramatically to natural progesterone, as I do to estrogen. But progesterone doesn't help me, even though I have adjusted the dose and taken it in many forms, including injections and suppositories made in England. I took it for the physical benefits, while I still had my uterus, but it didn't help my depression.

THE REST OF MY STORY

In December of 1995, I finally decided to do what my doctors had been urging me to do for years: have a hysterectomy. The main reason for my decision was that I had been taking estrogen on and off for over 20 years. I wasn't taking enough progesterone to balance the effects of estrogen because of the adverse side effects I experienced when taking even natural progesterone. I had been diagnosed with adenomatous hyperplasia for three years and, though this is not cancerous in itself, it can advance to atypical hyperplasia at any time. Because I continued to take estrogen, I could only expect that one day it could become cancerous.

I am now 51 years old, and I had put off the hysterectomy until I really felt I needed it. I was not in pain, so that wasn't an issue. I had a lot of nuisance symptoms, including bowel changes, shortness of breath, and badly splitting fingernails, but I didn't realize that they were related. I didn't feel great physically, but I was well enough to cope with a full-time job and a lot of other activities. I wasn't depressed, but sometimes I became very tired, which was nothing new.

I chose to have the surgery performed by a doctor I know, who kept up on the latest methods and could do a vaginal hysterectomy including removal of the ovaries. He was also

willing to attempt the surgery despite my history of adhesions. I told him, prior to surgery, that I had read the pros and
cons of taking out the ovaries. I knew, based on ultrasound
examination, that my overies were very tiny, partly as a result of the wedge resection surgery in 1970. I asked him to
make a judgement call based on how they looked; if he would
have to make an abdominal incision just to take out the
ovaries, and they didn't look too bad, he might leave them in.

I discussed with him my history of postsurgery bladder infections, and he said that he would insert an abdominal
catheter during the surgery (a tube going from the bladder
into a catheter bag). As a result of the catheter and intravenous antibiotics, I didn't get a bladder infection this time.

I told him that I could feel adhesions up as far as my stomach—that sometimes when I ate, my stomach pulled because
of them. I was also experiencing shortness of breath and wondered if adhesions were causing that. I suspected that he might
find a lot of adhesions, though I was hoping he wouldn't.

I felt very confident going into surgery and wasn't at all
nervous. When I came out of anesthesia, the surgeon told
me that he hadn't been able to do the surgery vaginally. He
couldn't get a laparoscope into my navel because of the adhesions, so he opened up my abdominal scar for the fourth time.
He said that things were as bad as I had said, and a lot worse.
The adhesions extended way up into my abdomen. My uterus
was stuck to my colon, and I had bowel obstructions in several
places. As with the previous round of surgeries, it was amazing that I had noticed relatively few symptoms.

My surgeon worked from my navel down and called in a
general surgeon to work from my navel up to my diaphragm.
It was a very extensive surgery, and they released all the
adhesions.

One advantage of having had similar surgery before was
that I knew what I had to do. I got up and walked the floor the
first night (due to the pain, not a wish for exercise). After that,
I recovered amazingly well. As I write, two weeks after
surgery, I feel pretty normal except for some strange pulling feelings in my abdomen. My split nails have already
disappeared.

As I look back over the years, I wish I had not had the first surgery for ovarian cysts in 1970; I don't think it was necessary. The primary reason for the surgery was to lessen my PMS symptoms, and it didn't work. But it has caused a lot of recurring problems with adhesions and may continue to do so.

I think that having a hysterectomy was inevitable for me. Estrogen was the only thing that lessened my depression over the years, and I don't feel that there was much choice about my taking it. I am grateful for the good years it has given me. I think that the hysterectomy is going to be good for me. It was good for my sister, and my mother says that she was never well until she had a hysterectomy.

Though Chapter 12 on hysterectomy describes the disadvantages of this surgery, a hysterectomy is a great choice for many women. Before I had my surgery, numerous women told me how much better they felt after theirs. As I mentioned elsewhere, I tend to counsel women whose experience after hysterectomy is negative. Many times this is because their hormonal support has not been properly managed by their physician. Sometimes it's more than that. Some women's health just breaks down after hysterectomy, and their hormones are extremely difficult to manage.

This illustrates the fact that some things are good for one particular woman and bad for another. The birth control pill can be a real blessing for some women and can cause tremendous problems for another. Drugs such as Prozac save lives every day, but some people have an extreme adverse reaction to taking Prozac. Similarly, a hysterectomy can be either good or bad depending on the individual's reaction.

I would recommend getting all the facts of your own case, researching the risks and options to the best of your ability, and treating hysterectomy as a later or last resort. But don't close your mind to it.

SUMMARY

Even today it is extremely difficult for many women to find help for their hormonal problems. A lot depends on whether a woman can find a physician who is both sympathetic and knowledgeable about these problems. These doctors do exist, but they are a relatively rare breed.

My own experience in trying to get help is illustrative. Over a period of 20 years, I lived in England, Australia, New Zealand, and the United States, and I had PMS in all four countries. I sought help everywhere I went. Over a period of several years, that meant visiting with numerous physicians, including six psychiatrists. I took most of the antidepressants available at the time, with no relief.

I knew instinctively that my problems were related to my menstrual cycle, because they started at ovulation and ended when I began my period month after month. But no one was really listening to me. In those early days of craziness, nobody believed that I had a hormonal problem, nor did they believe in the existence of PMS. They thought that I was manic de-pressive—but lithium and other psychotropic drugs didn't help. I had to read myself to health; fortunately, I was handed a few good books to help me on my way and found kind physicians who cooperated with me.

I learned back then, and repeatedly over the following 20 years, the amazing impact of estrogen on the mind. Its anti-depressant action on the hypothalamus and central nervous system via the estrogen receptors, and its catalyst action in as-sociation with other psychotropic drugs, is presently being studied. Researchers are finding that estrogen increases endorphin, serotonin, and dopamine levels, and it decreases MAOs, functioning much as an antidepressant would. Estro-gen aids memory, verbal coordination, and moods. I knew all that from experience by the time I was 29.

Other hormones also affect the mind. A lack of thyroid, progesterone, or even the male hormone testosterone can also cause depression. Some women have a positive reaction to natural progesterone and a poor reaction to estrogen. We are not all the same. The women who respond dramatically to natural progesterone often continue to have a favorable re-action to it over many years. I tell women that there are "es-trogen types" and "progesterone types." Sometimes a trial of each hormone is necessary to find out which hormone will help most. Sometimes the basic problem is the thyroid.

The type of hormone you take is very important. The type of synthetic progestin that is in the birth control pill is much more likely to cause depression than natural progesterone. Provera, a common part of hormonal replacement therapy in older women, is also a synthetic progestin, and many women react adversely to it. Synthetic progestins do not match the chemistry of the body's natural progesterone. They shut down ovulation and lower production of natural proges- terone, thereby causing a hormone imbalance. This can lead to an increase in weight and mood disorders. Women with a predisposition to hormonal problems may find their condi- tions worsened by using these synthetic substances.

This information on synthetic progestins has been avail- able for at least 20 years, but its significance has been con- stantly downplayed and overlooked. So when a woman goes on birth control pills or is given Provera at menopause and complains of depression, she is often not listened to—even though many doctors admit that women frequently complain and refuse to take synthetic progestins because of the emo- tional problems these medications give them.

Synthetic hormones are used for a variety of reasons— politics, economics, marketing, ignorance of other options, and product familiarity built up over years of medical tradi- tion when few options were available.

There is also a general lack of belief that PMS or hormonal depression at menopause really exist or that they can cause considerable suffering. (Doctors aren't alone in this; many women don't believe in these problems either—until they get them.) Why treat a problem or search for answers if you don't believe in it?

Physicians often give the impression that the only really important issues around menopause are the obvious physical ones. They pore over breasts and reproductive organs, cardiac vessels and bones, as with some cadaver—not seeing that there is a person behind the body, who may be struggling to stay sane. The emotional problems—depression, irritability, anger, anxiety, and paranoia—suffered by some women with severe hormonal problems are passed off as unimportant. For other women, it's their treatment-resistant skin problems, their horrendous hormonal migraines, or their seizures that are overlooked. Neurologists, psychologists, dermatologists, and other specialists often completely overlook a hormonal cause or connection.

In my case, my main symptom was suicidal depression, and it was very serious. My life, my personality, my sanity, my reason for living were at risk, and finding help was like digging for gold. Like many women, I feel angry that it was so difficult to find help when the information was already known, and the only options I had were antidepressants and tranquilizers, which didn't help.

Because of the tortuous path I trod in trying to find help, I began helping other women in 1982. I found that there are many women with hormonal problems who still have as much difficulty getting help as I did over 20 years ago. The beneficial effects of the right hormones—particularly estrogen, progesterone, and thyroid—on a woman's emotional and physical well-being are still highly underestimated. The impact of these hormones is as widespread as the cells they affect. Because these hormones are basic ingredients in the cell's production of enzymes and the production of energy, deficiencies can affect the whole body, though symptoms vary from woman to woman both in type and severity.

To put this in perspective, it is important to keep in mind that many women don't have hormonal problems. They have no trouble with their periods or pregnancies; they can take the birth control pill for 10 or 20 years, have tubal ligations or hysterectomies, and go through menopause with no problems. For them, it is not necessary to take hormones. Hormones are very potent; they can even alter the DNA. So I am not suggesting that they are for everyone.

But at the other end of the scale there is a large subset—millions of women with severe, incapacitating hormonal problems—who are finding it difficult to get any practical help.

This book is for them.

SECTION ONE

WHAT GOES WRONG?

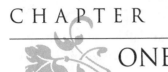

CHAPTER

ONE

WHAT'S WRONG WITH MY HORMONES?

A woman who feels emotionally or physically sick often senses that her symptoms are connected with her menstrual cycle, and that they began at a time of hormonal change. She may visit her doctor hoping to have her suspicions confirmed. Instead, the idea that her symptoms have a hormonal cause is more likely to be dismissed or ridiculed.

If the doctor tests her, the results may be normal and he or she is likely to assume that there's nothing wrong with her hormones. But the woman knows there's a hormonal link. She may have premenstrual syndrome or be experiencing side effects from the birth control pill. Her problems may have started with a pregnancy, or after a tubal ligation, at menopause, or after her uterus or ovaries were removed. She knows that the way she feels is not normal, but it's difficult to argue with a doctor who depends heavily on medical tests for diagnosis.

Hormonal problems are frequently difficult to discern because they present themselves so differently in different women, with symptoms varying dramatically in type and intensity. This is because the endocrine system affects the body at so many levels, from the brain to the individual cells.

Because the hormonal system is complex and intimately linked to so many body functions, women may experience any of hundreds of symptoms.

CASE HISTORIES

The following examples illustrate typical cases of people with a variety of hormonal problems. You will meet each of them again in more depth later in this book.

Barbara, 41 years old and a dental hygienist, began having problems six or seven years after her tubal ligation. She came to see me because she was having severe, incapacitating migraine headaches just before her period. In addition to the migraines, she had extreme itching on her head and skin, severe panic attacks and allergies, and diminished sex drive.

Cassandra, a 52-year-old writer and editor, was through menopause and taking a standard dose of hormone replacement therapy—0.625 mg of Premarin (conjugated equine estrogens) during days 1 through 25 of the calendar month, and 10 mg of Provera (medroxyprogesterone) during days 15 through 25 of the month, with no hormone supplements from day 26 through the end of the month. She was feeling listless and tired, especially on the days off the hormones, and on the days on Provera she felt very cranky.

Dana, a 36-year-old intensive care nurse and mother of one, had mild PMS and suffered from severe allergies. She came to me for an opinion because she wanted to get pregnant again, but she had difficulty carrying her pregnancies to term. There was a strong history of autoimmune thyroid disease in her mother's family, and she believed that this was her problem too. She was having a problem convincing some of her doctors of this, even though her only successful pregnancy had been carried while Dana took thyroid.

Jeannie, 39 years old and a minister's wife, began having problems after toxemia during pregnancy. After delivery, she had severe postpartum depression and no menstrual periods for three years. Her depression continued and deepened, and now she was having symptoms of menopause—extreme hemorrhaging with her periods, severe hot flashes, and night sweats. Her mother had similar problems at the same age and had her uterus removed at age 37 and her ovaries taken out shortly afterward. Jeannie was being treated with an anti-depressant—Parnate—and, because it wasn't working, her psychiatrist wanted to give her shock treatment.

Laura, 27 years old and another minister's wife, had two small children. She had severe hormonal problems that began in puberty. There was a strong history of thyroid problems on her mother's side of the family. Laura was diagnosed as hypo-thyroid at age 15, but took medication for only a year. Over the next 12 years, Laura had every hormonal problem in the book, including highly irregular and heavy periods, endo-metriosis, endometrial cancer, and postpartum depression after both births. She had repeated surgeries, including having her uterus removed, then one ovary, and then the other. Even though young, she was suffering from extreme estrogen deprivation.

Lynelle, 38 years old and a county public health nurse, was a single parent with two children. In her twenties, while in school, she had her first panic attack—severe enough that her mother had to come and look after the children. It's possible that coming off the birth control pill contributed to this. Later, after Lynelle contracted a number of upper respiratory viruses, the panic attacks returned and worsened. Episodes were mainly premenstrual. At the same time, her waist-length hair began to break off, and her periods became extremely heavy. Her symptoms were severe enough to occasionally take her to the emergency room.

Sandra, 47 years old and a sales representative, had the most severe case of PMS I have ever seen. Her problems with severe suicidal depression and PMS appeared to begin around age 37, after having a tubal ligation. In retrospect, we found out that she had multiple autoimmune and endocrine prob-lems, including Hashimoto's thyroiditis, diabetes mellitus, and adrenal and ovarian failure. She was also unipolar, meaning that she had recurrent seasonal depressions.

Robin, 41 years old, was a homemaker and mother of three. She always had PMS and had been given thyroid medication for a short time at age 16. She had postpartum depression after her second and third children and then seemed to go into a peri-menopausal state. There was a strong history of immune system and thyroid problems in her family. At one point, Robin was prescribed Prozac and had a severe physical reaction to it.

Mona, 40 years old and a nurse, began having horrible menstrual problems at puberty. Her periods were never normal. The flow was extremely heavy and she had severe cramps. She was later diagnosed as having endometriosis and polycystic ovaries. She had postpartum depression after a miscarriage at age 21. Subsequent pregnancies were a nightmare, and her uterus was removed in her late twenties. Cysts continued to form in her ovaries, and she had the ovaries removed some years later. Her hormone replacement was not adequate, and Mona suffered from extreme depression for which she had been given many different medications and a recent course of electroshock therapy. Nothing was working.

Ron, now in his sixties, developed chicken pox at age 20 while in the army and was put in quarantine where he also developed mumps. He was sick for several months. Told that he would never have children because of damage to his testes, he nevertheless later married and had five children! His problems began in his late forties when testosterone deficiency, caused by viral damage to his testes, began to affect his health. He developed severe allergies, osteoporosis, and cardiac arrhythmia, felt the cold intensely, lost weight, and experienced diminished sex drive.

These are real people, who kindly agreed to let me use their case histories (with changed names). They all have obvious hormonal problems, some genetic, some triggered by a hormonal event such as the birth control pill, pregnancy, a tubal ligation, a hysterectomy, or even a virus. They illustrate some of the myriad ways in which hormonal problems can affect different people.

HORMONAL DEPRESSION

According to Mark S. Gold, M.D., author of *The Good News About Depression*, mental depression is the most common reason why people seek medical treatment—even more frequent than the common cold. There are numerous reasons for being depressed, some physical and some in reaction to outside factors. An unhappy event can make a person sad and depressed. But that is not the same as having a depression that originates within the body.

There are also numerous possible origins of endogenous (biochemically caused) depression, including heredity, chemical imbalance, sickness, and injury. According to Dr. Gold:

> Depression can be a biological illness for which you need a doctor. It can be the first sign of a developing physical illness—perhaps even a deadly illness. Depression can be a side effect of virtually any prescription or illegal drug, or a symptom of another physical illness.[1]

He goes on in his book to list 75 diseases, including certain cancers, that manifest themselves as depression in their early stages. Dr. Gold's book will be very helpful to people whose main symptom is depression.

It is not within the scope of my book to discuss all of these forms of depression. Rather, I am limiting my discussion to depression that is hormonally caused. The reason it seems necessary to point out this hormonal link is that medicine has routinely overlooked or undervalued it.

Today, biopsychiatrists like Dr. Gold are more aware of these important hormonal links. They are cognizant of the copious literature that links thyroid disorders and emotional problems, and the fact that cortisol levels are often very high in depressed people. A few biopsychiatrists, such as Elizabeth Lee Vliet, M.D., are also familiar with the estrogen link with depression (see later chapter on this subject).

Women who have hormonal depression often sense its cause because the tides of their moods ebb and flow with predictable hormonal changes—before their periods, after childbirth, approaching natural menopause, after hormone treatment such as the birth control pill or Provera, or after surgery that affects the hormones, such as hysterectomy, oophorectomy, or tubal ligation.

As a rule, chronic depression can cause loss of appetite, insomnia, and low sex drive. Some women with premenstrual depression experience the opposite symptoms, including food cravings, sleeping too much, or premenstrually high libido. The depression caused by low-estrogen states approaching menopause or by hypothyroidism has more in common with chronic depression, however. So even hormonal depression can involve a mixture of symptoms.

Some women will be able to treat their depression with hormones with great success. Others will find that they don't work at all. Some women will have great success using antidepressants. Others will find that they don't work or that they produce adverse side effects. Some women will need a combination of hormones and antidepressants. There is no one regime that fits every individual.

I THINK THERE'S SOMETHING WRONG WITH MY HORMONES

Women frequently suspect that their problems are related to their hormones. But so often, when they ask about it, their physician acts as though hormonal problems don't exist or aren't important.

"This has nothing to do with your hormones." "Your hormones are normal." "You're too young." "You're working too hard." "You're under too much stress." "This is just part of being a woman." "You just have to put up with this." "There's nothing we can do." "When you have a baby it will go away." "We'll put you on the birth control pill." "I'll give you some Xanax." "I think you ought to see a psychiatrist." Often there's a patronizing pat on the head and the intimation that the problem is of no consequence and that the woman is neurotic.

Am I exaggerating, or is it really difficult to find help for these problems? The women I see often tell me that they have gone from one doctor to another with little practical help. Why is this so? The next chapter will discuss some of the reasons.

CHAPTER

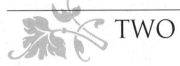 TWO

WHY IS IT SO HARD
TO FIND HELP?

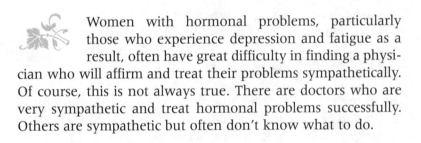 Women with hormonal problems, particularly those who experience depression and fatigue as a result, often have great difficulty in finding a physician who will affirm and treat their problems sympathetically. Of course, this is not always true. There are doctors who are very sympathetic and treat hormonal problems successfully. Others are sympathetic but often don't know what to do.

FEW DOCTORS BELIEVE IN
HORMONAL PROBLEMS

Generally, it is not easy to find a doctor who really believes that women can have extremely severe symptoms just because their hormones are out of balance. Comparatively few doctors recognize PMS as a legitimate physiological disorder, and they offer only limited options for treatment. In England, 25 percent of general physicians follow Dr. Katherina Dalton's suggestions for treating PMS, and natural progesterone suppositories and injections are available through the

41

National Health Service. Here in the U.S., a concerted effort has been made to discredit her work because of the difficulty researchers have had in duplicating her results. However, thousands of women can attest to the efficacy of natural progesterone.

I do not believe that natural progesterone is the answer for all women with PMS. I am one who did not respond to it. Nevertheless, I have seen many, many women who do very well on it over the long term, and I believe that women should have the right to try it. I also believe that natural progesterone is generally a better choice as a complement to estrogen than synthetic progestins such as Provera.

It is easier to find help for menopausal problems than for PMS. Researchers agree that menopause can cause real problems, and that estrogen deficiency in the later years of life can be devastating to physical health. Their concern is more with the physical results of hormone depletion—osteoporosis and heart disease. They aren't always sympathetic to the emotional problems that some women endure.

TREATMENT NOT UNIFORM

Nevertheless, there does not seem to be any uniformity in treatment at menopause or after hysterectomy, partly because some physicians still worry about the risk of cancer for women taking estrogen. Some doctors will only prescribe small doses of estrogen after removing a woman's ovaries, even if the woman still has obvious symptoms. Another doctor might prescribe four times the amount the first doctor prescribed. So doses are not always uniform, and if a woman does not respond to the usual brand and dose, the physician may not offer her other choices.

These days, most doctors will automatically give women some estrogen after their ovaries are removed. But if the patient has only her uterus removed, many doctors don't seem to take into account the fact that she may have estrogen depletion symptoms immediately or a few years down the line.

Many still believe that if a woman has only part of one ovary, she will have enough estrogen to get her through menopause. This is not necessarily true, despite the fact that some women seem to be fine after this surgery. When a woman loses her uterus, part of the ovarian-uterine artery that goes through the uterus is removed. She also loses the hormones that the uterus produces (prostaglandins, and possibly even estrogen; some researchers think that the uterus may make some estrogen). Her ovaries may subsequently shrink as a result of less blood flow and lowered amounts of hormones coming from her pituitary gland.

It is not uncommon to see a woman in her late twenties or early thirties who has had her uterus removed and is experiencing migraine headaches, joint pains, sweating, or depression. Often, her doctors shake their heads and don't know what's wrong with her. One young woman I know, whose uterus was removed at age 28, lost 10 percent of her bone mass within a year! Of course, this is not typical, but these and other menopausal symptoms are not uncommon in such young women who have had hysterectomies, even if they retain their ovaries.

PREMATURE MENOPAUSE
IS FAIRLY COMMON

The phrase "premature menopause," refers to women who cease having periods earlier than normal. But there are many women who could be called premenopausal who still have menstrual periods yet experience a decline of estrogen levels long before menopause. Such women have a very difficult time finding sympathetic treatment. "You are too young to be going through menopause," is the usual comment. Their hormone levels may appear normal, but they are experiencing typical physical and emotional symptoms of menopause.

When the topic of menopause is discussed, 50- to 60-year-old women are usually the focus. Since 7 to 11 percent of women go through premature menopause before age forty, according to Dr. Richard Bronson, physicians should not tell women that they won't go through menopause until they are about 50. There are too many exceptions. Women often start experiencing gradual ovarian failure and consequent estrogen decline in their mid-thirties.

A woman I saw recently began having night sweats at the age of 34 (see Jeannie's story in Chapter 7, Postpartum Depression). Her doctor said that if she weren't so young, he would have thought she was going through menopause. He put her on a series of psychotropic drugs that worsened her condition and turned her into a couch potato. When I saw her, her next option was shock therapy. The doctor's first thought was best; Jeannie's mother had gone through menopause at 37, and since this is often a hereditary pattern, it was no surprise that Jeannie was having hot flashes. After I saw her, she had a severe reaction to her antidepressant and was hospitalized. Taking her off the medication and treating her hormonally for menopause transformed her within a few weeks. I see so many similar cases of misdiagnosis with hormonal problems that I know this type of incident is common.

POSTPARTUM SUFFERERS NOT RECOGNIZED

Even less attention has been paid to women with postpartum depression (PPD), which has not received the attention in the U.S. that it has in Europe. Typical treatment in the U.S. is with antidepressants, not hormones. Dr. James Alexander Hamilton of San Francisco believes that PPD is a polyendocrine disorder, occurring because of the dramatic decline of estrogen, progesterone, β-endorphins, and cortisol within a few days of delivery. This sudden drop can make the pituitary gland sluggish and often leads to lowered thyroid levels as well. Dr. Hamilton believes that this problem should not be treated as a typical clinical depression, since it is obviously hormonally triggered. This is not to say that these women never benefit from antidepressants, but hormones may be more appropriate for this type of depression—especially if the problem is caught early.

THE CARING VERSUS THE CALLOUS

Because I am not a doctor or a biochemist, I can use only the information that doctors and biochemists generate, and I am grateful for it. I don't know as much as they do about how the body functions or about disease in general. However, I do know what hormonal problems are like and how it feels to have them. The criticisms I make of doctors are not an attack on their intelligence or their undeniable skill. I am pointing out an area in which there is frequently a gap in diagnosis and treatment, and one in which they have little training and sometimes little sympathy.

Medicine has, in general, been very slow to focus on women's problems. The available research is sometimes confusing, and there are large information gaps in the literature. Useful treatments are frequently not FDA-approved. Doctors who treat women for PMS and premenopause often step ahead of their colleagues and receive disapproval for using "unconventional measures." These pioneering doctors read up on the subject after they leave medical school, because hormonal problems are barely discussed there. Such physicians are to be commended, because they take a risk in treating these women's problems.

Through the years, I have worked with many caring physicians, and I am extremely grateful for the support they give women. I have met many idealistic physicians who enter medicine with the aim of alleviating suffering. They really listen to their patients and try to help them.

Having given accolades to the best of physicians, let me say that, because physicians are often oriented toward medical research, they sometimes treat their patients as scientific experiments and don't really listen to them. Because physicians are in charge of the prescription pad, they are part of the reason women find it difficult to get help for hormonal problems.

IS IT DIFFICULT TO GET HELP?

Is it an exaggeration to say that women find it difficult to get help? Yesterday a woman going through menopause called me on the phone. She'd had a hysterectomy some time ago and then started having menopausal symptoms. She was trying to get some answers about the need for estrogen and what the side effects would be. She had called the education department of every hospital in the Sacramento area and contacted physicians' offices and numerous women's organizations. She said she couldn't believe that there was no organization dispensing the kind of information she needed, and added, correctly, that there must be thousands of women in their fifties going through these problems. Why, she asked, aren't there women's groups everywhere dealing with this problem?

I have frequently asked myself the same question. This situation is improving as time goes by, but it continually amazes me that the whole area of women's hormonal problems is so neglected when: 1) the number of older women increases year by year; 2) these hormonal problems are so common; 3) there is sufficient information available to make diagnosis and treatment possible in most cases; and 4) the treatments are relatively safe and the results are usually spectacular.

What prejudices are operating to make it so difficult for women to recognize and get help for hormonal problems? The answers are multiple and complex and not restricted to the attitude of the physician. The material that follows lists some reasons:

Women's Attitudes

- Everyone tends to go by her own experience. We need to remember that a large group of women don't have hormonal problems, and they are as much in the dark about menstrual problems as men are. They can be most unsympathetic. Often I see a woman who had no problems until she had a tubal ligation. She used to think that PMS was just an excuse. Now that she has PMS, she's changed her mind! If women haven't experienced hormonal problems themselves, they don't believe in them. If they have mild problems, they believe a little bit. When women have very severe symptoms, hardly anyone else believes them.

- Among the women who don't have extreme hormonal problems are those who resent the largely male physicians telling them that they need hormones after menopause to be "nice" and "good-looking" until they die. Some women are violently opposed to hormone therapy, and this is fine. But it's a shame if they oppose hormone replacement therapy for all women, because some women are dying emotionally and spiritually for lack of it.

- Many women feel that PMS or menopause can be used as an argument to limit women who are trying to excel in their careers, competing against men for high-level jobs. Other women who wouldn't classify themselves as hard-nosed feminists resent the term PMS because it's one more argument that men can use to discredit women. Isn't PMS a large part of the evidence men use to label women fickle, changeable, moody, and incompetent? I can understand why these women are upset, and their observations are valid, but denying the existence of PMS and menopause won't make the problems go away.

- Women are extremely sensitive about their hormones, perhaps because of the association with their femininity and sexuality—their very being. They seem to treat this area of their lives as something apart from the rest of their body. While they willingly take other medications for depression, panic disorders, diabetes, or other chronic problems, they may reject hormone therapy because they don't want to feel that they are being controlled by their hormones.

- When I ask women how their grandmothers and mothers went through menopause, I often find that this topic was never openly addressed. Times are changing. Some women with problems are willing to talk openly about them, but the old taboos fade slowly and many women are still reluctant to discuss these subjects. When women become unreasonable, irritable, and angry, they are embarrassed by their behavior and try to pretend that the behavior never

happened. It's not always pretense. Many really have forgotten how badly they behaved!

- Women with severe hormonal problems are extremely vulnerable. They usually have very low self-esteem, and it is
  difficult for them to speak up for themselves and insist on
  being heard by their doctors (particularly in a situation
  with a male gynecologist while the woman is naked on the
  examination table). Women are often unable to communi-
  cate effectively what they are going through, since mental
  confusion and inability to think clearly are common hormonal symptoms. Their minds become confused and their
  thinking incoherent, and so these women appear to have a
  psychological rather than a hormonal disorder.
- Women often forget that medicine is big business and that
  they are paying the bill. They treat their physicians like
  gods and are afraid to differ with them. They don't assert
  themselves and demand better treatment.
- Many women today prefer to treat their hormonal problems by natural methods. This may be perfectly appropriate for some women, and, as a 30-year vegetarian who
  believes in a healthy lifestyle, I'm all for it. But there are
  many women whose quality of life will be greatly reduced
  if they don't take hormones.
- Women often don't like the idea of taking hormones.
  Hormones have had bad press, and as soon as the word
  "hormone" is mentioned many women think "cancer."
  Recent studies, however, support the idea that women are
  less likely to get cancer if they are on the right combination
  of hormones than if they are off hormones altogether.
- Many postmenopausal women think that taking estrogen
  is optional rather than important, and they often only take
  it for a short time while the hot flashes are extreme. They
  don't understand the effects of lack of estrogen in old age
  or know that once they go off estrogen, it will soon be as
  though they've never been on it. They don't know that
  current research supports long-term low-dose estrogen and
  progesterone therapy for most women.
- Another problem for postmenopausal women is that they
  don't wish to keep having periods by inducing them hor-

monally each month. They often don't know that there are ways to take hormones, which make it unnecessary to have a period (though these methods don't work for all women).
- Many women don't like the effects of the synthetic progestin part of hormone replacement therapy, because it makes them irritable and depressed. They often stop taking estrogen for this reason.

Men's Attitudes

- Men often find the topics of menstruation and menopause repulsive—a sexual turnoff—so, they talk about these subjects as a joke in a way that degrades women. Consequently, women tend to avoid discussing their problems in any real depth with their partners, and understanding breaks down. The personality changes resulting from PMS and menopause are a large, often unrecognized, factor in many divorces. Typically, women with hormonal problems become irrationally angry, and often there is a seed of validity in their anger, but the whole thing is blown out of proportion. The woman is, at the time, convinced that she is right. The man is perplexed and bewildered and likely to accuse the woman of being crazy, which leads to verbal and sometimes physical fights. When this occurs over a period of time, marriages break down.

Lack of Research, the FDA, and Insurance Companies

- Insurance companies often won't pay for doctor's visits where the diagnosis is PMS or menopausal problems because of a lack of conclusive research and lack of FDA approval for hormone treatments. This means that often insurance companies won't cover the cost of treatment. There is little incentive to open PMS and menopause clinics, because doctors know that it is difficult to make them financially successful. Indeed, most PMS clinics have a very short life span.
- For sexist, political, and economic reasons, women have been dreadfully discriminated against in medical studies. In

the past, men and male rats have been almost exclusively used in studies, even in studies of equal impact to both sexes—for example, heart disease. Women are physiologically quite different from men, and it is devastating to women's health when both sexes are viewed as biologically the same. When women are a few years past menopause, their incidence of death from strokes and heart disease rises dramatically and reaches the same level as that of men. Their capillaries are finer than men's, and death occurs more often with the first heart attack in women. Despite this, millions of dollars have been spent on research on heart disease in men, but very little on women. The subjects of menopause, osteoporosis, PMS, premenopause, and the effects of tubal ligations and hysterectomies have been thinly researched, resulting in huge information gaps. There is, however, enough information already gathered to help women with hormonal problems, though finding it is not always easy.

• There is, I think, a downside to the way researchers face this problem, though probably this attitude is unavoidable. In trying to be precise about the causes of PMS and the way it manifests itself, the plight of the individual living with these symptoms ceases to be important. One researcher participating in a panel on PMS mentioned that, in some ways, there has been no real progress in defining PMS in 50 years. What happens to the women with these problems in the meantime while the researchers search for definitions? Because of uncertainty on the part of researchers, many doctors are likewise hesitant to treat PMS; they want to understand the problem exactly before they will try to find solutions for it. Do we sufferers have to wait another 50 years to get treatment just because no one can say with certainty what causes PMS?

• The fact that the FDA has not approved the use of natural progesterone for PMS or after menopause fuels this conservative stance. Because of this, some doctors are reluctant to prescribe natural progesterone, and HMOs often won't pay for the prescription.

- It helps to realize that Provera, which has been used for many years as hormone replacement therapy, is not FDA-approved for use after menopause either. (The Depo-Provera injection is approved by the FDA for birth control only.) Nor are such drugs as Prozac and Xanax approved for treating PMS, but doctors use them all the time for this purpose.
- FDA approval impacts advertising: a drug cannot be advertised for a particular disorder unless it has FDA approval for that particular disorder. Lack of FDA approval, therefore, doesn't mean that a doctor cannot prescribe natural progesterone. A physician can prescribe a drug for a particular problem if doing so is considered common medical practice by the state board where the doctor practices.
- The FDA is slow when it comes to approving hormones. Perhaps this is due to the shadow of such drugs as diethyl stilbestrol, a synthetic estrogen that has caused birth defects into the second generation. In the past, the FDA seemed to speed up when it came to patrolling and controlling pharmacies that make prescription doses of natural progesterone available. Not too long ago, the FDA was trying to classify compounding pharmacies who produced large quantities of natural progesterone as manufacturers. They also wanted such pharmacies stopped from shipping hormones over state lines. If this had happened, prescription doses of natural progesterone would have become unavailable.
- More recently, there have been cuts in the staff at the FDA, and they are kept busy dealing with really dangerous drugs. Because of this, the staff is not spending time outlawing substances unless they are proven to be dangerous and cause major side effects or death.
- The FDA has said that progesterone is a relatively safe drug. But researchers in the U.S. have not been able to duplicate Dr. Katherina Dalton's studies in England, which demonstrated success in treating PMS with natural progesterone. Without the confirmation of its own studies, the FDA will not approve the use of natural progesterone for PMS. Approximately eight to ten studies have been done using natural progesterone treatment for PMS, concluding that

progesterone works no better than a placebo. These studies have all been criticized as inadequate for one or more of the following reasons:

1. The PMS patients were not properly screened for these studies, and, therefore, some participants did not have genuine PMS.

2. The progesterone was not given in sufficiently high doses. Dr. Dalton says that 400 mg is the normal dose in suppository form; the studies used no more than 200-mg suppositories.

3. The patients did not take the progesterone often enough. When patients took it in the morning and not again until evening, their symptoms came back by midday. This is because natural progesterone has a short half-life and only covers symptoms for five to six hours. The return of symptoms was seen as an indication that progesterone was ineffectual. But had the progesterone been given more often—for example, in the morning, at noon, and possibly again at night—the symptoms most likely would have been controlled.

4. There may have been a problem with poor absorption. Suppositories are made from different types of medium, some better than others. Some pharmacists believe that using oral capsules of micronized natural progesterone in oil would produce better results than suppositories.

Doctors' Attitudes

- I have been told by a number of physicians that the subject of hormonal problems, specifically depression, is not taught in depth at medical school. According to an acquaintance who works at a medical school, the curriculum is taught by the "butterfly method," wherein attention alights gently on each subject and quickly flies to the next.

- Women with the hormonal problems covered in this book tend to fall between the cracks of medical specialties. Family physicians are more likely to be helpful, because their scope is more general, and they are more likely to view the body as a whole.

- The training for the OB/GYN specialty centers on surgery and delivering babies. Training about the hormonal disorders I have described is not given in any detail. It is still fairly common practice in treating women with severe PMS to first give Lupron, which puts women into chemical menopause, to see how they fare, and then perform a hysterectomy and oophorectomy. I think this is a pretty drastic treatment, especially since hysterectomy frequently triggers hormonal problems. There may be a place for this option after all other avenues have been explored. While a hysterectomy initiates some women's hormonal problems, it helps other women. But it's a bit like playing Russian roulette. What it will do to a given individual is the question—and the answer won't be determined until afterwards. The surgery is performed on the assumption that if women don't have their ovaries, they can't ovulate and therefore won't have PMS. I don't believe this is a good enough rationale, because I have seen women who don't ovulate, who still have severe symptoms of PMS if not the strict pattern. Just be aware that hysterectomy or treatment with Lupron can produce PMS in someone who doesn't already have it. But balance that information with the thought that these procedures can solve problems for some women.
- Endocrinologists are the specialists who should treat these hormonal disorders, but they seem to deal with obvious thyroid, pituitary, adrenal, and pancreatic problems, as well as endocrine cancers, leaving the ovarian problems to the OB/GYNs.
- Women who have severe hormonal problems are frequently sent to the specialist who deals with mood problems: the psychiatrist. Their approach to treatment is to give psychotropic drugs and, occasionally, shock therapy—rather drastic forms of treatment, which often result in severe side effects and treatment failure.
- Doctors often unwittingly treat women impersonally. They sometimes give the impression that they are interested in the workings of the machine but not the person. I am grateful for the fine physicians I have met, but I talk to

women every day who are dissatisfied with the arrogant attitude of their doctors and the poor medical care they have received. To understand this point, every physician should read the book *The Doctor,* by Dr. Edward E. Rosenbaum.

- Doctors tend to underestimate or treat as superficial the hormonal problems that women experience. They are accustomed to life-and-death drama in the delivery room and in surgery. These other problems seem so inconsequential by comparison. But if these doctors could really get inside a woman's mind and find out what it feels like to want to put your fist through the wall—or worse, your husband or child—they might think differently.

- There is a popular TV doctor who takes the position that PMS doesn't exist and that menopause is not a disorder and shouldn't be treated. Of course, menstruation and menopause are part of the natural order and are not problems in themselves, but malfunction of the reproductive organs happens, as with any other system in the body.

- Doctors may acknowledge that PMS is a real problem, but controversy still exists about treatment. Some will suggest that women improve their diet (eliminate sugar, salt, and caffeine; take magnesium, vitamin B_6, primrose oil, and certain herbs); and get more exercise. But, generally, women with problems that do not respond to these simple changes have limited options for treatment apart from the birth control pill, Prozac, and other even more drastic alternatives.

- When doctors do feel free to prescribe hormones, they often use the birth control pill, which can cause depression in some women. Synthetic progestins do not work the same way natural progesterone does in the cell's receptors, and, by occupying the space that natural progesterone should use, they lower the body's levels of natural progesterone, often causing depression.

- There is a realistic fear of malpractice. There has been increasing litigation, and the cost of malpractice insurance—especially for OB/GYNs—has escalated dramatically. As a result, many OB/GYNs have stopped delivering babies, have become very conservative about treatment, and are forced to practice defensive medicine, using only approved prescriptions and procedures.

- Since the endocrine system and the way cells function are so complex and relatively little understood, doctors should think twice before worsening symptoms by doing anything that might interfere with the delicate balance of the endocrine system; including prescribing birth control pills, other synthetic progestins, or Lupron; or performing surgery such as tubal sterilization, hysterectomy, or oophorectomy.

Rather, it might be wise for a doctor to try the simplest natural hormones first—a small amount of oral estradiol taken daily with enough natural progesterone cyclically to make the necessary changes in the uterus and to relieve symptoms. If doctors would try this simple combination, with its great physical and emotional benefits and relative lack of side effects, on their patients suffering from moderate PMS and premenopause, I believe they would be convinced. This minimum treatment is all that many women would need.

SUMMARY

You can see that there is little recognition of these problems and relatively little research. The attitudes of the FDA and insurance companies are unhelpful, and the hands of physicians are consequently tied even if they want to treat these problems, which many don't. This is why it is frequently difficult for women to find help for their hormonal problems. In fact, many women are powerless to get help because the odds are against them one way or another.

The present situation in medicine will not change until women convince other women and their doctors that their problems are real. Women will have to demand treatment, realizing that their bodies belong to *them*, not to their doctors. And some physicians need to realize who pays the bills.

When I go to see my OB/GYN, Dr. Jones, I find his attitude quite refreshing. As he examines me, he explains what he's doing and why. If there's a problem, he tells me what it is, what he knows about it, and how it can be alleviated. He gives me options and lets me make educated choices. At the end, when I'm about to leave, he always says, "And is there anything else I can do to help you today?" I always leave his office in a wonderful frame of mind.

Not only is Dr. Jones well informed on hormonal problems, he knows how to treat his patients with dignity, respect, and kindness. He treats his patients as though we have enough intelligence to take part in decisions about our treatment. That is why women flock to him and are ecstatic about him as a physician and surgeon.

But many doctors are not like Dr. Jones. Those doctors should beware. There is a new generation of women who will not stand for the treatment they've been given in the past: male-chauvinistic, unsympathetic, uninformed, and—as far as results are concerned—useless and sometimes dangerous.

HOW CAN I FIND HELP?

There are a number of things you can do to help yourself.

1. Learn all you can about your problem. I have included a list of Recommended Reading at the back of this book. These days, there are many helpful books available on specific topics such as menopause. You might go to your local library and see what they have to offer. If your budget is limited, you might order a book you want through inter-library loan. If you live near a hospital medical library, you may be able to use Med-line to research a particular topic.

2. Marshall your family's medical history. Call your mother, sisters, and grandmother if you have them. Ask your aunts and cousins. Keep the information simple and clear. Often your mother's history and that of her female relatives can tell you a great deal about your own problems, because hormonal problems are often hereditary.

3. Write your own point-by-point medical history. Doctors don't have a lot of time to look through page after page of material. Help them with a summary of the peaks and valleys. List age, condition, treatment of problems, surgeries, age when on the birth control pill, eating disorders, and so on. Also, list normal events such as puberty, pregnancies (any problems), and age at menopause. Be brief.

4. Ask your physician for copies of your medical records for you to keep. Some doctors' offices don't like giving them out except to another doctor; I am not sure why, because we pay for the tests.

5. Find a sympathetic physician. Ask your friends. Ask a nurse. Call your local hospital and see if they have a referral line. Look through the yellow pages in your phone book. You might call several doctors' nurses, briefly explain your problem, and ask them a few questions about how the doctor might treat your condition before you pay a lot of money for a full consultation. This way, you may get a feel for the doctor's approach without putting out a lot of money for nothing.

6. You may be able to get a good referral from a national group such as the North American Menopause Society in Cleveland, Ohio, or from one of the pharmacies that compound natural hormones listed in the back of this book. Madison Pharmacy has a zip-coded directory of physician names, and can give you some local choices for a small charge. None are guaranteed, of course.

7. In choosing a type of physician, the following specialties may be a good choice: family physician, OB/GYN, endocrinologist, or internist. Your HMO (health maintenance organization) may only allow you to go to a family physician, in which case you have little choice. You might also do well going to a nurse practitioner or a physician's assistant; I know a number of these who do a great job. Often they will spend more time with you than a doctor would.

8. If you can find a few really good medical articles on specific subjects, many physicians will appreciate the information.

Even though some doctors get a little annoyed if their patient tries to tell them something, other doctors are open to learning new information. A physician in the medical office next door to my office told me the other day that women are coming in and asking for natural hormones frequently now. This will happen more and more.

9. Make the most of your medical appointment. You may need to make more than one appointment so that you have enough time to talk. Doctors these days are very pressed for time because of the restrictions placed on them by HMOs. Even if you have had a problem for a long time and feel angry with your doctor, it doesn't do any good to make him or her angry. You can tell your doctor how you feel while keeping your dignity.

Questions You Might Ask Your Physician

1. *Do you think that PMS is a real problem?* Your doctor might say "Yes, it is a real problem, but we don't know what causes it, and so there is no known treatment." You might provide information you have collected about the treatment you would like to try.

2. *What would you use to treat women with PMS?* Your doctor might suggest exercise, vitamin B_6 (always take it as a complex), magnesium, an essential fatty acid such as primrose oil, and restricting coffee. These are good suggestions and worth trying, but are probably not enough to help severe cases. Your doctor might prescribe birth control pills. (They help some, and make some worse. The type of pill is important. A slightly higher estrogen/lower progestin pill such as OvCon 35 or 50, Modicon, or Brevicon is less likely to cause depression.) Or diuretics. (Diuretics can be very harsh on the system and not too helpful. Probably spironolactone is the best diuretic, since it is an analog of natural progesterone.) Or Prozac. (Prozac helps some women. There are a number of studies showing that it does. I don't think it should be a first

treatment, since women with a family history of hormonal depression may need to take it for many years. It does help a lot of women, but some women have really bad side effects from Prozac.) Your doctor might suggest trying natural progesterone, and if your symptoms fit the classic pattern of PMS, you might go for it. (Information on PMS symptoms and treatment is given in Chapter 5). Estrogen taken in the last half of the menstrual cycle is also a treatment for PMS. The patch might help if progesterone doesn't.

3. *What do you think of hormone therapy?* Natural progesterone? (Remember that most studies indicate that natural progesterone is no better than a placebo, so some doctors will echo this.) *What about estrogen for PMS?* A number of nationally known physicians (see Chapter 11 on Estrogen and Depression) use estrogen for PMS.

4. *I have had hormonal problems for years; I have been diagnosed as depressed and have been treated with antidepressants which have not worked; I have read that hormones can help depression; would you be willing to try them on me?* Articles by Dr. J. W. W. Studd and colleagues of London, England, would be helpful, as well as the book *Screaming to Be Heard: Hormonal Connections Women Suspect and Doctors Ignore,* by Dr. Elizabeth Lee Vliet.

5. If your doctor does not specialize in your type of problem, ask: *"Do you know anyone who specializes in these problems? Do you know what their approach is? Would you be willing to give me a referral?"*

6. *My mother and sisters have thyroid problems; my tests have always been normal, but I think I may have a thyroid problem (describe specific symptoms); would you be willing to do extra tests?* (The extra tests are listed in Chapter 8 on the thyroid.)

7. *I'm only 39, but I feel as though I'm going through menopause (describe specific symptoms); my mother stopped having periods at age 41 and so did my grandmother; I've heard this can be hereditary; would you be willing to test me?* There is a hereditary predisposition for some women to go through

menopause earlier than the norm. If you mention this, your doctor will probably pay attention to it.

8. *I am having side effects from a particular hormone; would you be willing to try a more natural form of estrogen (progesterone, thyroid) on me?*

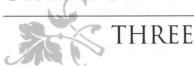

THREE

HOW YOUR
HORMONES WORK:
THE ENDOCRINE SYSTEM

HELPFUL DEFINITIONS
FOR THIS CHAPTER

Endocrine System: The system of glands and other structures that produce internal secretions called hormones, which are released directly into the bloodstream, influencing metabolism and other body processes. Included are the hypothalamus, pituitary, thyroid, parathyroid, adrenal glands, ovaries (in women), testes (in men), pancreas, and so on.

Gland: A body of cells specialized to secrete or excrete materials. Endocrine glands secrete many chemicals and hormones directly into the bloodstream. Exocrine glands, by contrast, carry their secretions externally—for example, the sweat and salivary glands.

Hormones: Chemical messengers, sent out by the endocrine glands, which control or stimulate hundreds of vital processes and act on almost every cell in the body. Hormones influence how we grow, our sexual development and sex drive, sleep patterns, and mental alertness. They affect our personality and behavior, height and weight, speed of movement, and gender and sexuality.

Hypothalamus: A part of the brain adjacent to the pituitary. It has many functions and contains the centers for appetite, sex drive, thirst, and sleep. It controls the autonomic, parasympathetic, and sympathetic nervous systems, the immune and endocrine systems, and many other body functions.

Autonomic and sympathetic nervous systems: Concerned with regulation of cardiac muscle, smooth muscle, and glands.

Parasympathetic nervous system: Stimulates the heart, smooth muscle, and glands of the head and neck, as well as the tissues of the chest, abdomen, and pelvis.

Immune System: Specialized cells and molecules whose primary function is to distinguish what is self and what is not self in order to defend the body against foreign living things or substances.

Autoimmune disease: A condition in which the body's defenses mistake the body's own healthy tissue for an enemy and attack it.

Autoantibody: An antibody formed in response to, and reacting against, one's own tissue. These will damage different tissues, glands, or organs, depending on the type of autoantibody produced.

Pituitary gland: Also called the hypophysis. Located at the base of the brain in the sella turcica and attached by a stalk to the hypothalamus. It has two main lobes: 1) the anterior lobe, secreting several important hormones which regulate the proper functioning of the thyroid, parathyroid, adrenals, ovaries, and so on (also produces prolactin and growth hormone), and 2) the posterior lobe, whose cells serve as a reservoir for oxytocin and vasopressin, releasing them as needed.

Prolactin: Stimulates maternal behavior and secretion of breast milk. Inhibits ovarian hormones at times during the menstrual cycle and lactation.

Growth hormone (somatotropin): Hormone that accelerates body growth.

Oxytocin: Stored in the posterior pituitary. It induces active labor, increases the force of contractions, helps contract the uterine muscles after delivery of the placenta, controls postpartum hemorrhage, and stimulates milk ejection.

Vasopressin: Stored in the posterior pituitary. It constricts blood vessels, raises the blood pressure, increases peristalsis (the undulating motion of the intestines during digestion), exerts some influence on the uterus, influences resorption of water by the kidneys, and helps concentrate urine. Used as an antidiuretic.

Thyroid gland: An endocrine gland that consists of two lobes, one on each side of the trachea (windpipe), joined by a narrow bridge. The thyroid gland produces the thyroid hormones thyroxine, also known as tetraiodothyronine (T4), and triiodothyronine (T3), which require iodine for their manufacture. These are essential for proper growth and development and for regulating metabolic rate. If thyroid-deficient, infants can have arrested growth and can develop cretinism with severe retardation, dwarfism, and other deformities. The thyroid also secretes calcitonin.

Parathyroid glands: Small disk-shaped glands that usually are found on the back and side of each thyroid lobe. Most people have four of these, but the number can vary. Parathyroid hormone raises the amount of calcium that circulates in the blood, while the thyroid hormone calcitonin lowers it.

Metabolism: The sum of all the physical and chemical processes by which living organized substance is produced and maintained (anabolism). Also the transformation by which energy is made available for the uses of the organism (catabolism).

Basal metabolism: The minimal energy expended to maintain respiration, circulation, peristalsis, muscle tone, body temperature, glandular activity, and the other vegetative functions.

Adrenal gland: A flattened body above each kidney, consisting of a cortex and a medulla. The cortex makes steroid hormones, and the medulla makes epinephrine (adrenaline) and norepinephrine.

Cortex: The outer, firm layer; the larger part of the adrenal gland. It secretes various hormones including mineralocorticoids (aldosterone), glucocorticoids (cortisol, also known as hydrocortisone and cortisone), androgens, 17-ketosteroids, and progesterone.

Aldosterone: An adrenal hormone involved in the regulation of electrolyte and water balance, resulting in retention of sodium and loss of potassium.

Cortisol: An adrenal hormone involved in metabolism of carbohydrates, fats, and proteins, alteration of connective tissue response to injury, inhibition of inflammatory and allergic reaction, and many other actions. Helps fight infections.

Medulla: The central portion of the adrenal gland. It synthesizes, stores, and releases catecholamines (epinephrine and norepinephrine).

Adrenaline (epinephrine) and norepinephrine: Adrenal neurotransmitters involved in a person's "fight-or-flight" response when in danger or under emotional or physical stress. They are also released in response to low blood pressure, low blood sugar, cold exposure, low oxygen levels, and other stressful circumstances. Both hormones have similarities, causing the heart to beat faster, increasing alertness, and providing energy. However, norepinephrine is a powerful vasopressor, constricting the muscle tissue of the capillaries and arteries, whereas epinephrine both constricts and dilates various blood vessels to bring more blood to the muscles to provide extra strength, if needed.

Ovaries: The two walnut-sized female sex glands located near the uterus. The ovaries contain a woman's lifetime supply of eggs and produce the hormones estrogen, progesterone, and testosterone (as well as other androgens).

Follicle stimulating hormone (FSH), luteinizing hormone (LH), estrogen, progesterone, and testosterone: see Chapter 4 on the menstrual cycle for definitions.

Uterus: The hollow, muscular organ in female mammals that houses the embedded and fertilized egg and nourishes the embryo and fetus. Its cavity opens through the cervix into the vagina below and into a uterine tube on each upper side.

Cell: The basic unit of living organisms, consisting of a nucleus (sphere-shaped body at the center of the cell) surrounded by cytoplasm (viscous, translucent fluid) enclosed in a cell membrane or plasma membrane. There are trillions of cells in the body. Biologists group them according to their similarities, and there are approximately 300 different types. There are specialized cells to control digestion, breathing, excretion, circulation, and reproduction. Other cells in the nervous and endocrine systems coordinate and integrate the functions of the other systems. Most cells contain certain common organelles (little versions of organs within the body). Like a separate little universe or a little body, each cell functions as a tiny factory, keeping the whole body working at peak performance.

Cell membrane or plasma membrane: The membrane around the cell that is semipermeable (it allows entry of some substances and excludes others).

Cell receptor: Hormone molecules are often too large to pass unaided through the cell membrane, so the cell contains receptors to facilitate this. A receptor is a molecule on the surface or within a cell that recognizes and binds with other specific molecules, enabling the visiting molecule to produce a particular effect within the cell. As an example, there are cell receptors for each specific steroid hormone. When a hormone molecule attaches to a cell receptor, the receptor acts as a transmitter and passes information into the DNA (genetic material) found at the center of the nucleus of the cell. This transmission of information results in many important chemical events. This is why hormone function is so vital. The sex hormones have pivotal functions in the cell and act as both supervisor and janitor.

HOW THE ENDOCRINE SYSTEM WORKS

The endocrine system consists of a number of glands which produce hormones. These glands include the hypothalamus, pituitary, thyroid, parathyroid, ovaries, testes, adrenals, and pancreas. You can see the location of the endocrine glands in

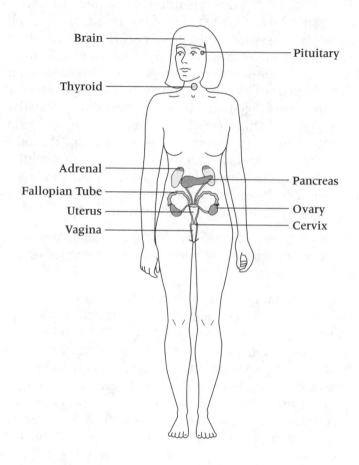

Figure 1   Female Reproductive Anatomy

Figure 1. Like the spine, the position of these glands is quite central in the body, and their role is very important.

Hormones are chemical messengers that pass information through the bloodstream, traveling from gland to gland and gland to cell. The nervous system also conveys information, but hormones do it in a much more concentrated and efficient way. If you didn't have an endocrine system, you would need a more complex nervous system with much more "wiring."

The hypothalamus and pituitary constitute the "head office" of the endocrine system and control myriad hormonal and immune system functions. These glands are located close together in the brain, at each end of an organ about the size of a tonsil. They control the hormonal system like a sensitive conductor leading an orchestra.

The brain begins the endocrine processes by sending out a variety of releasing and stimulating hormones into the bloodstream. Like an arrow winging its way to the bull's-eye, these hormones travel to various target glands—for example, the thyroid, the ovaries, the adrenals, the pancreas, and the mammary (breast).

These target glands, in turn, produce other hormones that travel to many of the body's cells. There they enter the cell receptors, combine with the DNA in the cell nucleus, and work to maintain the healthy functioning of each cell.

There are also individual feedback systems to the brain for each hormone so that the brain knows what is going on in the body at any time and can adjust its own output of hormones.

Four Levels of Function

To express it simply, you could say that there are four main working levels: 1) the brain (hypothalamus and pituitary); 2) the glands (thyroid, ovaries, adrenals, pancreas, and so on); 3) the many cells affected by hormones; and 4) the feedback system to the brain. The bloodstream is the go-between that carries messages back and forth.

More About the Hypothalamus

The hypothalamus is a tiny gland in the limbic area of the brain. It acts like a radar station, catching and fielding all the outside impulses entering the brain. It has many functions.

The hypothalamus controls the endocrine system, producing releasing hormones that target the pituitary. It also controls the central nervous system, the immune system, and the sympathetic and parasympathetic nervous systems. So it controls many of our unconscious actions, including the regulation of body temperature, hunger, thirst, and sex drive. It also contains the sleep center and helps the body handle stress.

More About the Pituitary

The pituitary has its own specific functions. In addition to producing stimulating hormones that go to the glands, it produces growth hormone, prolactin, oxytocin, and vasopressin. Prolactin is elevated during pregnancy and controls lactation afterward. One of the functions of prolactin is to inhibit the ovarian hormones, which it does after pregnancy. Estrogen and progesterone levels plummet to almost zero after delivery, which can cause a menopause-like postpartum depression in some women; they may experience drying of the vagina, fatigue, hot flashes, low sex drive, headaches, and depression. This inhibiting function of prolactin can also affect the thyroid, contributing to either a temporary or permanent condition of low thyroid after pregnancy.

Prolactin is also present during the menstrual cycle, and elevated levels of prolactin can inhibit progesterone levels. One of the theories about the cause of PMS is that some women have too high a level of prolactin, though tests do not support this thesis. Still, high prolactin levels may be one cause of PMS. Women who have inappropriate leakage from the breast (galactorrhea) may have high prolactin levels, and sometimes this is due to a tumor in the pituitary, which is usually benign. Pituitary swelling can also be caused by hormonal imbalance in the target glands.

The pituitary is also a major producer of endorphins—neurotransmitters which help people have that "great to be alive" feeling. Researchers have found that women with PMS have only 25 percent of the endorphin levels that normal women have premenstrually. The β-endorphins also drop drastically after delivery of a baby. And women going through menopause also have lower levels of endorphins. Taking estrogen and natural progesterone raises the endorphin levels.

Releasing and Stimulating Hormones

The hypothalamus puts out *releasing* hormones, including TRH (thyroid releasing hormone) for the thyroid, CRF (corticotropin releasing factor) for the adrenals, and FSH-LHRH (follicle-stimulating hormone, luteinizing hormone releasing hormone) for the ovaries. These are chemical messengers that go to the pituitary gland and cause it, in turn, to produce *stimulating* hormones. These stimulating hormones (including TSH for the thyroid, ACTH for the adrenals, and FSH and LH for the ovaries), then travel to their respective target glands.

Any time one of these glands doesn't function properly, it tends to throw out the production of the other glands, because they are all closely related and their functions are interdependent.

How the Thyroid Gland Functions

The hypothalamus puts out a hormone called TRH (thyroid releasing hormone), which travels to the pituitary which, in turn, sends out TSH (thyroid stimulating hormone). TSH goes through the bloodstream and targets the thyroid gland, where several types of thyroid hormones (thyroxine) are produced. Two main kinds are tetraiodothyronine (T4) and triiodothyronine (T3). The thyroid gland also indirectly produces calcitonin, a hormone that helps regulate calcium in the bloodstream. The various hormones produced in the thyroid gland enter the bloodstream and make their way to the cells where they are responsible for many different functions. For instance, the thyroid gland controls the body's temperature and metabolism.

The body has a thyroid feedback system to the brain. When you are cold and your blood levels of thyroxine are low, the feedback system notifies the hypothalamus to send out more TRH and start the process again. When blood levels of thyroxine are high, the hypothalamus switches off the production of TRH.

Low thyroid (or hypothyroidism) is the most common thyroid malfunction. When your thyroid function is low, you tend to feel the cold excessively. Your bodily functions, movement, coordination, thinking, and speech slow down, and you may feel exhausted, anxious, and depressed. You may find that you have little sex drive and have frequent sinus and upper respiratory infections. Or you may have menstrual disorders, with cramps and heavy menstrual flow. By contrast, hyperthyroidism speeds the body up and can create extreme nervousness, agitation, and wakefulness; menstrual flow tends to be light.

How the Adrenal Gland Functions

The hypothalamus sends CRF (corticotropin releasing factor) to the pituitary, which triggers the pituitary to produce ACTH (adrenocorticotropin hormone). ACTH travels to the adrenals, which produce several kinds of hormones: adrenaline; glucocorticoids, including cortisol (hydrocortisone); mineralocorticoids, including aldosterone; and androgens, including dehydroepiandrosterone (DHEA) and androstenedione (both of which are converted to testosterone and dihydrotestosterone).

Adrenaline is the fight-or-flight hormone that helps to control stress. Cortisol is the hormone that helps control infections and allergies. Aldosterone helps regulate fluids and electrolyte balance. Androgens, including testosterone and DHEA, are considered "male" hormones, which women also produce (just as men have low levels of female hormones). Men have 20 to 40 times the amount of androgens that women do.

Androgens break down in the fat cells into estrone, a weak estrogen. Women who are overweight, particularly with fat deposited around their middle (android obesity), have higher levels of androgens. As a consequence, they have higher levels of unbound estrogens. This type of estrogen has been linked to increased risk of breast cancer.

The adrenal gland has many necessary functions; without the cortex, a person cannot handle stress and will die.

How the Ovaries Function

The hypothalamus secretes FSH-LHRH (follicle-stimulating hormone, luteinizing hormone, releasing hormone). This travels to the pituitary, which, in turn, produces FSH and LH.

Traveling through the bloodstream at different times of the month, FSH and LH produce estrogen and progesterone—the two main female hormones in the ovaries. FSH causes the production of estrogen in the first half of the menstrual cycle and develops the egg for fertilization. LH causes ovulation, the production of progesterone, and lower levels of estrogen during the second half of the cycle.

Estrogen has many functions in the female body. It stimulates the breast tissue. It also builds up the lining of the uterus to house a pregnancy each month. Without estrogen, skin, hair, bone, muscles, mucous membranes, the vascular system—in fact, just about every tissue in the body—begin to dry and deteriorate.

Progesterone supplements and balances the effects of estrogen in the breasts and uterus. Like estrogen, its function is ubiquitous and its influence on the body is very calming and sometimes depressive. The ovaries also produce testosterone and other androgens, which help sex drive, muscle strength, and mental clarity, and provides a feeling of well-being.

After menopause, the ovaries still produce hormones, though the quantities and types change.

Down at the Cellular Level

The target organs—the thyroid, adrenals, and ovaries—produce hormones, and the hormones enter the bloodstream heading for the cells.

There are trillions of cells in the body. Biologists group them according to their similarities, and there are approximately 300 different types. Each cell functions as a microfactory, keeping the whole body working at peak performance.

Hormone molecules are unable to directly enter the cell nucleus. However, these molecules can enter their specific cell receptors, and information is then transmitted into the cell nucleus. Inside the cells are tiny specific receptors for each hormone. The hormone molecule is like a key; the receptor is like a lock. A particular hormone molecule must be recognized by the receptor and "fit" into it. Then it must "open" it, just the way a key would open a lock. When this happens properly, the receptor is enabled to transmit information into the cell's DNA. This leads to important chemical changes.

To respond properly to a progesterone molecule, the progesterone receptor first needs "priming" by estrogen. When estrogen is produced in the first half of the cycle, progesterone receptors increase in number. There is a switching back and forth of both hormones. At times progesterone increases estrogen levels, at other times it inhibits them, depending on the phase of the menstrual cycle.

Universal Effects

Hormone receptors are more prevalent in the cells of certain organs, such as the limbic area of the brain, which controls the emotions, and the breasts and uterus. (These hormones also work in other organs in the body, but by other methods than via receptors). When the endocrine system doesn't work properly, hormone levels can change. When hormones are at a low level, their receptors decline in number. Everywhere that these cell receptors are missing or nonfunctional, deficiency symptoms are likely to occur. This applies to all the hormones. Thyroid and cortisol, for instance, affect virtually every cell in the body.

Individuals with hormonal problems may have widely different symptoms, affecting many parts of the body. This is because the hypothalamus controls so many body systems, and, at the cellular level, there is such a widespread dispersal of cell receptors.

The Gate Theory

If the body were dependent on nerve impulses to control the function of every cell, it would need many more nerves and use more energy than it presently has. Controlling the cells by hormones is a much more efficient and economical process.

Cells contain enzymes made of protein molecules that take raw material (organic molecules coming into the cell) and make it usable within the cell or prepare it for export to other needy cells.

To protect the cell, there are protein "gates" protruding from both sides of the cell wall. These "gates" have several functions. They release waste products from the cell and help to retain nutrients. They also act as sentries, blocking or admitting any invasive substance that tries to enter the cell.

There are exceptions that bypass the gate or sentry, however. The main steroidal hormones—estrogen and progesterone in women, testosterone in men, and thyroid in both sexes—can go in and out of the cell wall at will and can enter many different types of cells. They do not have to pass through the "gates."

According to Dr. Norman Farb's unpublished manuscript on the gate theory:

> Steroids (sex hormones) have a peculiar capability. They do not need a gate in the cell wall to allow them to enter the cell. Once inside the cell, they connect with their receptor, pass through the nuclear pores and reach the site of the nucleus that contains the genes (the DNA). The binding of the hormone with the gene somehow enables the cell to maintain itself, to repair and rebuild the gates on the cell wall and the enzymes. Without this maintenance, the cell deteriorates and ages, with effects on the entire organism.

The steroid hormones, therefore, largely control the health and well-being of the cell. When the steroid hormone levels are low, repair and rebuilding of the gates and production of important enzymes cannot take place, nitrogen is thrown out of balance, and the cell breaks down. Waste products accumulate; invaders have open access; nutrients leak out of the cell; and the connective tissues are affected. Because hormones increase or decrease the rate of activity of the cell, a decrease in the number of receptors means that the cell will no longer function properly.

The Body's Switching Mechanism

When estrogen levels drop, the number of estrogen receptors also diminishes. Taking estrogen not only increases the level of estrogen in the blood; it also increases the number of receptor sites, making estrogen more available to the cells.

Estrogen also increases the number of progesterone receptors and primes them to work, while progesterone can both increase and decrease estrogen receptors depending on the phase of the menstrual cycle. This switching back and forth between estrogen and progesterone is a strong argument for giving some women both hormones for PMS and pre-menopause.

The Feedback System to the Brain

The body has many feedback systems which send information to the brain. Each hormone has a feedback system to the brain, able to notify the hypothalamus about what is happening hormonally in other parts of the body. If the feedback system indicates that the body is low in certain hormones, the hypothalamus will increase its production of releasing hormones, and the whole process begins again.

Body Rhythms

It's not only the type and amount of hormones sent out that makes the endocrine system work. There are also delicate body rhythms that switch back and forth.

Dr. Dean Black mentions that our bodies pulse with rhythm.[1] Most major systems in the body have two distinct types of function that constantly switch back and forth with opposite effects. Dr. Black cites the brain, which has a right and left half, as an example. The left half notices things, the right gives them meaning, and the two sides switch back and forth.

The nervous system can be divided into the sympathetic and parasympathetic halves. One controls the world without; the other controls the world within. We repeatedly swing back and forth, between the outside and inside world.

The hormonal system also has two components: the catecholamines and the endorphins. In general, the catecholamines arouse us, and the endorphins calm us. Again, there is a constant swinging back and forth between the two. The immune system also has two opposing components: its aggressive immune cells and its calming suppressor cells. The body has two general types of processes—the catabolic and the anabolic—which alternate between breaking apart and combining, freeing energy and recovering it.

The menstrual cycle is another example. Estrogen builds up the lining of the uterus, and progesterone breaks it down when pregnancy doesn't take place. Estrogen dilates the blood vessels; progesterone constricts them. Estrogen produces progesterone receptors and primes them to work. Progesterone can switch the estrogen receptors either on or off. These events are constantly happening, back and forth and on and off.

To the rhythm principle, Dr. Black adds synchronization, a principle of physics which demonstrates that stronger rhythms can "capture" weaker rhythms and coordinate them. The hypothalamus synchronizes the many disparate rhythms in the body and makes them march to one tune in team formation.

When women have hormonal problems, the rhythm and the synchronization of their menstrual cycle are thrown out of gear. It's as if members of an orchestra were playing discordant notes at different tempos. Treating hormonal problems includes restoring the body's rhythms.

Dr. Black makes the point that PMS is a "dynamic" disease, characterized by abnormal body rhythms, rather than by a simple chemical deficiency that can be measured. Dr. Black says that this may be why the results of many PMS research studies have been inconclusive and why the usual double-blind approach has not worked.

How the Glands Interrelate—The Team Effect

All the glands controlled by the pituitary not only have individual functions, they also strongly influence each other and function as a team. The thyroid sends a releasing hormone to the hypothalamus that starts the whole menstrual cycle rolling. Women with thyroid problems frequently have menstrual problems as a result. The thyroid both exerts control over the adrenals and is supported by the adrenals.

In the adrenals, androgens break down into weak forms of estrogen and progesterone, so the adrenals function as back-up sex organs supporting the ovaries. They have a particularly important role after menopause, when the ovaries shut down their major production of estrogen. After menopause, women are supplied with estrogen through the breakdown of androgens, produced by both the adrenals and the ovaries.

If a woman loses one or both ovaries, her estrogen levels are obviously going to be affected. But the adrenals also play an important role. Many women function well after menopause, until they experience a shock or trauma such as a car accident or the death of a close family member, which may bring on adrenal exhaustion and begin typical menopause symptoms.

You can easily see the team effect. When one gland doesn't work properly, the others may be affected to one degree or another.

More Than One Problem

When the level of one hormone is low, there is a tendency for others to decline in sympathy, and hormonal problems can become very complicated. Thyroid, estrogen, progesterone, and other hormones are closely related in function, opposing, augmenting, and balancing each other.

Women can have autoimmune and polyendocrine disorders, in which there are problems with the immune system. Sometimes more than one gland is affected, and more than one hormone is low or malfunctioning. These disorders are rare. But the extreme cases possibly illustrate what is going on at a minor level in women with multiple hormonal symptoms.

The Endocrine System Is Complex

When one looks at the complexity of the endocrine system and the menstrual cycle, it is not really surprising that they can break down, just like any other part of the body. The surprising thing is that some physicians almost act as though the endocrine system doesn't exist.

Women's hormonal and immune systems are much more intricate than men's because of ovulation and pregnancy. Men may have their own hormonal cycles, but they do not have the dramatic rise and fall of hormones that women experience during their menstrual cycles. Pregnancy creates the need for a stronger immune system, since the fetus is a foreign object that normally would be rejected by the body. The complexity of the female immune system enables a woman to carry a baby to term.

Because of the complexity of the female immune system, women have by far the greater proportion of autoimmune system diseases, such as lupus and rheumatoid arthritis.

Likewise, women can easily have problems with menstruation because their cycles are so intricate. Problems often begin at puberty, and some women lose their health after a particular pregnancy.

HOW HORMONE IMBALANCE AFFECTS BLOOD SUGAR

The pituitary gland produces growth hormone, and one of its functions is to produce glucagon in the pancreas. Insulin is also produced in the pancreas under the indirect control of the pituitary, and glucagon and insulin control blood sugar levels. Because the pituitary is involved in the production of all these hormones, blood sugar levels can easily be affected when thyroid and sex hormones don't work properly.

PMS is an illustration of this. Progesterone, the hormone dominant after ovulation during the second half of the menstrual cycle, and gamma globulin (which carries the blood sugar), share receptor sites in the cells. When progesterone levels are low, blood sugar levels tend to be low because one of the functions of progesterone is to metabolize sugar. Conversely, during pregnancy, when progesterone levels are very high, some women develop gestational diabetes, a high blood sugar condition which may be temporary or may herald the onset of permanent diabetes.

Dr. Katherina Dalton states that treatment for low blood sugar in women with PMS is essential. These women need to eat more frequently premenstrually, because of the erratic fluctuation of their blood sugar levels. Tests may not show any problem, but such women are functionally hypoglycemic. When blood sugar levels drop below a certain level, it can cause shock, and adrenaline is quickly produced to counteract this. Since blood sugar levels drop much more quickly premenstrually, adrenaline spurts out sooner.

When this occurs, women may often find that they have headaches, become suddenly irritable and tired, or have angry, violent episodes, especially when they haven't eaten for a long time. Once the blood sugar level drops, it can take a week to rise to normal levels again. Though it may seem a minor point, following a hypoglycemia diet by eating complex carbohydrates every three to four hours can result in significant improvement. Hormone therapy alone, without such a diet, may be a treatment failure; both treatments may be necessary for success.

There is also a known connection between blood sugar problems in women—both hypoglycemia and diabetes—and low thyroid problems. Nathan Becker, M.D., has said that 75 percent of female diabetics are also hypothyroid.

At menopause, when estrogen is low, women are also subject to unpredictable fluctuations in blood sugar levels.

The message is: when the hormones malfunction, changes in blood sugar are inevitable, and attention to diet is extremely important.

HOW HORMONE IMBALANCES AFFECT BRAIN FUNCTION

Recent studies have suggested that a disruption of certain neurotransmitters in the brain is responsible for PMS. Neurotransmitters are just different types of hormones—chemical messengers passed from one point to another in the brain by the firing of neurons. They are responsible for the process of thought. When they don't function properly, people may become depressed, psychotic, or schizophrenic. Doctors use anti-depressants to change thinking by chemically altering the neu-rotransmitters in the brain.

There are about 100 known neurotransmitters. Re-searchers know much about only four of them: serotonin, dopamine, norepinephrine, and the endorphins. Neuro-transmitters in the brain help trigger and control the produc-tion of sex hormones. And, at the same time, sex hormones such as estrogen increase the levels of these neurotransmitters and improve memory and mood. So sex hormones and brain neurotransmitters are intimately related, triggering each other. This is important because it explains why many women with hormonal disorders have severe emotional problems, and why some find improvement with the use of antidepressants, others with hormones.

HOW HORMONE IMBALANCES AFFECT THE IMMUNE SYSTEM

The immune system is programmed to destroy foreign pro-teins that it doesn't recognize. Hormones are made of protein and, sometimes, when your hormones drop significantly or fluctuate wildly, the immune system sensors lose their mem-ory bank for these hormones. This may result in the produc-tion of antibodies and white blood cells, which can fight and destroy a person's own hormones.

This is particularly true of the thyroid—the most common endocrine gland that builds up antibodies. Thyroiditis can re-sult from this, and while the usual thyroid blood levels may appear normal, a high antibody count may indicate a problem. Women may have normal thyroid levels, yet the thyroid hor-mone may not work in the cells. Thyroid antibodies can de-stroy thyroid hormones. This can happen at three levels: in the thyroid, in the bloodstream, and in the cell receptors. Also, some people are resistant to their own thyroid hormone.

Antibodies can also build up against the ovaries and adren-als. Not only does your body sometimes fight the hormones it makes, it may also fight the hormone supplements you take.

So, sometimes, women taking estrogen, progesterone, or thyroid experience side effects though they really need these medications.

RARE EXAMPLES OF SEVERE HORMONAL IMBALANCE

There are two relatively rare disorders which may illustrate the type of disease process occurring in milder hormonal problems: Sheehan's syndrome and polyglandular autoimmune syndrome (PAS).

In Sheehan's syndrome, there is partial or complete destruction of a mother's pituitary gland after severe shock (usually from hemorrhage) in giving birth. The resulting physical shock can cause hypopituitarism (low pituitary function) in the mother, which in turn leads to low levels of other hormones (especially cortisol and thyroid). This disease causes multiple endocrine problems. It involves autoimmune changes as the drastic drop in hormone production after delivery affects immunity. One of the symptoms of Sheehan's is psychosis.

In the polyglandular autoimmune syndrome (PAS), there is an autoimmune process going on in the body which causes one endocrine gland after another to fail over a period of years. The majority of affected individuals are female. When a number of family members have the same problems, there appears to be a genetic basis for the disease. Schmidt syndrome (autoimmune low adrenal and low thyroid function) was the disease originally termed "PAS," but the definition has been expanded to include any combination of a number of autoimmune problems. These include adrenal insufficiency, thyroiditis, hypoparathyroidism (low parathyroid hormone levels), and failure of the ovaries in women or testes in men. Sometimes a person with PAS may also have one or more of the following: diabetes mellitus, pernicious anemia, chronic autoimmune hepatitis, vitiligo (a skin disease characterized by whitish areas, sometimes with borders the color of a sun tan), myasthenia gravis (a disease causing abnormal muscle weakness or fatigue), hyperthyroidism, or malabsorption syndrome (such as celiac disease, which is a wheat intolerance that causes damage to the upper intestine, or sprue, a chronic tropical disease caused by long-term ingestion of infected food and characterized by diarrhea, emaciation, and anemia) and systemic candidiasis (yeast infestation). The most significant feature in the lab test results of people with PAS is low levels of circulating hormones and the presence of antibodies to one or more endocrine gland. The gland may appear normal at first, but over time its functioning becomes increasingly low.

DISEASE MODELS

These are very rare diseases. I have only seen one or two women who ultimately turned out to have Sheehan's syndrome, and a few who were diagnosed with polyglandular autoimmune syndrome. I am interested in these two disorders because they are models that illustrate the kind of disease process that could be at work in some women with complex hormonal problems.

Both diseases are polyendocrine disorders, meaning that they involve a failure of more than one endocrine gland as a result of either physical trauma (Sheehan's syndrome) or heredity, stress, and environmental factors (PAS). These are different diseases with different causes, but there are similarities between them. For instance, adrenal and thyroid failure are central to both diseases and are also linked with failure of the sex hormones.

Both diseases illustrate the teamwork of the glands: when one gland is affected, others are often impacted. They both illustrate the complexity of hormonal problems and the involvement of the immune system.

The Link with Thyroid

Both Sheehan's syndrome and PAS involve thyroid failure and illustrate links with other hormonal problems—Sheehan's with thyroid and postpartum depression, and PAS with thyroid and early menopause. In the polyglandular autoimmune syndrome, autoimmune thyroiditis is linked with early ovarian failure, which can lead to premature menopause. Note that menopause before the age of 40 commonly occurs in women with some type of autoimmune disease. Though PAS is very rare, autoimmune thyroiditis is amazingly common in women (approximately one in eight women have it). While not all women who have thyroiditis will experience menopause before the age of 40, it may be one cause of a long and difficult perimenopause; the autoimmune process may also be causing early damage to the ovaries over a period of years.

Hormonal Problems Are Not Always Simple

These two rare diseases show us that hormonal problems are not simple. This is why researchers still don't know exactly what is happening in PMS—not because it's a non-event or just an excuse that women use to misbehave. Rather, it's because PMS is so complex and elusive that it has thus far defied specific measurement and absolute explanation.

SUMMARY

Interference with the hormonal system at any level can cause a woman to experience chemical changes and alterations in her rhythm and synchronization, with resulting symptoms of hormonal distress. This explains why there are many causes for PMS and other problems. They can arise from genetic tendencies, from the use of the birth control pill or other hormones, from hypothalamic or pituitary problems from pregnancy, miscarriage, or abortion, from anorexia or bulimia, from surgery such as tubal ligation or hysterectomy, or from conditions such as ovarian cysts, polycystic ovaries, endometriosis, or uterine fibroids. They can also occur as a result of immune system breakdown from chemical poisoning or viral problems. Stress and lifestyle also play their roles.

Knowing how the endocrine system works at different levels enables women to understand how important hormones are to health and well-being and why hormonal problems can be complex and can give rise to so many different symptoms.

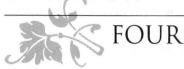

CHAPTER

FOUR

THE MENSTRUAL CYCLE: HOW YOUR HORMONES WORK

HELPFUL DEFINITIONS
FOR THIS CHAPTER

Menstrual Cycle: The number of days between menstrual periods. Days are counted from day one of the flow of one period to day one of the flow of the next period.

Menstrual Flow: The number of days of menstrual bleeding.

Ovulation: The time when the egg leaves the ovary and travels down the fallopian tube to the uterus. Usually takes place midcycle (day 10–16; the average is day 14), in a 28-day cycle. Time of highest fertility. Sex drive often peaks then.

Units of measure:

NANOGRAM: One billionth of a gram in weight(10^9). Abbreviation: ng.

PICOGRAM: One trillionth of a gram in weight (10^{12}). Abbreviation: pg.

INTERNATIONAL UNITS: Measurements of the activity of a substance, not its weight, expressed as so many international units

(IU) per milliliter (ml) of fluid. One thousand International Units is abbreviated mIU.

GRAIN: 64.8 milligrams, or 0.0023 ounce.

MICROGRAM: one millionth of a gram. Abbreviation: mcg.

Follicle-Stimulating Hormone (FSH): A pituitary hormone which is at high levels before puberty (because estrogen is low). As estrogen levels rise around puberty, normal FSH levels drop. Mid-cycle levels are typically about twice the base level. FSH levels begin to rise as estrogen levels drop about a decade before menopause.

Levels of FSH:

NORMAL ADULT FEMALE: 5 to 20 mIU/ml. Varies depending on when during the cycle the blood test is done (the day blood is drawn needs to be noted).

TOO LOW: less than 5 mIU/ml. Can indicate that a girl has not yet reached puberty; can indicate hypothalamic or pituitary failure in premenopausal women; can be suppressed by high doses of estrogen.

HIGH: 40 mIU/ml to 200 mIU/ml. Causes: postmenopause, after removal of ovaries; ovarian failure. When FSH is over 20 mIU/ml, menopause may occur within five years. But factors other than low estrogen can elevate FSH, and women with elevated FSH levels can still occasionally be fertile. See *Levels of LH.*

Oocytes: These are immature eggs stored in the ovary from before birth. Each month, a rise in FSH brings a number of eggs (about 20 to 1,000 per cycle) to the surface of the ovary. Most eggs produce estrogen, atrophy, and die. One or two are chosen to mature and become the "egg of the month."

Follicle: A unit containing an egg surrounded by a layer of granulosa cells that produce estrogen. Each egg or oocyte is contained in a follicle.

Follicular Phase: The first half of the menstrual cycle, from day one of the flow until ovulation. Named for the time when a number of follicles in the ovary are being stimulated to maturity. Estrogen, the main female hormone, is dominant.

Luteinizing hormone (LH): This is a second stimulating hormone from the pituitary gland. It surges in mid-cycle after estrogen levels suddenly plummet from their highest levels. The LH surge causes the "egg of the month" to exit the ovary and enter the fallopian tube.

Levels of LH:

NORMAL ADULT FEMALE: 7 to 14 mIU/ml: The rise in FSH levels experienced by women entering perimenopause precedes the rise of LH by almost a decade. While LH remains normal, ovulation is possible. Therefore, FSH tests alone as an indication of menopause are not always conclusive since FSH levels can fluctuate greatly during the perimenopausal years. (This is particularly true in women with autoimmune problems that are temporarily affecting their ovaries. In such cases, interpreting a high FSH level as menopausal may be premature.) FSH levels can drop at times, allowing women to become pregnant. LH levels rise abruptly at menopause and so should also be tested for along with FSH. When LH levels rise to about a third of the level of a woman's postmenopausal FSH level, menopause is considered complete.[1]

Corpus Luteum: Literally means "yellow body." Describes the yellow patch left behind when the chosen egg exits at ovulation. The corpus luteum produces progesterone and estrogen during the last half of the cycle and also supports pregnancy.

Luteal Phase: The second half of the menstrual cycle, from ovulation until the next flow. Usually lasts 10–16 days, but there are exceptions. Named because the corpus *luteum* is present at this time. Progesterone, the second female hormone, is dominant.

Hormones

Estrogen   The main female hormone, estrogen has about 300 known functions in women. For reasons related to proportion of body fat but not fully understood, estrogen levels rise just before puberty and cause sequential (but variable)

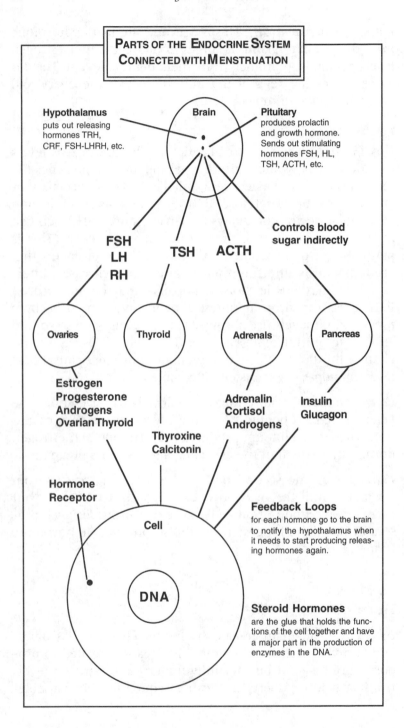

PARTS OF THE ENDOCRINE SYSTEM
CONNECTED WITH MENSTRUATION

Hypothalamus
puts out releasing
hormones TRH,
CRF, FSH-LHRH, etc.

Brain

Pituitary
produces prolactin
and growth hormone.
Sends out stimulating
hormones FSH, HL,
TSH, ACTH, etc.

FSH
LH
RH

TSH　ACTH

**Controls blood
sugar indirectly**

Ovaries　　Thyroid　　Adrenals　　Pancreas

**Estrogen
Progesterone
Androgens
Ovarian Thyroid**

**Thyroxine
Calcitonin**

**Adrenalin
Cortisol
Androgens**

**Insulin
Glucagon**

**Hormone
Receptor**

Cell

Feedback Loops
for each hormone go to the brain
to notify the hypothalamus when
it needs to start producing releasing hormones again.

DNA

Steroid Hormones
are the glue that holds the functions of the cell together and have
a major part in the production of
enzymes in the DNA.

changes as they rise. Over a two-year period, the female child will develop breasts, grow pubic and underarm hair, change shape from being a child to an adult female, experience a thickening of the vaginal wall, develop an endometrial lining in her uterus (womb), begin to menstruate, and later begin to ovulate. These changes reflect a progression toward fertility. Apart from its primary functions in maintaining the menstrual cycle and pregnancy, estrogen has many secondary effects throughout the body (breasts, bones, brain, vascular system, etc.).

Estrogen levels vary greatly throughout each cycle. One major function of estrogen is to promote thickening of the uterine lining. Estrogen is at its lowest level around the onset of menstruation and at its highest level just before mid-cycle. To permit successful ovulation to occur, estrogen needs to be at a certain, consistent level for five hours. After the high, the estrogen level suddenly drops as the follicles fade away and the brain puts out a mid-cycle surge of LH (luteinizing hormone). This surge causes ovulation.

Estrogen levels rise again in the luteal phase, but not as high as before ovulation.

As the number of available eggs diminishes during a woman's thirties, forties, and fifties, estrogen levels drop. Though menopause is a natural process, it can become problematic for many reasons, and women commonly experience estrogen deficiency symptoms.

Estradiol (the main human estrogen):

NORMAL ADULT LEVELS: In the early follicular phase and late luteal phase of the menstrual cycle: 30 to 150 ng/ml.

IN THE LATE FOLLICULAR PHASE: 100 to 500 ng/ml.

PERIMENOPAUSAL: greater than 20 ng/ml.

MENOPAUSAL: 40 to 200 ng/ml.

Progesterone Progesterone has been called the "secondary female hormone," but it is primary during pregnancy, as its name implies ("gest" refers to gestation, otherwise known as pregnancy). Apart from its role in the menstrual cycle and pregnancy, like estrogen it affects several systems in the body.

For instance, there are many progesterone receptors in the brain, where progesterone functions as a natural anesthetic similar to anti-anxiety medication. Because of its calming effect, even natural progesterone can make some women with a predisposition to depression worse.

Progesterone is virtually absent during the first half of the menstrual cycle, but its levels rise in the luteal phase. It fluffs up the lining of the uterus, thickened by estrogen, like a nest. It fills the lining with protein and starch in provision for possible pregnancy. If conception doesn't take place, progesterone levels eventually drop. This initiates the breakdown of the uterine lining and brings on the menstrual flow.

If conception takes place, the corpus luteum remains throughout pregnancy and only fades about one week postpartum. The corpus luteum in the ovary maintains the pregnancy until the placenta takes over and supersedes previous hormone production. While estrogen and other hormone levels rise dramatically during pregnancy, pregnancy is largely sustained by progesterone production for at least the first seven weeks. In the case of a woman who experiences frequent early miscarriages, pregnancy support with natural progesterone is sometimes given until the twelfth to sixteenth week.

Progesterone Levels:

NORMAL MENSTRUATING ADULT LEVELS: greater than 10 ng/ml during the mid- to late-luteal part of the cycle.

Testosterone   Testosterone is called the male hormone because it appears in much higher levels in men (500 to 1,500 ng/ml), and it produces a male's secondary sex characteristics. Women also produce some testosterone. Testosterone increases bone and muscle strength, sex drive, and a feeling of energy and well-being. The stroma, a part of the ovary, produces most of the testosterone in a woman. The levels are fairly consistent throughout the menstrual cycle, with perhaps a slight mid-cycle surge which increases sex drive at ovulation.

It is important to a woman's sexuality and overall health that she have enough testosterone. While the normal adult female range is given as 20 to 85 ng/ml, it is probably ideal to have a woman's testosterone levels between 35 and 50 ng/ml. Many women in their late thirties and forties are very low in testosterone (often less than 10 or 20 ng/ml).

OVERVIEW OF A WOMAN'S REPRODUCTIVE LIFE

After looking at the bigger picture of how the endocrine system functions, we can now focus on how the menstrual cycle works. The menstrual cycle spans the years during which a woman is in her reproductive prime. It is a process with a beginning, a peak, a decline, and an end.

The ovaries, from birth, contain the entire supply of a woman's eggs, and a pair of ovaries only functions for approximately 50 years at the most. Once they are depleted, reproduction is no longer possible and estrogen declines sharply, leading to menopause and the end of menstruation. Even before a female baby is born, all the eggs she will ever have are present in her two ovaries. Estimates vary, but there are six to seven million eggs present in the female baby by the middle of her mother's pregnancy. At the time of birth, about 80 percent have already died off (a process called atresia), and a baby may have between 500,000 and 5,000,000 eggs in her ovaries. These continue to die off and, by puberty, the numbers are down another 80 percent to between 200,000 and 300,000 eggs.

Every time a woman ovulates, not one or two, but between 20 and 1,000 eggs are used up. Most produce estrogen and die; only one or two eggs per cycle will fully mature. The more frequently women ovulate, the more eggs they use up. In previous generations, women had more pregnancies and fewer periods.

As women age, they tend to use up eggs more rapidly, and between the ages of 38 and 44, the average woman uses up about 50,000 eggs. Women go through menopause when the eggs in their ovaries run out, causing the hormones to drop to a much lower level. This process can be gradual or it can be quite abrupt. There is also some chemical timing in the brain that contributes to menopause.

Loss of Follicles or Eggs over a Lifetime

Age	Average # Follicles	Range		
6–9	484,000	258,000	to	755,000
12–16	382,000	85,000	to	591,000
18–24	156,000	39,000	to	290,000
25–31	59,000	81,000	to	228,000
32–38	59,000	15,000	to	208,000
40–44	8,300	350	to	28,000

—Thierry Hertoghe

After menopause, the ovaries still produce hormones—mainly androgens—and the adrenal gland acts as a backup.

Age of Menopause

The average age of women going through menopause naturally is 51.4 years. But, possibly because of differences in the numbers of estrogen cells and eggs a woman is born with, some may stop their periods and go through menopause earlier than normal (about eight to eleven percent before age 40). Some women may stop their periods at as early as 28 or 30 years old, and it is often the case that their mothers and grandmothers did, too. At the other end of the scale, about five percent of women still menstruate in their early sixties.

Different Now Than Before

In previous eras, women had many more pregnancies and about 40 or 50 menstrual cycles over a lifetime. Women today have about 400–500 cycles, with ovulation taking place many more times. The number of eggs and estrogen cells used up is accelerated, and the pituitary and ovarian hormone levels may begin to fluctuate earlier. Removal of one ovary reduces the hormone-factories to half and may lead to pre-menopausal symptoms. Removal of both ovaries puts women into instant menopause, and women with only part of an ovary or a fallopian tube removed may also start symptoms prematurely.

Some women have a gradual descent into menopause, experiencing subnormal hormone levels at a relatively early age. This may cause chronic hormone deficiency symptoms, manifesting themselves as PMS and premenopause. These symptoms can last from as early as the thirties (for a few women, even younger) to the time when a woman actually stops menstruating (averaging in the mid-forties or early fifties) and sometimes beyond.

The Normal Menstrual Cycle—How It Works

The menstrual cycle occurs every 28 to 29 days on the average, with day one being the first day of flow. FSH (follicle-stimulating hormone) is produced mainly during the first part of the cycle, toward the end of menstrual bleeding. Produced by the pituitary gland, FSH goes through the bloodstream to the ovaries and causes hundreds of eggs to rise to the surface of the particular ovary selected to ovulate that cycle. FSH also stimulates estrogen cells that produce estrogen, so estrogen levels soar to their highest just prior to ovulation and then suddenly drop.

The first part of the menstrual cycle up to ovulation is called the follicular phase, when estrogen is dominant. Progesterone, the second female hormone, is almost absent at this time. During this phase, the endometrial lining in the uterus gradually builds up like a nest, preparing to receive and nourish the egg in the event that fertilization and pregnancy occur.

Meanwhile, in the ovary, just before mid-cycle, one or two eggs have developed to become the "egg(s) of the month." The others die off, and the estrogen levels drop precipitously. As this happens, LH (luteinizing hormone) is released into the bloodstream by the pituitary in a mid-cycle surge that causes

Different Hormonal Levels Throughout the Menstrual Cycle

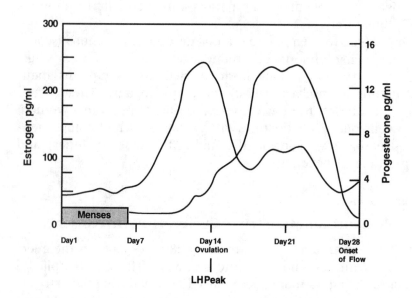

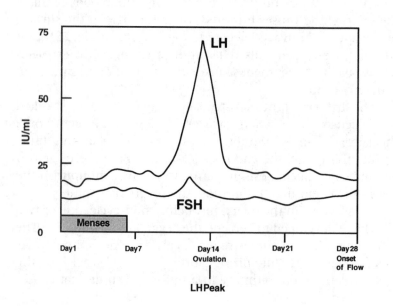

ovulation. The "egg of the month" is catapulted out of the ovary into the waiting, undulating fallopian tube.

At the place on the ovary where the egg has been released, a yellow patch called the corpus luteum is formed. This patch produces a high level of progesterone, the second female hormone, during the second half of the cycle. Progesterone is low or even absent during the first part of the menstrual cycle, but very high during the second half, beginning when women ovulate. Estrogen continues to be produced during the second half of the cycle.

When a woman is young, the second curve (postovulation) of estrogen is about as high as the first (preovulatory) curve. But, as women enter their thirties and forties, the tendency is for the first estrogen curve to rise and the second estrogen curve to drop. (However, in some women, the first curve can also begin to drop.) Women with high preovulatory curves will have heavier bleeding because the estrogen overstimulates the endometrial lining. Conversely, women with lower preovulatory curves will have lighter bleeding. As some women approach menopause, they may have both tendencies, depending on which ovary is functioning during a particular cycle.

The first half of the cycle is estrogen-dominant because progesterone is absent. The second half of the cycle, after ovulation, is progesterone dominant. Estrogen is present, but progesterone levels are usually higher. When a woman does not become pregnant, her progesterone levels drop precipitously, and the lining of the uterus sloughs off causing her to menstruate, ending the cycle. Then the cycle begins all over again with the rise of FSH.

How Hormone Levels Change with Age

As the eggs are used up month by month, hormone levels start to change. A gradual lessening of the ovaries' supply of eggs and estrogen cells causes the ovaries to notify the pituitary gland to send more FSH. Higher levels of FSH overstimulate the few remaining eggs and estrogen cells. The high levels of estrogen produced cause greater thickening of the endometrial lining of the uterus, resulting in heavier periods.

In other cases, FSH may become lower, producing less estrogen in the ovaries and a thinner lining of the endometrium. This will cause periods to be lighter. Some women may have irregular spotting because they do not have enough estrogen to "hold" the endometrium intact, and the lining keeps sloughing off. Some women may experience both extremes—heavy or light bleeding—in alternate months.

Women may begin to notice symptoms of premenopause in the first half of their menstrual cycle, particularly between the fifth to eighth or tenth day of the cycle (the time when estrogen normally rises). The symptoms may be subtle; she may feel a gradual emotional and physical decline with symptoms such as low-grade depression, fatigue, low self-esteem, anxiety, insomnia, heart palpitations, muscle tightness in the neck, dizziness, hot flashes, drying of the vagina, or general muscle or joint pain. Women suffering from depression or panic attacks at this time of life should ask themselves whether the cause might be hormonal.

Beginning in their mid-thirties, some women will not ovulate every month and will skip periods. When that happens, the corpus luteum may not form. Even if it does, it may not produce adequate levels of estrogen and progesterone in the second half of the cycle. During this time (the luteal phase), hormone levels will be low. This is why PMS, which occurs after ovulation, may begin or worsen around age 35.

SOME WOMEN HAVE HORMONAL PROBLEMS EARLY IN LIFE

There are all sorts of reasons why the hormonal cycle can stop working at its best. Some women have a hormonal system that doesn't function normally from early in life, and often they are subclinically hypothyroid or have congenital PMS. Symptoms may begin around puberty or after a pregnancy, and tend to worsen as a woman ages.

PMS may begin after some hormonal event—being on the birth control pill, going off the pill, being pregnant, or having a tubal ligation, hysterectomy, or surgery on their ovaries or fallopian tubes. Other women who have such physical problems as endometriosis, one or more cysts on their ovaries, fibroid tumors, scarring of the ovaries or fallopian tubes as a result of an infection, and so on, may have disruption of their hormones. So do some women who have anorexia, bulimia, or amenorrhea (having no periods). Some of the same triggers can bring on premature menopause with estrogen deficiency.

Autoimmune dysfunction is another factor. Sometimes, in illnesses such as lupus erythematosus, myasthenia gravis, multiple sclerosis, Hashimoto's thyroiditis, and Graves' disease, the same autoimmune antibody process triggering the disease finds similar tissue in the ovary and partially destroys it. These diseases are much more common in women than in men. Women with these problems may tend to go through menopause or have symptoms of ovarian dysfunction earlier than normal.

Because the hypothalamus also controls the immune system, women with hormonal problems frequently have allergies and respiratory problems, such as bronchitis or asthma.

SUMMARY

It should come as no surprise that when the endocrine system and the menstrual cycle are out of synchrony, a large variety of symptoms is produced, and women feel both physically and emotionally sick as a result.

Often, one gland is the main problem. When each hormone malfunctions, certain patterns and symptoms are produced. And with a little help and information, many women can figure out for themselves what is happening to them. We will expand on this in later chapters.

The menstrual cycle *is* natural, but many women have been taught that menstrual problems are also natural. They have been told for generations that pain and discomfort are simply to be endured. The truth is that the endocrine system and menstrual cycle are very sensitive and can easily be disrupted, just like any other system in the body. In some cases, the problem is not easily solved.

HORMONAL PROBLEMS

CHAPTER

FIVE

PREMENSTRUAL SYNDROME

Every month before her period, Mary becomes depressed, irritable, and angry for no apparent reason. She screams at her children and finds fault with her husband. Things that wouldn't bother her most of the time become huge in her imagination, blown all out of proportion.

Initially, Mary thought she was just a moody, unstable person. The up-and-down moods among the females in her family had often been a topic of conversation. So, understandably, Mary blames her symptoms on her environment. She thinks that her feelings and reactions are just learned behavior aggravated by daily stress. Underneath, she's convinced that if she exerted just a little more willpower, she could control her behavior.

But she's noticed that these symptoms occur cyclically; sometimes she has them and sometimes she doesn't. Her symptoms are intensifying now that she's reached 35. Sometimes she thinks her menstrual period has something to do with the way she feels, though her symptoms seem to last two or three weeks out of the month. "I only have one good week a month," she complains. Her symptoms worsened with her last pregnancy, and after she had a tubal ligation, her problems seemed to become even more severe.

Her doctor says that it's all in her mind, but Mary knows it's more than that. She has a week or so each month when her symptoms disappear, and she feels normal and emotionally stable. Then, at ovulation, it's as though a switch is thrown, and she's back into having symptoms. "It can't be my imagination," she insists. She's become very hard to live with, and every month she wants to run away. She has little feeling of self-worth, feels she is a failure, sometimes thinks she's going insane, and thinks she may be better off living alone.

In addition to her emotional symptoms, Mary has some physical problems. Her skin breaks out before each menstrual period. Her breasts swell, her head aches, and her joints are stiff. She has premenstrual hot flashes and occasional panic attacks, too. But her emotional symptoms, depression and anger, worry her more than the physical ones.

"It's the close relationships that are difficult," she confides. "I get so angry with my husband and the kids over nothing. I feel a complete loss of self-control. I can see afterward that I've overreacted, and I keep reminding myself of this, but it never helps at the time."

Mary doesn't really want to kill herself, though she often thinks about doing it. She says she wouldn't mind being killed in a collision in order to end her life without the responsibility of doing it herself. "I sort of panic inside because I don't know how much more of this I can take," she says. "I sometimes think that if it gets just a little bit worse, I'll do myself some damage. It's very frightening and very hard to explain."

Her husband can't understand what's going on, and he's getting fed up with it all. He says she's like two people; part of the month she's on top of the world like the girl he married, the other part she's impossible.

"She cries a lot when she's not shouting," he says. "Sometimes I wonder how much longer I can stand it."

"He's so logical," says Mary, "and I'm often irrational. I can't get him to understand how I feel. But you can't blame him. I don't understand it either."

Mary's problems are probably hereditary, since her mother and sister also have mood swings. Mary's symptoms begin after ovulation and end toward the end of her period. The week after her period, she feels fine. Mary has classic premenstrual syndrome.

Only a Mother Could Love Her

Only a woman who has severe premenstrual syndrome (PMS), or someone who has to live with her, really understands how traumatic this experience can be. Possibly 40 to 60 percent of menstruating women have some degree of PMS. Five to ten percent of them experience incapacitating problems. Their physical and emotional symptoms can interrupt family life and lead to problems at work, loss of jobs, divorce, child abuse, violence, alcoholism, drug abuse, depression, and even suicide.

Simply stated, such women have a variety of symptoms that appear like clockwork before their menstrual period each month and disappear after their period. Some women only have symptoms for a short time prior to menstruation. These symptoms disappear when the flow begins. Other women may be overwhelmed by symptoms beginning shortly before ovulation and lasting well into their menstrual flow, causing these women to say they have only "one good week a month."

A woman may find that she has one bad month, then one better month, alternately—or a worse month every third month. This is probably because ovulation tends to occur in alternate ovaries in consecutive cycles, although it sometimes occurs more than once in a row on one side. A woman may know which side the troublesome ovary is on if she feels pain when she ovulates on that particular side.

THE DEFINITION OF PMS

PMS is characterized by a clustering of symptoms in the premenstruum (before the period) and an absence of symptoms in the postmenstruum (after the period). The *timing* of the symptoms is more important than the *type* of symptoms. But there are *common* symptoms. The important factor in women with classic PMS is that these symptoms are cyclical.

What Are the Symptoms of PMS?

Irritability, lethargy, and depression are known as the "PMS triad," and are almost always present. Other emotional symptoms include feeling out of control, feeling worthless, a desire to escape, sporadic crying, uncontrollable rage, paranoia, sadness, anger, anxiety, phobias, and guilt.

There may be many physical symptoms, such as headaches and migraines, flu-like symptoms, recurrent yeast infections, food cravings, and, occasionally, epileptic seizures. Some women report eye problems such as conjunctivitis, sties, visual disturbances, and tunnel vision; skin problems such as acne, boils, herpes, and hives; or respiratory problems such as hoarseness, asthma, and tonsillitis. Dr. Katharina Dalton has identified about 150 symptoms of PMS. Nobody has them all. Some women have only emotional symptoms and no physical symptoms. Occasionally, a woman will have migraine but no emotional symptoms.

Some Common PMS Symptoms

Acne	Addiction	Aggression
Alcoholism	Allergies	Arthritis
Asthma	Backache	Bloating
Blurred vision	Boils	Bronchitis
Clumsiness	Colds	Colitis
Confusion	Conjunctivitis	Constipation
Crying jags	Depression	Dizziness
Epilepsy	Exhaustion	Eye problems
Fainting	Fatigue	Fear of crowds
Fibrocystic breasts	Flu-like symptoms	Food cravings
Forgetfulness	Headaches	Heart palpitations
Hemorrhoid flare-up	Herpes	Hives
Hot flashes	Hyperventilation	Increased sex drive
Insomnia	Irritability	Joint pain
Leg heaviness	Lethargy	Loss of control

Low blood sugar	Low self-esteem	Migraines
Mood swings	Muscle pain	Muscle weakness
Nausea	Nervousness	Numb extremities
Panic Attacks	Paranoia	Physical violence
Rage	Recurrent colds	Recurrent infections
Rapid heart rate	Sinusitis	Sties
Suicidal tendencies	Tender breasts	Tension
Tonsillitis	Yeast infections	Weight changes

There Are Different Patterns

Notice below some common patterns of PMS symptoms (A, B, C, and D). Note that some women do not fit these classic patterns.

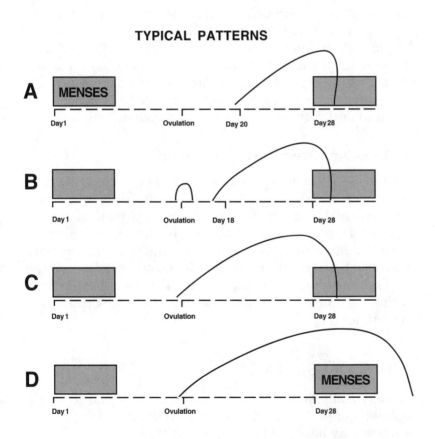

TYPICAL PATTERNS

The Importance of Record Keeping

Many physicians ask patients to chart their symptoms for at least two months before beginning treatment for PMS. Keeping a calendar chart that shows the timing of symptoms in relation to your menstrual period will show a clear pattern if you have classic premenstrual syndrome. It is also helpful to fill in a day-by-day journal of your symptoms and feelings.

More Than PMS

Many women have symptoms that recur before each menstrual period and disappear after it, but there are those in an even more complicated predicament. They may have PMS combined with some other problem, such as postpartum depression. Perhaps they are heading toward menopause and are experiencing estrogen-deficiency symptoms. Possibly they have a related adrenal or thyroid deficiency. Sometimes a chronic yeast infection or allergies makes PMS worse. In these cases, the timing of symptoms may vary from that in a clear case of PMS, and such women will not benefit as much when their PMS is treated alone. They need additional treatment to deal with their other health problems.

PMS Is Not Premenstrual Magnification

Contrast PMS with symptoms of chronic illness that may worsen premenstrually, which Michelle Harrison, M.D., calls premenstrual magnification. For instance, chronic migraines, chronic depression, chronic asthma, or chronic epilepsy may occur at any time and do not appear to be connected with menstruation. However, all chronic diseases tend to worsen around the time of menstruation. Sometimes these non-hormonal problems will not respond to hormone therapy, but sometimes they do.

WHAT CAUSES PMS?

Nobody really knows the exact cause of PMS, and there are many theories. No doubt, PMS is a multifactorial problem; a woman may have multiple causes for her PMS.

MENSTRUAL CHART

Day	Jan	Feb	Mar	Apr	May	Jun	Jul	Aug	Sep	Oct	Nov	Dec		Example		
1																
2																
3																
4																X
5																X
6																X
7															X	X
8															X	X
9															X	X
10														X	HX	HX
11														X	HX	HX
12														X	HX	HX
13														X	M	M
14														X	M	M
15														HX	M	M
16														HX	M	M
17														M	M	M
18														M		M
19														M		
20														M		
21														M		
22														M		
23																
24																
25																
26																
27																
28																
29																
30																
31																

Filling in the Chart—Use X for general symptoms; use appropriate initials for severe symptoms such as headaches (H), depression (D), seizures (S), etc. Write an M for menstruation or a P for period on the days you menstruate. See sample chart on right, where the woman is having regular monthly cycles with 5 or 6 day periods. This chart can still be filled in with symptoms, even if menstruation is absent, as in prepubertal girls or postmenopausal women, who still have cyclical symptoms.

Dr. Guy Abrahams believes that poor nutrition is a cause of PMS. He suggests that a diet high in animal fat, high in calcium in proportion to magnesium, and lacking in certain vitamins, such as B_6, may cause or worsen PMS. S. Thys-Jacobs, M.D., has postulated that women with PMS have transient hyperparathyroidism at ovulation caused by a deficiency of a vitamin-D liver metabolite, leading to imbalance of the calcium/phosphate ratio in the cells and disturbing the parathyroid.

Some believe that PMS is a hormonal problem, related to low levels of progesterone. Yet there are women who do not ovulate and, therefore, do not produce any progesterone, and still do not get PMS. Other researchers believe that PMS is related to low levels of estrogen. Still others believe that the cause of PMS is related to the ratio of estrogen to progesterone. One useful theory is that PMS is a half-menopause. Some women, for whom the problem is cyclical, have low levels of progesterone. Other women may need some estrogen, especially as they age. But note that rigorous studies investigating the differences in blood tests between women with and without PMS have not shown much difference.[1]

Others have postulated that PMS is a thyroid disease. It is true that women with thyroid problems, particularly low thyroid, often have PMS, and there does appear to be a link between the two conditions. But not everyone who has a thyroid problem has PMS, and not everyone who has PMS has a thyroid problem.

Those who promote evening primrose oil as a remedy for PMS say that women who have PMS have high levels of prolactin, the hormone that causes lactation after pregnancy and is also present during the menstrual cycle. One of prolactin's functions is to lower progesterone levels. This theory of high prolactin as the major cause of PMS does not hold, since many women with high prolactin levels do not have PMS, and many women with PMS have apparently normal levels of prolactin.

There is some evidence that women with PMS have lower than normal levels of DHEA, an adrenal hormone, which indicates that an adrenal gland dysfunction may be involved.

Women with PMS have some disruption of the neurotransmitters in the brain. Neurotransmitters are brain chemicals that send messages or impulses through the nervous system. Premenstrually, endorphin levels in women with PMS are only 25 percent of the levels in women who don't have PMS. Levels of serotonin, another neurotransmitter in the brain, are also known to be low in women with PMS. One of the functions of neurotransmitters is to oversee and regulate hormone function. Some researchers theorize that it is the disruption of these brain chemicals that throws the pituitary hormones out of synchrony.

There is no doubt that PMS often results when the hypothalamus and pituitary glands become disturbed for some reason. Because the pituitary gland produces hormones that go to a variety of target organs, several glands may be affected (e.g., ovaries, thyroid, adrenals).

Women with polycystic ovaries and endometriosis frequently also have PMS, and treatment for these specific conditions often helps their PMS.

Added to the problems, which appear to start primarily in the brain, are cases of PMS which seem directly triggered by surgery. For example, some women get PMS after having a tubal ligation, a hysterectomy, or surgery on their ovaries or fallopian tubes.

While the pituitary gland produces hormones in the ovaries, there are also hormonal feedback systems to the brain from the ovaries. So you might say that the pituitary gland speaks to the ovaries, but the ovaries also speak back to the brain. In the case of a tubal ligation or other abdominal surgery, the progesterone feedback system to the brain may be interrupted in some way, triggering PMS.

Present research indicates that women with PMS may have fewer progesterone receptors than normal women.

The birth control pill frequently triggers or worsens PMS, as does the use of synthetic progestins such as Provera. Provera can cause women to feel irritable and depressed and may compound PMS.[2]

Others believe that some women who have PMS may have chlamydia, a sexually-transmitted infection, or other infections. Some say that intestinal parasites can indirectly cause PMS. When the body produces antibodies to these parasites, the antibodies attack organs such as the ovaries and cause hormonal upsets. Others believe that PMS is a candida, or yeast-related, disease, and others think that women with PMS are allergic to their own hormones.

These are just a few of the current theories about the causes of PMS, which is probably a multifactorial problem.

PMS—A Half Menopause

Norman Beals, Jr., M.D., and Norman Beals, Sr., M.D., spent a combined total of more than 60 years helping women with hormonal problems, and came to the conclusion that PMS is like a half-menopause. What they mean is that menopause is the time when ovarian hormone levels drop drastically, and PMS is an early beginning of this process. In some women, progesterone levels are functionally lower than they should be; in others, estrogen is depleted; and in others, both hormones are running low at the same time.

Progesterone is only produced by the ovaries in significant quantities after ovulation. If progesterone levels are lower than normal, a woman is likely to have PMS symptoms which occur only in the second half of her menstrual cycle. Women with symptoms of PMS that are severe enough to treat hormonally often respond to natural progesterone therapy. But sometimes natural progesterone alone just doesn't work.

Because estrogen levels can also be low in the luteal or second phase of the cycle, and because estrogen helps stimulate the production of progesterone receptors, women with PMS may do better on estrogen than on natural progesterone. Estrogen may be particularly helpful for women with severe depression as the presenting symptom. These women may benefit from using the estrogen patch for a week or two before their periods.

Estrogen may also be the answer for those (usually older) women whose PMS symptoms extend to or recur at the end of the menstrual cycle (approximately days five through eight). Normally at this early time in the cycle, estrogen levels should be rising, but in a premenopausal woman this rise may be blunted. She may have such symptoms as insomnia, panic, fatigue, vertigo, or headaches and muscle cramps in the back of her neck—all at the end of her period. This woman might benefit from extra estrogen at this time.

In summary, some women do well on progesterone. Other women feel better on estrogen. Others do best on a combination of the two.

Not All Agree

Some experts who treat PMS don't agree with the theory that PMS can be related to estrogen deficiency. In the past, some experts have claimed that many women with PMS have excessive estrogen levels, and many claim that women can't be estrogen-deficient if they still have periods. But other doctors believe that a woman can have menstrual periods despite having lower-than-normal levels of estrogen.

Many physicians disagree with the suggestion that PMS is caused by a hormone deficiency at all, because the hormonal blood test results of women with PMS are often normal.[3] This may be partly because it is difficult to separate free and bound hormones in serum. Free hormones are biologically active and available to the body. Bound hormones can't be used until they are broken down. Therefore, the usable amount of a hormone may be much lower than the blood test suggests. This is why saliva tests, which reflect only "free" hormones, are more reliable indicators.

Medical researchers generally admit that PMS is a valid complaint, but suggest that progesterone works no better than a placebo and that there is no known cure.

Don't Let Differences of Opinion Disturb You

- Some doctors believe that women with PMS have high estrogen and low progesterone levels.
- Some doctors believe the opposite: that progesterone levels are high and estrogen levels low in women with PMS.
- Other doctors believe that either progesterone or estrogen levels or both may be low.

- The majority of physicians believe that PMS is not caused by a hormonal deficiency at all.

Don't be afraid of these differences of opinion. While the range of opinion among experts may be tremendous, many women can still find treatment that will help.

Practical Help for Women Is Available

Despite the differences of opinion about the causes of PMS and menopausal distress, the description of PMS as a progesterone deficiency or a half-menopause, and estrogen deficiency as the other half-menopause, is useful even if simplistic. And, practically, treating women with a combination of estrogen and progesterone often works.

Many women with classic, severe PMS or postpartum depression do benefit from natural progesterone if given correctly according to the protocol suggested by Dr. Katherina Dalton.

Some women, who do not fit the classic PMS patterns, may also benefit from taking estrogen for PMS. Others, with a low thyroid profile, may find that adding a little thyroid medication makes a big difference in the way they feel.

WHAT ACTIVATES PMS?

While the exact cause of PMS is still undetermined, there are known factors that can initiate or heighten symptoms.

Family History Is a Risk Factor

Among susceptible women, it is common to find other family members with PMS—particularly on the maternal side. Each woman in the family will probably begin her own PMS initiation at puberty, or even a couple of years earlier.

In such families, PMS is a lifetime battle, sometimes severe at onset, sometimes starting mildly and worsening with age. When these especially susceptible women encounter any hormonal crisis, their PMS may worsen. Menopause may be the end of PMS symptoms, but some women continue to have cyclical problems long after they stop menstruating.

Some women who have never had a family history of PMS may also experience symptoms after taking the birth control pill or having a pregnancy, a tubal ligation, or a hysterectomy.

Sometimes stress or poor diet can trigger PMS, and it tends to begin or worsen as women age—particularly from age 35 onward.

Birth Control Pills Tend to Intensify PMS

Most women with a history of PMS would be wise to avoid oral contraceptive pills for at least two reasons. First, they contain synthetic progesterone, which can depress the pituitary gland and stop it from producing its own progesterone.

Second, while synthetic progestins replace progesterone in some of its functions, they do not work as well in the progesterone receptors throughout the body and in the brain. These receptors are very precise and will only accept the real thing. Synthetic progestins are like keys that fit the progesterone receptors but cannot open their "locks" or make them function.

This is why PMS will frequently worsen in women who take some types of birth control pill. The pill is a major cause of PMS and a reason why PMS is now widespread. On the other hand, the new birth control pills contain a low dose of synthetic progestin, and some women with PMS do seem to feel better on the low-dose pill.

Hormonal Problems Are Common After Tubal Ligations

Some women who have had a tubal ligation (also called a tubal sterilization), in which the fallopian tubes are tied to prevent conception, may later experience symptoms of PMS, premenopause, or both. Though some research suggests that women have no side effects from tubal ligations, there are many women who disagree.

Physicians who believe that side effects result from tubal ligation have different opinions on why this is so. Some think that these adverse symptoms are due entirely to the surgery. Others feel that the onset of PMS-like symptoms may be partially due to life stresses at the time of surgery or to the hormonal upheaval of pregnancy and delivery, frequently occurring at the same time the tubes are tied.

Dr. Niels Lauersen estimates that 15 percent of women who have tubal ligations will experience side effects such as heavy bleeding, increased pelvic pain, or post-tubal-ligation syndrome (with symptoms of PMS or premenopause).[4] Another source suggests that up to 60 percent of women will experience premenopause within six to seven years after surgery, depending on the type of tubal ligation performed.[5]

This means that a woman who has a tubal ligation at age 30 may find herself having subsequent hormonal problems, either immediately afterward or by about age 36. Some researchers have suggested that older methods of performing tubal ligations may damage the ovarian artery that runs close to the fallopian tube. The surgery lessens or cuts off the blood flow to the ovary, causing a decrease in pituitary hormone stimulation to the ovary and a lessening of either estrogen or progesterone production, or both.

Dr. Sandra Cabot, an Australian physician and naturopath, in her book *Don't Let Hormones Ruin Your Life*,[6] has a chapter called, "Surgical Sterilization May Be More Than You Bargained For." She states: "It is a pity that women undergoing or considering tubal ligation as a method of contraception are not always advised of all its possible long-term effects." She describes the different types of tubal ligations and concludes that the use of falope clips and filschie clips are the safest techniques. She mentions that blocking the blood supply to the ovarian artery causes high blood pressure in the ovary, which can result in damage to the ovarian tissues. This may lead to poor ovarian function and affect the normal production of estrogen and progesterone.

For more information, see Chapter 12 on tubal ligations and the Recommended Reading section near the end of this book for a list of publications by Dr. Cabot on hormonal problems.

PMS and Hysterectomy

Some women who didn't previously have PMS may start noticing cyclical problems after a hysterectomy, even when only the uterus was removed. So it's surprising that doctors often suggest a hysterectomy as a cure for women with PMS.[7] Women sometimes think that losing all their reproductive organs and not menstruating would be absolutely wonderful, and, indeed, some women are lucky in their response to this surgery. Surgery may sometimes stop their PMS symptoms.

On the other hand, a hysterectomy may make the problem a lot worse, compounding it by adding estrogen-deficiency symptoms. Curing PMS by having a hysterectomy is a lot like playing Russian roulette, and the odds are not always good; some women have infinite difficulty adjusting their hormone treatments afterward. Often, the main reason for this is that their doctors don't work with them to balance their hormones.

Serious research papers have suggested hysterectomy and oophorectomy as a cure for very severe PMS. This is a drastic solution and a last resort, because it can worsen the problem instead of curing it. The theory behind this suggestion is that if women don't have ovaries, they won't ovulate, and they can't possibly have PMS, which is not true. Women can have cyclical PMS-like symptoms even if they don't ovulate (for example: girls with PMS who cycle a year or two before puberty but don't ovulate or menstruate; older women with PMS who have amenorrhea and don't ovulate; women with PMS who have had hysterectomies; and some rare postmenopausal women who don't have periods but still have cyclical PMS-like problems into old age).

Did a hysterectomy help or hinder your mother? This may be a guide for you. And, if you have the surgery, will your doctor be willing to help you find a hormone supplementation balance that works for you? Generally, if you already have severe hormonal problems, the less you do to irritate your hormonal setup the better. Having said all this, I must add that there is a definite place for hysterectomy. I have just had a hysterectomy after putting it off for ten years, and it does not seem to have adversely affected my moods.

An excellent book on this subject is *Hysterectomy: Before and After*, by Dr. Winnifred Cutler. Also read Chapter 12 on hysterectomies in this book.

The Connection Between PMS and PPD

Women with PMS are prone to having a hormonally-induced postpartum depression after pregnancy and tend to experience characteristic pregnancies. One group feels exceptionally well in the second or third trimester (after the first twelve- to sixteen-week period of nausea). This is because their progesterone levels are very high after the sixteenth week. The other group may have difficult pregnancies, with toxemia, depression, migraines, or other complications. A history of toxemia or pre-eclampsia (a pregnancy-related condition that can result in coma and convulsions if left untreated) is very common in women with PMS.

Women with both types of pregnancies have an increased tendency to have postpartum depression. This can be mild to severe, lasting from a few days or a couple of weeks, to months, or continuing for years. And some women have postpartum depression that never seems to lift.

Just as there are different types of depression in general, different types of depression are experienced after childbirth. Symptoms of postpartum depression (PPD) range from the relatively mild and short-lived "baby blues" to very severe and possibly long-lasting psychosis. Some women may need treatment with antidepressant or antipsychotic medication. However, a lot of women can find relief without these heavy-duty drugs by using various hormone treatments for a few weeks to months.

Although PMS and PPD are often linked, there are women who have one and not the other—some who have no PMS but difficult PPD, and others who are the opposite.

Also, note that if a woman has postpartum depression after one child, it does not necessarily mean that she will have it after the next, though it does increase her chances. On the other hand, there are some women whose postpartum depression worsens with each child.

Read Chapter 7 on postpartum depression for more detailed information.

PMS and Endometriosis

Endometriosis occurs when tissue identical to that found in the uterine lining (called the endometrium) grows on organs and structures outside of the uterus itself. The following description is from *Consumer Reports:*

> Endometriosis is not malignant but it mimics cancer in the way it spreads and attaches itself to other organs, most commonly the ovary, bladder, and bowel. This wandering tissue retains its uterine function and each month it bleeds in response to hormonal influences just as the uterus does. Also, as in the uterus, this tissue releases prostaglandins which in the uterus help the uterus to contract. The action of these hormones causes a general menstrual pain in some women. The same pain is also found at the local sites of the misplaced tissue during menstrual periods. The bleeding at these sites may cause adhesions between organs which can lead to chronic pain and infertility in endometriosis sufferers.[8]

Endometriosis is mainly found in the abdominal cavity, for instance on the outside of the uterus, the ovaries, the fallopian tubes, the bowel, the bladder or other organs, such as the kidneys or appendix. But it has been found occasionally in the lungs, brain, and, rarely, in strange places such as the surface of the underarm. Endometriosis can be widespread, yet the patient can be symptom-free. Another patient might have tiny amounts of endometriosis, yet experience extreme pain. Adenomyosis is a form of internal endometriosis, in which the endometrial tissue grows into the muscles of the uterine wall, usually after a difficult delivery.

Endometriosis is not fully understood, but it is an autoimmune phenomenon. One known cause of endometriosis is exposure to the pesticide dioxin. Endometriosis has also been linked with candida (yeast infections). Some women develop endometriosis at the site of surgery after having their tubes tied. The endometrial tissue can apparently travel through the incision and adhere to the outside of the tubes.[9] Retrograde bleeding, in which menstrual blood travels through the fallopian tubes into the abdominal cavity and back again, has also been blamed. Retrograde bleeding is not uncommon during menstruation, as frequently observed during abdominal surgery. But not everyone who has retrograde bleeding gets endometriosis. There may be a history of endometriosis in some families, with each generation developing it as they get older.

There seems to be a high incidence of endometriosis in women with PMS, though, to my knowledge, this has not been researched. Joel Hargrove, M.D., and Guy Abrahams, M.D., have noted that endometriosis is present in at least 50 percent of cases in which severe cramp-like pain is a major symptom of PMS.[10] Dr. Nils Lauersen has also treated many women who have PMS and endometriosis simultaneously.[11] Pain and infertility are the two major reasons why women seek help for endometriosis.

Early Warning Symptoms of Endometriosis
* Menstrual cramps that become progressively worse as time passes;
* Ovulatory pain (*mittelschmerz*);
* Painful intercourse;
* Infertility for unknown reasons;
* Bladder infections (yet tests for bacteria repeatedly come out negative);
* Severe shifting pelvic pain a few days before and during menstruation;
* A history of rupturing, bleeding cysts;
* Nodules on the uterus that can be felt by the physician;
* On examination, the cervical os (the dimple at the opening of the cervix) not being aligned with the vagina and the anus, indicating that the uterus may have adhered to other organs (this can also be due to surgical adhesions);
* A sudden chronic bout of mid-cycle or menstrual pain (which could also be due to other causes).

Note that abdominal laparoscopy may be necessary for diagnosis.

Relief for Endometriosis   Endometriosis often begins at puberty, and women find that they have a long-term progressive problem that requires skillful management over a period of many years. Different types of endometriosis need different treatment, depending on the extent of involvement and the presenting symptoms. For instance, if a woman is trying to become pregnant, the birth control pill would not be a good choice for treatment.

Most of the time, a young woman with endometriosis who is not having problems with infertility will just be offered pain management or the birth control pill. Women who have endometriosis who wish to have children are usually advised to have them early, as infertility is a common consequence of endometriosis. If a woman is having trouble becoming pregnant, she may be offered a course of Danazol, followed by laser surgery to remove the endometriosis lesions. If a women is in extreme pain and fertility is not an issue, she might be offered Lupron or Synarel to put her in chemical menopause and cause regression of the lesions. The last-resort treatment is hysterectomy with removal of the ovaries. None of the treatments is symptom-free, and none guarantee freedom from a return of the endometriosis. Even hysterectomy cannot remove the microscopic lesions in the bloodstream and attached to other organs that are left behind.[12] Hormone replacement therapy does not reactivate endometriosis in the majority of women,[13] but there are exceptions.

Though endometriosis can be a difficult disease to manage, there is a silver lining for many sufferers. Some women with severe pain and infertility find miraculous relief as a result of one or more of the solutions described previously. Sometimes when PMS and endometriosis exist together, treatment of the endometriosis brings relief from the PMS. John Lee, M.D., and Christiane Northrup, M.D., both recommend the use of Pro-Gest® cream for endometriosis,[14] and I have found a number of physicians who use the birth control pill to help the endometriosis lesions regress and to minimize pain, with prescription natural progesterone during the second half of the cycle to lessen the symptoms of PMS. There is no research done on this, but it may be worth trying to see if it helps.

SUMMARY

Women who are going through PMS can lead pretty miserable lives for part of every month. They are often embarrassed by their behavior, and when their mood improves as their menstrual flow begins, they will sometimes deny that the awful symptoms ever happened. They have an irrational hope that next month will be different, but they often find that the same old process repeats itself when the second half of the cycle rolls around again. Because this denial mechanism is so strong, many women don't seek treatment until their symptoms are chronic and the effect on their life is serious.

If you have PMS, I encourage you to read the treatment section at the end of this chapter and then take action. Your life and the lives of those who love you and live with you can be greatly improved.

CASE HISTORIES

Lynelle's Story

Lynelle is an intelligent, fun-loving 38 year old, and a single parent with two children. After an extremely difficult marriage, she divorced and returned to school to train as a nurse so that she could support her family.

While in school in 1985, she began to experience a series of anxiety attacks. These seemed to wax and wane in intensity in the coming years. Sometimes they were fairly well under control. At other times, they were severe. The worst episodes were initiated by having a virus or a bout of bronchitis. More than once, Lynelle had to take time off work and ask for help from her mother because she was unable to take care of herself and her children. Lynelle was given Xanax, and the anxiety problem lasted for a couple of months. At times, she was unable to drive because the motion made a rushing feeling come over her. She also had to make occasional midnight trips to the emergency room when her heart started beating out of control.

Lynelle went to many physicians over the next few years, including several family physicians, gynecologists, two endocrinologists, two psychiatrists, and a cardiologist. She had a lot of tests done during that time, and the consensus was that her problem was due to being overweight and under stress. She was told more than once that her problem was psychiatric, even though many of the symptoms were physical. A family doctor put her back on Xanax. She took the Xanax, but it didn't solve her problems, so he sent her to a psychiatrist who told her that there was nothing wrong with her, and that she was just doing too much. Not satisfied, Lynelle went to another psychiatrist who wouldn't treat her until she stopped taking Xanax. This was an impossible situation, because as soon as she stopped taking Xanax, her symptoms worsened.

One physician in the Bay Area suspected that Lynelle's thyroid gland wasn't functioning properly. At the time, her blood tests indicated that she was hypothyroid, but the doctor felt that the birth control pill she was taking influenced her thyroid test results, and he did not treat the condition. He told her that she was very ill and experiencing a type of nervous breakdown.

A family physician checked Lynelle's thyroid gland, and performed several unusual tests including a gastrointestinal series (upper GI), an examination to determine whether she had an adrenal tumor, and a Doppler Echogram to check for mitral valve prolapse. The test results were all normal. The physician put her on Inderol for her high blood pressure and left her on Xanax.

This same family physician sent her for a full workup by an endocrinologist. He told Lynelle that she was hypertensive and overweight, and that her problems were all stress-related.

By this time, Lynelle had begun to chart her symptoms and found that they were related to her menstrual periods. She went to another endocrinologist, who checked her thoroughly again. By this time, she had accumulated five thyroid tests. Two out of five indicated abnormally high thyroid levels. The endocrinologist said that the majority would rule. I met Lynelle around this time. I thought that she might have Hashimoto's thyroiditis, because she had high, low, and normal thyroid test results. The weight gain, her hair breaking off and falling out, her PMS and heavy bleeding, excessive feelings of cold, heart irregularities, high blood pressure, and other symptoms were all typical of a thyroid disorder. Her current family physician agreed to prescribe natural progesterone for her.

Lynelle then went to a female physician who examined her and found a lump on her ovary. A sonogram showed a number of cysts on her right ovary. She referred Lynelle to a gynecologist, who felt the cysts and suggested that Lynelle have an exploratory laparoscopy (a surgery in which a small incision is made through the navel, through which a scope is inserted into the abdominal cavity to examine the pelvic area).

Lynelle was nervous about having an anesthetic because of her high blood pressure and palpitations, but eventually gave in and had the procedure done. The surgeon removed a cyst on her left ovary (not the right), and mended a hole in a liga- ment on the right side which may have been responsible for Lynelle's pain.

Lynelle felt fine for a month. But then she began having very heavy bleeding and horrible clots with her periods. If she stood up during her period, she would immediately hemor- rhage, and the heavy bleeding would last for days. She then took a synthetic progestin for three months. During that time, she had to go to the emergency room for the bleeding, so her doctor increased the progestin dosage.

Lynelle was offered a laser ablation, a hysterectomy, or shots of Depo-Provera. She refused all these options.

Four months after the laparoscopy, Lynelle's anxiety episodes returned. She would experience an irregular heart beat, up to 120 beats a minute, lasting for three hours at a time, frequently in the middle of the night. After each episode, she would feel as though a truck had run over her.

At this point, Lynelle went to a cardiologist and was diag- nosed as having mitral valve prolapse. This doctor changed the type of synthetic progestin that Lynelle was taking, and then doubled the dosage. This helped, but milder heart palpitations still recur occasionally.

Once the heart palpitations were under control, and the high doses of synthetic progestin lessened her bleeding, Lynelle was able to begin taking low doses of natural proges- terone (100 mg taken orally every night during the second half of her menstrual cycle). This helped keep her moods sta- ble, and her bleeding remained manageable for several years. She probably would have felt even better on more natural progesterone, but as a single parent, she couldn't afford it.

What's Happening Now   After two years, Lynelle stopped taking natural progesterone when she started having very heavy bleeding again about a year ago. She was referred to a female gynecologist, who ran various tests and put her on Provera.

Lynelle continues to take 10 mg of Provera during days one through twelve of the calendar month, and it has controlled the bleeding. However, Provera makes her irritable, so she is going to go back on double her former dose of natural progesterone (this is still a low dose). She continues to have episodes of tachycardia (rapid heartbeat) and arrhythmia (irregular heartbeat) occasionally. She thinks that they are seasonal (spring and sometimes in the fall). She also still takes an extremely low dose of Xanax.

Generally, Lynelle is feeling much better than she was when we first met three years ago. She says that her physicians feel they have checked into the thyroid issue thoroughly, but she still wonders if thyroid is part of her problem. I think it is.

I asked Lynelle if she felt that doctors had listened to her. She said, "Generally, no. Medicine is a profession just like any other field; some physicians know a lot, and others are inept. You could put four administrators or four cooks on a panel and get varying answers to the same question. It's the same with doctors.

"Most people think, fallaciously, that doctors know everything. After all, they've gone to medical school, and they have a license. Not only do the patients think the doctor knows everything, many doctors are convinced they know everything, too. Or, at least, they believe they have the capacity to know everything.

"They don't listen," she continued. "They just make conclusions from the blood work and the physical examination. If they can't see the cause of the symptoms, the problem doesn't exist. It doesn't really matter how sick you feel. If they can't measure or define the problem, they blame it on stress or on emotional problems that twist the patient's perception of what is going on. If a person also happens to be overweight like me, they are even more prejudiced. The fact is that, though I went on Weight Watchers that time and lost forty-five pounds, I put it all back on, and since then, I have been unable to lose weight on any diet."

Lynelle continued, "I think there is a difference between male and female personalities in medicine. A man is a man, whatever his profession, and a lot of men have big egos. You don't try to tell them anything in their area of expertise, or they will be offended. Women are better at listening, generally. Sometimes, however, medical training changes that. The medical profession has traditionally been negative toward women. Some women during their training have almost taken on the personality of the male to survive.

"Of course," she concluded, "listening takes longer. Most physicians have the pressure of financial survival—costs of insurance, rent, telephone, and personnel. They cannot spend more than 10 minutes with each patient. They have to make a decision about what is going on very quickly, and this is hard when symptoms come and go as they do with me. But, though I still don't know exactly what's going on, I'm fortunate that natural progesterone removes the worst of those dreadful episodes I kept getting."

Sandra's Story

When I first met Sandra, she was on the verge of suicide. Her eyes were almost swollen shut, and she had tunnel vision. She was having migraines and occasional seizures, and the muscles in her back were in knots. She turned out to have the most complex case of severe PMS that I have ever seen. Her history is abbreviated here, because she can't remember it all in sequence.

Sandra was molested by her father for several years. Beginning at the age of 10, when she commenced her periods, she rarely ovulated. She was told that she would never become pregnant; when she did become pregnant, her physician was amazed, because he felt that she never had adequate ovarian function. The pregnancy was very difficult, and after a hard labor she was told that she should never become pregnant again. A year after the delivery, she had a tubal ligation, and then went into a severe depression.

Sandra went to a psychiatrist who put her on an antidepressant called Sinequan. She believes that this made her even worse. She felt depersonalized, as if she was floating above her body watching herself. After the tubal ligation, Sandy not only became constantly depressed, she also started having PMS. This was relatively short in the cycle, lasting about four days each time, but it was very intense. Sandra frequently left home for a few days to spare her family from her verbally and physically violent anger.

When I met her, ten years ago, Sandra had been enduring depression and PMS for nine years, and the situation had worsened during the previous 18 months. She had been to many doctors, and two of them said that she had severe PMS. In pursuing this possibility, she came into contact with me. I had just started counseling women and was really out of my depth when I talked to Sandra. I have seen many women since with severe problems, but none as bad as hers.

Sandra told me later that she had been planning suicide when she saw me, and that if I had so much as blinked in disbelief, she would have carried through with her plans. I arranged for her to see a gynecologist the next day. I happened to be in the gynecologist's office the day Sandra came and talked to her, but she was in such a state that she didn't know I was there. She has no memory of that day or even of going to the doctor's office. Dr. J. gave her a double shot of progesterone, a great leap of faith because he had just started using progesterone as a treatment, and because her problems were so severe. The shot made Sandra feel better immediately, and the effect lasted about six hours before fading, but it gave her the conviction that her problem was indeed hormonal, and it encouraged her to keep trying.

Dr. J. told her that he could feel a mass on her left side. I sent Sandra to an internist, Dr. C., because she had more experience with progesterone therapy. Dr. C. had another gynecologist examine Sandra, and he was unable to find any growth. They both presumed that Dr. J. was wrong. Actually, he was right. There were two pedunculated (on stalks) dermoid cysts. The problem was that they were floating in the abdomen and had changed position. The cysts weren't identified again for three years.

Sandra's problems were very complex. During at least three consecutive Septembers, she was admitted involuntarily to a psychiatric ward for suicidal depression. Physically, she looked terrible—white, gaunt, as though she were dying, with eyes nearly swollen shut and muscles in knots. She also had migraines and occasional seizures. She had terrible, protracted daily crying jags that began and ended suddenly.

Sandra became so desperate that she called every PMS center she could find in the U.S. A receptionist for a group in Las Vegas told her about Dr. B., a hormone expert in Southern California, to whom they sent their most perplexing patients.

Sandra went to Los Angeles and stayed there for a month to receive treatment from Dr. B. He treated Sandra with estrogen and thyroid, but her response to estrogen was always initially poor. After each estrogen treatment, she would go immediately into depression, but later her mood would improve.

A genius with diagnosis, Dr. B. told Sandra what he thought was wrong with her: she was manic-depressive and had Hashimoto's thyroiditis, diabetes mellitus, and thalassemia (a genetic anemia found among Mediterranean people; she is Greek). He thought she might have a dermoid cyst because of her poor response to estrogen (dermoid cysts can produce hormones and interfere with hormone replacement therapy). She also had some sort of infection; her white blood count was extremely high. Later, doctors thought that the infection had been caused by the floating cysts irritating the organs in the abdominal cavity. On all counts, Dr. B. proved to be correct.

When Sandra went to a psychiatrist to pursue treatment for being bipolar, she was given lithium. She had a severe reaction but realized later that she had actually been reacting to an antibiotic that she was taking concurrently. At the time, she blamed it on the lithium and stopped taking it. This was unfortunate because her depression became much worse.

A few years later, Sandra started having extreme abdominal pain; one day it was so bad that she rushed to the emergency room. When a scan was done, the cysts were seen floating around and pushing against her liver and kidneys. Shortly afterward, her uterus, cervix, ovaries, and fallopian tubes were surgically removed. Despite being on estrogen, progesterone, and thyroid, she went into a deep depression with long, uncontrollable crying jags and was put in a psychiatric ward.

Eventually, a psychiatrist said that Sandra was classically unipolar (meaning that she had recurrent physiological depressions), and she was put back on lithium, which helped to finally stabilize her. After this, she found out that several aunts and cousins in her family had suffered from suicidal depression; there had been a veil of silence in the family, which was a great mistake, as it caused her years of agony. Lithium slurred her speech and caused her to be somewhat forgetful. But it stopped her terrible crying jags and the debilitating depression.

During this time, Sandra trained as a medical assistant and held a full-time job in a hectic practice. A very intelligent and capable woman, she showed incredible courage through the protracted experience she endured. It was a constant temptation for her to give up and commit suicide. She survived because of a rare inner strength and determination.

Although her symptoms appeared purely hormonal, it seems that she inherited a tendency toward depression which was always triggered by some hormonal event. Her problem was a combination of depression and autoimmune and hormonal breakdown. Each element required treatment for full recovery. Elsewhere in the book, I discuss polyglandular autoimmune syndromes, and I believe that Sandra has this type of problem. She says that she needed both lithium and hormones, and that they made a great difference to her.

Because psychiatrists, as a group, don't believe that hormonal problems cause depression, they usually treat only one side of the problem, and frequently have limited results with antidepressants because they don't address the hormonal issue.

What's Happening Now Considering how severe her problems were in the past, Sandra is doing very well. She is working full time and going to school at night. During the last three years, she has been using the Estraderm patch. She needs to change it every three days in order to avoid crying spells. From the 23rd to the 25th day of her menstrual cycle, she wears two patches through her PMS time. She doesn't take natural progesterone because it doesn't affect how she feels. She doesn't take testosterone, because it makes her too aggressive and sexually aroused.

She is also taking 0.175 mg of Synthroid daily, with no side effects. She was taking 2 mg, and her doctor lowered the dosage. He wants to lower it again because her tests show that her thyroid level is too high. Sandra won't let him lower it, because she knows she has to keep a very careful balance.

When she was on lithium, Sandra's hair became dry and brittle and almost all fell out. Her psychiatrist switched her to Tegretol, and she prefers it. She has clearer thinking when on Tegretol than when on lithium. She mentioned that lithium often affects the thyroid gland, but since she was already taking thyroid medication this has not been a problem for her.

Sandra takes 200 mg of Tegretol in the morning, and 300 mg at night, to control her unipolar depression. If she misses two doses, she has immediate facial changes, begins to slow down mentally, starts to move more slowly, and gets depression and mood swings. Her husband says that she goes into slow motion. She thinks slowly, talks slowly, and walks slowly. Her doctor tells her that this is a phenomenon associated with depression in which the motor skills are affected. It takes two days to build up to an effective level of Tegretol after she misses two doses. Her response is rapid and severe.

Sandra says that she would like to use the estrogen implant again; it helped her a great deal when she used it before.

Sandra remembers being given shots of Deldumone, which is a hormone injection made up of three-quarters testosterone and one-quarter estradiol. She says that, before she was on lithium, 2 cc of Deldumone would miraculously resurrect her from a terrifying depressive drop to full normalcy within eight hours. The effects would last only four days before she would bottom out again. She couldn't continually take Deldumone because the amount she needed would have given her a beard! When she went on lithium, it leveled her out dramatically.

Though Sandra is doing well now, she definitely feels that she is held together with medication. She has the flu more frequently than she should, but her energy level is good. I told her, "You've come a long way, baby!" I had seen her a number of times before treatment, and her symptoms at that time were horrendous. We commented that her case history would have been a lot longer if she hadn't lost much of her memory!

Sandra also takes Diabeta, which stimulates the pancreas to process excess sugar. She is getting close to having insulin-dependent diabetes. Her father has diabetes at age 70. If she walks for exercise, and watches her intake of fat, she can usually keep her blood sugar level under control. (Women with diabetes have more problems balancing their blood sugar levels than men, especially after menopause. Because of the high incidence of heart attacks in diabetics, it is felt that postmenopausal diabetic women should take estrogen.)

I have seen many women who are either bipolar or who have recurrent unipolar depressions like Sandra. These depressions are often seasonal, occurring either in September or February/March. If you have recurrent depressions, you may have the unipolar side of this problem. Many people resist being labeled as bipolar (manic-depressive) or unipolar. Yet, this is one of the easiest mental disorders to treat. For Sandra, taking lithium and then Tegretol with estrogen and thyroid was a lifesaver.

I identify strongly with Sandra and am sure that I have mild manic/depressive swings (cyclothymia). I was diagnosed as manic-depressive years ago, but it was not classic (based on the monthly cycle), and treatment with lithium was of no help. The hormones I take have helped me much more and are adequate most of the time. I can live with what's left over (I have seasonal swings, but they are not extreme). Realizing that the feelings I have are common among bipolar and unipolar people, and understanding the biochemical nature of these swings, is very comforting to me. It helps me understand why I am the way I am. And that takes the sting out of the problem.

I find it is not uncommon for women with hormonal problems to also be manic-depressive. This disease takes a number of forms and can be divided into six categories:

Bipolar I: Both major depression and mania (exaggerated gaiety and physical overactivity).

Bipolar II: Major depression alternating with hypomania (a less severe form of mania).

Bipolar III: Cyclothymia: mild depression alternating with hypomania. In the past this was considered a personality disorder.

Bipolar IV: Depression and, usually, no mania. These patients have recurrent bouts of extreme depression. Occasionally, certain antidepressants will trigger mania.

Bipolar V: Depression with no mania, but mania is seen in blood relatives.

Bipolar VI: Mania with no depression. This is a very rare condition, which can lead to psychosis and delusions. It is believed that bipolar VI patients will ultimately end up severely depressed.

Symptoms of mania include: roller coaster highs, irrepressible optimism, feeling great, feeling that anything is possible, overenthusiasm, grandiosity, garrulousness (overtalkativeness), insomnia and staying up all night, bursts of energy, pacing the floor, overresponsibility, taking on huge projects (and often succeeding!), overspending, domineering behavior, hypersexuality, supercreativity. Many famous statesmen, artists, and writers have been manic—that is how they have accomplished superhuman tasks.

Symptoms of depression include: bleak outlook, no mental or physical energy, suicidal thoughts, a feeling that everything is black and that the world is coming to an end, irritability, and long, physically-triggered weeping spells.

While mania feels good to the people experiencing it, and they often resist treatment, the flight comes to an end, and they can plummet to the opposite extreme. The resulting depression is such a terrible contrast that these people are at great risk for suicide.[15]

Some women with PMS and postpartum depression have a combination of hormonal dysfunction and manic-depressive or unipolar disorders. Depending on the severity, treatment for the specific problem may be helpful, as it was for Sandra.

DETAILED TREATMENT FOR PMS

Treatment for PMS varies according to the severity of each woman's problems. Many women with PMS may be able to control their symptoms with simple lifestyle changes. Others may need hormones.

Patience in Seeing Results

Many women find it difficult at first to commit to the lifestyle changes necessary for success in treating PMS, because they don't see immediate results. It is important for them to realize that their symptoms have been out of control for a long time, and it may take several months to show improvement. While some women experience dramatic results in an amazingly short time, others have to wait three or four months for the direction and momentum of their symptoms to change and for treatment to become effective. It is important to realize that what you do now will directly affect how you feel later.

Exercise and Relaxation

Daily physical exercise is almost always beneficial to general health. Some experts feel that exercise helps relieve PMS, because it increases endorphin levels in the brain. Premenstrually, women with PMS have lower levels of endorphins than normal women. Some women find exercise helpful; others don't. Still others with PMS don't have much energy to expend on exercise.

Women should also relax as much as possible during the premenstrual week, avoiding stress. Dr. Susan Lark's book, *The PMS Self-Help Book,* has excellent chapters on exercise and relaxation (see Recommended Reading).

Nutrition

The type of diet often recommended for women with PMS is high in unrefined carbohydrates and low in fat, refined sugar, and animal protein. (See Chapter 17 on diet.) It features lots of fresh fruits and vegetables. According to Dr. Guy Abrahams, a diet high in animal fat and high in calcium in proportion to magnesium may cause or worsen PMS.[16] He recommends foods with a magnesium-to-calcium ratio of at least 2:1, such as grains (the ratio in millet is 8:1). All unprocessed foods contain magnesium in varying amounts. The highest concentrations are in whole seeds (nuts, legumes, and unmilled grains) and green vegetables. Fish, meat, milk, and most fruits (except bananas) are poor sources of magnesium.

Abrahams believes that the reason women in Japan have little PMS is that they have a low intake of animal fat. Conversely, women in Ethiopia, who consume a lot of milk and other animal products, have a high incidence of PMS. Likewise, in the West, women who eat a lot of animal products are more prone to PMS.

Hypoglycemia Diet   Physicians who prescribe progesterone treatment often feel that eating regularly is almost as important as the hormone therapy. Women who have PMS frequently have functional hypoglycemia—erratic blood sugar levels—premenstrually.

A woman who experiences functional hypoglycemia may have sudden attacks of irritability. She may lash out in anger, and may have sudden pounding heart, anxiety attacks, or migraine. Many of the violent outbursts common to PMS are due to this drop in blood sugar level. Often, when asked, such women will admit to not having eaten for several hours.

Progesterone plays a major role in regulating blood sugar levels. This is due to the intimate link between progesterone and gamma globulin (they share receptor sites in many cells). Gamma globulin carries blood sugar through the blood stream, and low levels of progesterone interfere with this function. This is one reason why women with PMS have functional or transitory low blood sugar for a time before their menstrual periods.

Says Katharina Dalton, expert on PMS:

> . . . scientists have shown that progesterone receptors do not
> work in the presence of nor-adrenalin. Nor-adrenalin is re-
> leased when the blood sugar levels drop, such as when there
> has been a long interval without eating any carbohydrates.
> This means that in the treatment of both PMS and post-
> natal depression not only must attention be given to raising
> the blood progesterone level by the administration of pro-
> gesterone, but it is essential to prevent any release of nor-
> adrenalin by ensuring that the women are eating small
> portions of starchy food at three-hour intervals. As the nu-
> tritionists would say, one must encourage sufferers to be
> 'grazers,' eating at frequent intervals, and not 'gorgers,'
> only eating three times a day.[17]

Since premenstrual hypoglycemia is only a temporary
phenomenon, the results of tests for hypoglycemia are often
misleading.

Eat Small, Regular, Frequent Meals   After ovulation and
until the end of their symptoms, women with PMS should eat
frequent small meals (as many as six a day) approximately
every three to four hours to prevent low blood sugar attacks.
These meals should include a portion of some complex carbohydrate (starchy food). Women need eat only half a slice of
bread, a few crackers, a potato, or a small portion of rice. This
will help keep the blood sugar levels constant.

Because refined sugar makes the condition worse, women
are advised to cut down on refined sugar or remove it from
their diets. It is also advisable to stop smoking and cut caffeine
and alcohol out of the diet. Caffeine, alcohol, and nicotine initially cause higher glycogen levels (sugar stores) in the liver,
sometimes followed by a drastic drop in blood sugar level. The
higher levels at first induce a "sugar high," but this is followed
by a "downer" when the levels drop.

Eating regularly and avoiding foods or substances that adversely affect blood sugar levels is particularly important for
women who have sudden rages, panic attacks, or drastic mood
changes.

Vitamins, Minerals, and Herbs   It is more important to eat a
hearty, healthy diet than to take processed vitamins and minerals that do not provide the same balance as vitamins found
in natural foods. Still, some women seem to benefit from taking vitamins, particularly B-complex with vitamin B_6.[18] However, the FDA warns against taking B_6 to excess, and Dr.
Katherina Dalton cautions that taking doses even as low as 50
mg daily may cause peripheral neuritis.[19] Once women become sensitive to B_6, she says that even the low dose of B_6 in
packaged cereals may cause overdose symptoms. But others
disagree with this.

Vitamin E has also been found to be helpful.[20] Its antioxidant properties help prevent deterioration of the ovaries
and support fertility. It also helps resolve fibrocystic breast disease and reduce PMS symptoms.

Women who get muscle cramps and joint pain may benefit from taking a trace mineral supplement. Magnesium, calcium, and potassium work together to alleviate these specific
symptoms. You might take the recommended daily number of
capsules that contain 500 mg of magnesium to provide suitable doses of the other elements.

Women with PMS are considered potassium-users. This is
because premenstrual changes in adrenal production of aldosterone disrupt the sodium-potassium balance, causing sodium
to be retained in the tissues and potassium to be excreted in
the urine. Sometimes prescription potassium, such as K-Lyte,
is needed. Klorvess is a similar product with no sugar in it. You
don't want to overdose on prescription potassium, as it can affect the heart and blood pressure. A lower dose of potassium
is also available in salt substitutes and certain effervescent
antacids. When muscle cramps are extreme, taking the appropriate hormone with the trace minerals is probably the only
way to stabilize mineral balance.

Herbs such as vitex (agnus castus), yellow dock root, burdock root, wild yam root, licorice root, fo-ti, pau d'arco, astragalus, dong quai, ginger, oatstraw, comfrey, nettle, raspberry
leaf, squawvine, motherwort, horsetail, and red clover can all
be helpful. I suggest that you find an experienced herbologist
who grows and prepares organic herbs, rather than buying old

herbs in a store. See Recommended Reading at end of book for books by Rosemary Gladstar.

Vitamin D and Calcium   Women with PMS may have transient hyperparathyroidism at ovulation. In a small, controlled study of women with PMS by S. Thys-Jacobs, M.D., and M. J. Alvir, M.D.,[21] calcium metabolism was checked by blood draw at six points throughout the ovulatory cycle. In both the PMS group and the control group, calcium levels declined significantly when estrogen levels increased at mid-cycle. However, in the PMS group, parathyroid hormone levels were elevated 30 percent above normal during ovulation. In the control group, levels of parathyroid hormone did not vary during the whole menstrual cycle.

Significant differences between the groups were noted in the levels of calcium and of the vitamin D liver metabolites (products of metabolism) 25-hydroxyvitamin-D_3 (25D) and 1,25-hydroxyvitamin-D (1,25D). One woman with PMS was treated with oral elemental calcium and cholecalciferol (vitamin D_3) daily for three months, with resulting amelioration of her symptoms. The mid-cycle rise in parathyroid hormone declined with replacement of 25-hydroxyvitamin-D_3.

Dr. Robert Fredericks, an endocrinologist in Reno, Nevada, can explain this phenomenon. He says that vitamin D is actually a hormone. In the past vitamin 25 D has been given little attention, while vitamin 1,25 D was thought to be the most significant metabolite.

Dr. Fredericks says that some steroid hormones like estrogen and testosterone have received most attention because of their profound cosmetic and sexual effects. Metabolites such as 25 D may actually be more influential than these steroids in energy metabolism. He says that since 25 D probably evolved earlier, its effects may be more fundamental in the overall balance of energy regulation and behavior.

Dr. Fredericks orders a calcium tolerance test to better understand individual variations in the regulation of energy metabolism. The testing allows him to tailor an individual treatment approach to address the identified imbalances. His recommendations often include special vitamin D metabolites, other hormones, and minerals, such as calcium, phosphorus, and magnesium, as well as conventional medications.

L-*Tryptophan*   Two female physician's assistants in central California compared their life experiences to see what they had in common and whether the comparison would give them a clue about the cause of their PMS. The only common factor that they could find was that they both wet the bed until puberty. So they decided to study current research on the cause of late bed-wetting. They found that children who were late bed-wetters had low levels of serotonin in their brains.

The substance melatonin is normally produced from serotonin overnight. Apparently, in late bed-wetters, the low levels of melatonin kept them from experiencing rapid-eye-movement (REM) sleep. They seemed to stay so deeply asleep that they were not awakened by the urge to urinate.

These two women concluded that some PMS was related to low levels of serotonin and melatonin. Based on a questionnaire sent to 300 PMS sufferers, they found that, although the national average for late bed-wetters (male or female) was 1 to 2 percent of the general population, among PMS sufferers the percentage was much higher. In fact, among women with the most severe PMS, there was approximately a 36 percent incidence of late bed-wetting. Apparently, whatever caused late bed-wetting was related to PMS in some women.

The two women discovered that lower melatonin levels directly affected the mechanism of ovulation, causing it to occur a couple of days earlier in women with PMS than in those without PMS. Because of this, they theorized that PMS was not a hormonal problem but a sleep disorder—specifically a serotonin-deficiency disease. They reasoned that taking L-tryptophan,[22] an amino acid then available at health food stores, might correct the PMS condition. Many women have found L-tryptophan helpful, although the theory behind its use is probably too simplistic to cover all cases of PMS.

In 1990, an outbreak of problems caused by taking L-tryptophan capsules caused the FDA to withdraw it from the market. It was later found that the adverse reactions were caused by a contaminated batch of L-tryptophan from Japan. Even though the problems were not due to the L-tryptophan itself, the FDA has not reissued approval. This has been seen as very political.[23] The time may come when L-tryptophan will be back on the market, perhaps under prescription. The suggested dosage was one or two 500-mg capsules daily, with the dose raised premenstrually as necessary; limit, five capsules per day.

L-tyrosine[24] is supposed to have a similar action to L-tryptophan, and L-phenylalanine may also help alleviate depression. Both these amino acids are available in health food stores.

Evening Primrose Oil   Great claims have been made for the success of using evening primrose oil in treating PMS.[25] Advocates for evening primrose oil say that either women's sensitivity to their own normal levels of prolactin, or prolactin's action in reducing progesterone levels, causes PMS.

Evening primrose oil contains an essential fatty acid (EFA) also found in mother's milk. This EFA is a precursor of prostaglandin E_1 (different than the prostaglandin thought to be responsible for many menstrual cramps). It supposedly inhibits blood levels of the hormone prolactin. Apart from producing lactation after childbirth, one of the actions of prolactin is to reduce levels of progesterone. Black currant, linseed, and borage oil apparently contain the same EFA.

Some women use evening primrose oil alone for relief from PMS. Others take it with progesterone to help relieve such specific symptoms as swollen breasts, bloating, and acne. The suggested dosage for Efamol, the best-known brand, is six capsules daily for a couple of months and, from then on, three capsules daily.

Restrict Salt and Fluid   The sodium-potassium balance is altered in women with PMS because, just before menstruation, the body cells absorb sodium more readily, which attracts fluid. Bloating is a universal problem in women with PMS, and the pressure of retained fluid causes many symptoms. All women with PMS should cut down on salt premenstrually. Be careful of how much salt you consume in packaged and canned goods, and how much you add to your cooking or at the table.

Avoid Alcohol and Recreational Drugs   Many women, because of depression or stress prior to their periods, will try to
use alcohol or drugs to alleviate those symptoms. In this way,
they may also develop a habit of alcohol or drug abuse. Some
recovering women alcoholics and addicts who seek treatment
for PMS report that their past drinking or drug-using pattern
was always cyclical, and that their drinking or drug-using
bouts paralleled their premenstrual stress.

The rate of PMS among women alcoholics is substantially
higher than in the general population of women. Women
seem to have an added craving for alcohol premenstrually because their blood sugar levels are low. Many women also have
a lowered tolerance to both drugs and alcohol premenstrually.
Women, in general, handle alcohol less well than men because
they have significantly less of the enzyme that breaks down
alcohol in the stomach. Female alcoholics also get alcohol-
related liver diseases earlier than men.

Alcohol may make you feel relaxed initially. It first stimulates the nervous system, but then depresses it; it also raises
the levels of glycogen in the liver, sending blood sugar levels
up dramatically, only to drop drastically shortly thereafter.
Because changes in blood sugar level are so much a part of
PMS, avoiding any substance that exacerbates the problem is
most important.

Alcohol also tends to produce violent feelings. Many in-
stances of physical violence toward either a husband or children stem from a combination of PMS and alcohol abuse. It is
sensible for women with PMS to cut down on or, preferably,
eliminate alcohol entirely.

Some women with severe PMS may be tempted to use
recreational drugs to alleviate the misery of their symptoms.
However, the use of cocaine and amphetamines will further
aggravate the endorphin depletion common in women with
PMS, in addition to undermining their general health. The
habitual use of drugs such as heroin can stop menstruation
altogether. I once met a 17-year heroin user who did not menstruate during most of the time while she was using heroin,
and who went into menopause after she went off of it at the
age of 34.

Restrict Caffeine Intake   Caffeine, like alcohol, stimulates the central nervous system and then depresses it, raising the glycogen level and then dropping it. This can cause women to become irritable and worsens their PMS symptoms. Some women who are prone to headaches may find caffeine helpful at first, but the headache generally returns when the caffeine wears off. These women may develop the habit of drinking coffee or taking other drinks or pills with caffeine in them. PMS sufferers are advised to either remove caffeine from their diet or reduce their intake drastically.

Eat Chocolate, but Not Too Much   According to Debra Waterhouse, women need a little chocolate.[26] Chocolate contains magnesium, which is one reason why women crave it, and it increases levels of serotonin, the brain hormone that improves one's mood.

However, chocolate contains theobromine, which is similar to caffeine. It also has a high fat and sugar content, which tends to worsen acne.

There's no harm in eating one or two pieces of chocolate a day, if you have the willpower to resist eating a lot more. The problem is that women with severe chocolate cravings before their periods have great difficulty limiting themselves to one or two pieces—they're more likely to eat one or two pounds!

Diuretics

Diuretics are widely prescribed for PMS because of bloating, but are generally not very helpful. They are usually unsuccessful in alleviating the emotional symptoms connected with PMS. While diuretics cause some excretion of fluids from the body, using them is like dipping a teaspoon into a sea of fluid. If they are strong enough to rid the body of enough excess fluid to alleviate bloating, they also tend to cause excretion of minerals like potassium into the urine.

Herbs that may be helpful for their diuretic action are: *uva ursi,* buchu, chickweed, and cleavers.

Spironolactone, an Exception   Spironolactone is a diuretic that blocks the production of certain substances in the adrenal glands believed to cause or worsen PMS symptoms. Spironolactone is chemically similar to progesterone and functions like a hormone. Some women with mild-to-moderate PMS symptoms, including acne, may benefit from taking spironolactone alone. The usual dose is 25 mg three or four times a day, taken during the time when a woman has symptoms. Women with a history of breast tumors may wish to talk to their physicians about using this diuretic, because it has been associated with increased breast tumors in beagles (a breed of dog which commonly has such tumors, anyway).

Spironolactone also helps some women with hirsutism, but the doses used to treat this are much higher—400 to 600 mg daily. It is when Spironolactone is prescribed at such high doses that it is more likely to have severe side effects.

Women who use progesterone, and who have problems with excessive fluid that the progesterone does not alleviate, may wish to take spironolactone as well. You will need a prescription for spironolactone from your physician.

Antiprostaglandins

Research shows that some menstrual cramps are caused by prostaglandins (natural hormone-like substances in the body). Antiprostaglandins have been helpful in treating this type of cramping.

Some physicians treat PMS with antiprostaglandins because they think that PMS and menstrual cramps are the same thing. If a woman has both PMS and cramps, antiprostaglandins may certainly help the pain.

Women who have uterine fibroids often have a swollen uterus. The uterus produces prostaglandins and, when in a swollen state, it often produces higher levels, which may affect the hormonal cycling of the ovaries and cause PMS. If this is the main cause of PMS, antiprostaglandins may be helpful.

Bromocriptine

If a woman has hypophysitis (a swollen pituitary) or a pituitary tumor causing a surge in prolactin production, she may have symptoms of PMS. Where surgery is not indicated, medication with Parlodel (bromocriptine) to reduce the levels of prolactin may remove the symptoms of PMS. However, bromocriptine is not, generally, a treatment for PMS, and it has very strong side effects.

Progesterone Therapy

In severe cases, when PMS interferes with a woman's quality of life and when symptoms fit within the classic patterns of PMS, patients often respond well to cyclical progesterone therapy; it replaces a needed hormone, just as insulin helps some diabetics. While the exact cause of PMS is unknown, progesterone seems to be involved because symptoms occur at the time when progesterone is normally high. When this hormone is supplied, the symptoms often disappear completely.

Note the Different Types of Progesterone   Progesterone is erroneously used as a generic name for all those substances that function similarly to progesterone. Many artificial hormones called progestins have been synthesized in the laboratory. These substances are derived from progesterone but may take on the characteristics of other hormones, including the male hormone testosterone.

It is important to know the difference, since synthetic progestins often affect PMS sufferers adversely, while natural progesterone usually does not. Birth control pills, which contain synthetic progestins (not natural progesterone), are often given as a treatment to women with PMS. Most PMS sufferers should avoid them. (However, OvCon 35 often gets a better response than others since it has the lowest progestin content.) Provera, the trade name for medroxyprogesterone (a synthetic progestin) lowers both the ovarian and the pituitary production of progesterone.[27]

Information on how to obtain natural progesterone can be found in Appendix 2. The nonprescription creams tend to be weaker than the prescription progesterone, but they work well for some women with milder problems.

Transdermal Creams—Pro-Gest® The suggested protocol for using Pro-Gest® natural progesterone cream for premenstrual syndrome is taken from the Pro-Gest® package insert.[28] Note that everyone is different. Some women require more or less progesterone cream to alleviate their symptoms. But here is a starting protocol:

Don't use the cream from day 1 of bleeding to day 14 of the cycle.

Days 14–18:	$^1/_8$ tsp twice per day
Days 18–23:	$^1/_4$ tsp twice per day
Days 23 till period begins:	$^1/_2$ tsp twice per day
Then start again.	

The cream can be applied to your abdomen during cramps. You can rub it on the back of your neck or on your temples if you have a migraine. Absorption is especially good on the back of the hands.

Prescription Natural Progesterone—Pharmacy Warning When you receive your progesterone from the pharmacy, the package may contain a warning about possible side effects. You should understand that natural progesterone and synthetic progestins are classified in the *Physician's Desk Reference* as the same substance. While they are all similar in composition, there are small physical differences that have a profound impact on some women's moods.

The warning you receive from the pharmacy describes the possible side effects of all substances classified as progestational agents, whether natural or synthetic. Some women who have used progesterone-like drugs, which are often more like the male hormone testosterone, had a higher incidence of babies with birth defects. Natural progesterone is not known to produce birth defects.

A Typical Protocol for Taking Progesterone If a woman has a regular 28- to 30-day-cycle, she probably ovulates on about the fourteenth to sixteenth day. She may know this for a fact, since many women have ovulatory twinges or definite pain in their ovaries. Some have changes in their vaginal mucus. Others feel the onset of their symptoms.

If a woman has symptoms that begin with ovulation, she should begin taking her progesterone two days ahead of the time when she expects her symptoms to begin. So, if she has a 28-day cycle, she would begin taking her progesterone on the twelfth or fourteenth day. Because of variations in the length of cycles, the starting date may vary. When women have very irregular cycles, they would have to begin the progesterone at the first sign of symptoms.

To begin with, she could take a 100- to-200-mg dose first thing in the morning, and again between noon and 2:00 P.M. Often, twice a day is enough, and taking the second dose five to six hours after the first may keep the progesterone level high enough to see a woman through the whole day. But if the symptoms return at dinner or late evening, a woman could take a third and even a fourth dose of progesterone. Some pharmacists make a time-release capsule that lasts longer.

As the symptoms worsen toward the onset of menstrual bleeding, a woman might find that she needs to raise the dose at that point. Raising it any earlier may bring on overdose symptoms such as drowsiness and euphoria. But keep in mind that Dr. Dalton believes it is important to take enough progesterone around ovulation to avoid having problems premenstrually, and raising the levels of progesterone close to the time of bleeding may delay menstruation.

Women should take their progesterone faithfully every day, trying not to vary it too much, since varying the dose or skipping doses may cause irregular bleeding and mood swings.

When to Stop Taking Progesterone   We recommend that a woman take progesterone from day 14 of her cycle until menstrual bleeding begins, even if her period is a little late. This is to avoid a drop into symptoms that commonly occurs if the progesterone is stopped abruptly on the 26th day to bring on a period. Always stop taking progesterone by gradually decreasing the dose over a couple of days (cut the dose in half for a day or two, and then stop taking it).

In a given menstrual cycle, a woman should stop taking progesterone at the time when her PMS symptoms would normally stop: when her period begins, two or three days into her period, or at the end of her period. When a woman goes on progesterone, PMS symptoms may be delayed. If, prior to treatment, you had symptoms until the first or second day of your flow, and now that you are taking progesterone they seem to return during your period, you may take progesterone as long as necessary. In most cases, however, you should stop taking the progesterone by the end of your period. In that case, no progesterone would be taken until the twelfth or fourteenth day of the next menstrual cycle. There are exceptions to this rule; some women just feel better taking progesterone all the time, and it doesn't seem to alter their menstrual cycle.

Cancer Is Not a Known Side Effect   Many women are reluctant to take progesterone due to a fear of cancer in connection with taking hormones. Dr. Katherina Dalton makes the following points in her book *Depression After Childbirth:*

- Progesterone has been used since 1934 and carefully monitored since 1948 without any serious side-effects.
- Progesterone is used to treat vaginal cancer in daughters of women who took DES (diethylstilbestrol), a synthetic estrogen used to prevent miscarriages in the fifties and sixties.
- Natural human material is generally not cancer-producing. Insulin, for example, has been in use for over 50 years with no evidence of cancer production. The use of thyroid hormones produces no cancer risk. Thyroxine is given at birth to cretins and continued throughout their entire life.
- The body can convert active hormones into inactive ones for waste disposal. In the case of progesterone, it is changed to pregnanediol, which is excreted in the urine or feces.
- By contrast, synthetic steroids and other drugs such as diethylstilbestrol are not normally found in humans; the attendant risk of cancer may result either directly or indirectly from the breakdown products formed when they are excreted. The body does not have the necessary chemicals

to convert the synthetic progestins into the same inactive agents, and they are not disposed of in the same way as progesterone.[29]

Side Effects of Progesterone   Even when taking the correct progesterone therapy, some minor side effects may occur. They are frequently temporary problems:

- **Spotting or breakthrough bleeding** at mid-cycle and in the premenstruum (the several days before menstrual bleeding begins). Spotting may occur at ovulation if progesterone has been taken too early in the cycle, or if the uterine lining is already thick. If you start spotting premenstrually, you may stop taking the progesterone to allow your period to begin, but your PMS symptoms may return. Often spotting is a temporary problem and, after a few cycles of taking progesterone, will go away. Breakthrough bleeding sometimes indicates low estrogen levels that cannot maintain the endometrium and easily slough off. It may indicate the need for estrogen.

- **Lengthening or shortening of the menstrual cycle.** Sometimes the cycle lengthens or shortens on progesterone. It typically lengthens, with the period being delayed.

   If either occurs, you might adjust your progesterone dosage in consultation with your physician; often the cycle will stabilize after a few months. You may stop taking the progesterone earlier to avoid a lengthier cycle, but we do not advise this as often symptoms will return (and it often doesn't work). You could also cut the dosage in half and see if that brings your period on. Once your period begins, you may go back on progesterone during your period if your symptoms return and it helps.

   If you take progesterone too early in your cycle (more than two days before ovulation), you will be more likely to have mid-cycle or early bleeding. Usually, women only take progesterone during the second half of their cycles, but for some reason there are women who feel better taking it all month. These women may opt to put up with breakthrough bleeding just to feel better.

- **Missing a cycle.** Occasionally, a woman may completely miss a cycle or two when she first goes on progesterone. This is nothing to be concerned about.
- **Initial heavier or lighter bleeding.** Women going on progesterone may experience changes in bleeding. Their first period may be very heavy. But, in general, the flow can become either heavier or lighter. The color of blood may also change. There is no need to worry about these temporary changes, which tend to adjust themselves after one or two cycles. Very rarely, a woman may lose the lining of her uterus all at once. It will look like a lump of liver; while this may be frightening, it is not usually considered serious. If the lining is built up, it is good to get rid of it. If you are concerned, consult your physician.
- **Increase or decrease in food cravings.** Usually, progesterone will help decrease food cravings, but a few women may find that progesterone makes them hungrier. Generally, progesterone tends to normalize the appetite.
- **Increase or decrease in sex drive.** A few women find that progesterone lowers their sex drive, which can be disappointing. But if they have been sexually overstimulated because of PMS, they may be happy about a return to normality.
- **Sore breasts or fleeting joint pains.** When beginning progesterone therapy, women may get relief from their PMS but may have sore breasts or fleeting joint pains instead. (I have read that joint pain is a side effect. I have never heard of anyone having it.) A few women feel faint. Younger women and those who have had no children may feel euphoric or have restless energy or mild cramps. However, women who have had children are accustomed to having higher levels of progesterone in their system for most of the nine months of pregnancy. For them, overdose is unlikely. We advise women to ignore these minor symptoms as they will probably disappear after a couple of cycles.
- **Allergic reactions** may occur to the substance containing the progesterone or to the progesterone itself. Some women are allergic to the wax in the suppositories; they should switch to another form of treatment. Other women

get redness and swelling around injection sites, if they get shots. Typical symptoms of an allergic reaction can occur, including rapid heart rate and panic attacks. Some specialized allergy clinics can desensitize women to this allergy. Sometimes this reaction is due to antibodies produced by the body against progesterone.

- **Worsening of symptoms.** A small minority of women experience increased PMS depression from taking progesterone. They will be unable to take it, but may benefit from estrogen, with bimonthly or quarterly use of progesterone to protect the lining of the uterus. Some researchers will feel that this is not enough progesterone. However, I have found that many OB/GYNs with years of experience follow this practice. These women need to have their uterine lining checked regularly to avoid adverse changes.

Pointers for Success in Treating PMS with Natural Progesterone

1. **The Right Diagnosis**
PMS symptoms occur cyclically some time between ovulation and menstruation. Women who have symptoms for only a short time, about two or three days before their period, will feel normal for three and a half weeks out of the month. But other women can have symptoms for up to three weeks a month and only have one week without symptoms. When additional problems with low thyroid, menopause, and postpartum depression are involved, the PMS pattern may be less clear. Also, if a woman does not have PMS but has a chronic disease such as non-hormonal depression or headaches that occur at random times during the month and worsen at menstruation, she may not respond to progesterone therapy. Such variations and complications make it necessary to ensure that the diagnosis is correct.

2. **The Right Hormone**
Women must be certain that they receive natural progesterone and not one of the many synthetics which may erroneously be called progesterone. The reason that most

women with a PMS history do not tolerate the birth control pill well is because of its synthetic progesterone-like
hormones.

Natural progesterone is made from Mexican or South
American wild yams or soybeans, and matches the chemical composition of the progesterone in your body. While
synthetic progestins are similar to natural progesterone in
composition, they are not completely alike.

Synthetic progestins function similarly to progesterone
in the uterus. They both cause the lining of the womb to
thicken. When the levels drop, the lining of the womb
sloughs off. However, synthetic progestins do not function
like progesterone in the progesterone receptors found in
the brain and elsewhere throughout the body. In fact,
these artificial hormones lower the natural progesterone
levels in the blood, thereby worsening PMS.

3. **The Right Dosage**

The prescribing physician will determine the starting
dosage based on the severity of a patient's symptoms—
giving a lower starting dose for women who have never
been pregnant, more for women who have been pregnant. The average frequency for taking progesterone
ranges from one to three times a day, and may be increased if symptoms persist.

Your physician will determine your progesterone
dosage, but you will probably have to experiment to find
the correct amount for you. Correct dosage is an individual matter, and women's needs differ tremendously. This
is partly because women vary in their ability to absorb
and metabolize progesterone.

Different quantities of progesterone are put into different forms of medication—oral capsules, oral tablets,
sublingual tablets, suppositories, rectal fluid (a liquid
progesterone suspension that is placed in the bowel), injections, and so on. A single oral capsule may contain 25,
50, 75, 100 or more mg of progesterone and can be taken
under the tongue or swallowed. An oral tablet may have
100 to 400 mg of progesterone, and again it can be taken
either under the tongue or swallowed, depending on the

way it has been formulated. Absorption is sometimes better under the tongue, so dosages are lower when the tablet is intended to be taken that way. Suppositories, used vaginally or anally, vary from 25 mg to 400 mg. A single dose of rectal fluid ranges from 2 cc (100 mg) to 4 cc (200 mg). The intramuscular injection in oil ranges from 1 or 2 cc (50 or 100 mg) and upward.

The normal practice is to take a single tablet (or other form) from one to three times a day. However, it is possible that an individual who is sensitive to medication needs only a quarter of a normal dose. And some women who need more can take the equivalent of up to six doses a day (e.g., in the case of suppositories, 6 × 400 mg = 2400 mg per day).

When women take more progesterone and do not feel a corresponding benefit, there may be an absorption problem and alternative routes should be investigated.

4. **The Right Frequency**

Progesterone is taken at least twice a day; I suggest 7:00–8:00 A.M. and 1:00–2:00 P.M., then an added dose in the evening if necessary. Women who begin taking progesterone should feel a beneficial effect within an hour, and feel it wear off after four to five hours (though some time-release forms of progesterone last up to 12 hours; ask your pharmacist about this). This is why it is best not to take it morning and night if only two doses are taken; the medication will wear off by the afternoon, and symptoms will return. This experience of feeling the symptoms leave and then return helps women determine how much they need. They need freedom to experiment with adjusting their own dosage.

If the dosage is raised during the cycle, it should stay at the higher dose until the symptoms would normally cease at the end of the cycle. For some women, symptoms stop at the beginning of their period; for others, symptoms continue to the very end of their period. The dosage should not be alternately raised and lowered, as this can cause spotting and bring back symptoms. An exception to this is when the patient has severe symptoms at ovulation

but slight improvement later, lasting until the last part of
the cycle (B pattern; see chart on PMS symptoms). Then
progesterone can be effectively raised and lowered to
cover symptoms. High doses may be needed prior to ovulation, then the dose may be decreased for a few days and
then increased premenstrually.

Don't stop taking progesterone suddenly or miss days
during the last part of your cycle. This can cause breakthrough bleeding or a return of your symptoms.

If you use vaginal or anal suppositories, do not take
more than a single dose at one time. If you need more,
take it more frequently rather than in larger quantities.
Allow a minimum of an hour between doses if using suppositories, because there is relatively little absorption of
doses higher than 400 mg in suppository form. Also, using
more than one suppository at a time may hinder absorption because of the amount of wax in the suppository.

5. **The Right Form of Medication**
Women vary in their ability to absorb progesterone and
may need to experiment to get full benefit. If they have a
correct diagnosis and experience some relief from taking
progesterone, they should pursue becoming as symptom-
free as possible.

Progesterone may be taken in a variety of forms: oral
capsules of oil that are swallowed; oral tablets made of
powder; compressed wax suppositories, which can be
used either rectally or vaginally; a rectal fluid used with a
syringe; powder capsules taken under the tongue (somewhat bitter and ineffective); pellets surgically implanted
into the fatty tissue of the abdomen or hip; sublingual
drops; or creams and oils that can be rubbed on the skin.
As a last resort, daily intramuscular injections or a booster
shot at ovulation can be given into the fatty tissues of the
buttock.

In England, Dr. Dalton uses suppositories, injections,
or implants. Europeans are accustomed to suppositories,
and take well to using progesterone this way, but this is
not true in the United States, where women tend to find
the use of suppositories distasteful. Dr. Dalton believes

that the oral route involves a completely different process that counteracts the effect of progesterone, and until recently she never had much success with it. However, at a seminar in San Francisco in 1992, so many positive results were reported from the use of oral micronized progesterone that Dr. Dalton began trying progesterone capsules in oil in England with marked success. Many women in the U.S. find that taking oral progesterone works as well as using suppositories.

Some women become sleepy and feel somewhat "drunk" or euphoric as a result of taking oral progesterone. If this persists, they need to switch to using suppositories or the rectal fluid, or, in the most severe cases, injections. Taking progesterone with food may help.

Oral capsules and tablets   In the past, natural progesterone was not taken orally because it was destroyed by the action of the stomach. Then, a fairly effective oral progesterone capsule in oil was produced, and, more recently, a micronized oral tablet (some pharmacies also make a lozenge). One pharmacist says that the micronized oral tablet is longer-acting because the compression of the tablet allows more gradual absorption; its smaller particles have a greater surface area which also makes for better absorption.

Another pharmacist says that the powder-only tablet is still largely destroyed by the stomach, and that very large doses would be needed. When the sublingual capsule is in oil, the progesterone is absorbed through the lymphatic system, and doses can be lower.

Suppositories   These may be made with one of several bases: glycerinated gelatin, cocoa butter, or polyethylene glycol. Progesterone absorption has been found to be significantly higher using the polyethylene glycol. If a woman uses suppositories vaginally, she will need to wear a pad, as the melted wax leaks. In the rectum, the sphincter muscle holds the suppository in place so that it does not leak. However, it can stimulate a bowel movement, so it should be used only after a bowel movement if possible. Some women find that the rectal suppositories cause gas or diarrhea. Women seem to tolerate the cocoa butter/ fatty-acid based suppositories better rectally.

Rectal fluid   The rectal fluid is usually absorbed better than suppositories, and is almost half the price. Rectal fluid can also be made with a variety of bases, and absorption can vary. For best results, do not insert the syringe higher than an inch into the rectum. Past a certain point, the fluid is absorbed into the colon, passes into the portal system (the blood vessels that take foods from the stomach and toxins from the bowel to be porcessed by the liver), and is destroyed.

Sublingual Tablet   A number of smaller compounding pharmacies make a hard gel sublingual tablet which often contains sugar to mask the mild bitterness of progesterone. This can cause cavities in the teeth so you might ask if the form you are going to take contains any sugar (sublingual capsules usually don't). Bajamar Pharmacy has an excellent sublingual tablet of natural progesterone which contains a burst of orange instead of sugar. It is absorbed within a couple of minutes.

Sublingual powder capsules   These work well on their own for women who don't need a lot of progesterone. They are also often used as a booster with either suppositories or rectal fluid for women who tend to have sudden attacks of anger or depression. Taking progesterone under the tongue works quickly, but it may cause blood levels of progesterone to rise and fall suddenly. That's why some women need to use it with another form of progesterone that will last longer in the bloodstream.

The powder tends to clump under the tongue but is eventually swallowed. Keep it at the back of your mouth under your tongue as long as you can, but don't expect it to dissolve. You will gradually swallow it, but try to keep it there as long as you can for maximum absorption. For the same reason, don't drink beverages for about an hour after taking these powder capsules. Once you swallow the progesterone, it is not as effective. As mentioned before, sublingual capsules may cause "progesterone drunkenness," especially if more than one capsule is used. If this effect occurs regularly, cut the dose in half or try another form of progesterone.

Powder capsule as a suppository   Women who are allergic to wax may use the powder capsule as a suppository, using KY Jelly to lubricate it first. If you use the powder capsules vaginally, be aware that they are gritty; the grit does not come out easily, and both men and women may find it abrasive during intercourse.

Injections   Women with severe PMS or postpartum depression may benefit from daily intramuscular injections of progesterone, or, in the case of PMS, a booster shot of progesterone around ovulation, followed by daily use of another form until menstruation. In the U.S., the injectable progesterone is prepared by Rugby (50 mg per ml) in a peanut-oil base, which can be very irritating, possibly causing redness, swelling, and even abscesses. Women who receive these shots on a regular basis may develop scar tissue.

If a woman develops an abscess, she should check with her physician. But if the injection site is slightly red or swollen, I have found that charcoal compresses are helpful. Crush two or three charcoal tablets, add a little water, and spread it on gauze; put it over the injection site, and tape it on overnight. Charcoal draws out any swelling or infection that might be present. It is very messy, but effective.

This information is not meant to confuse or discourage. It is meant to show the various ways of taking progesterone and the difficulties some may find with each method. You need to be versatile and to understand that both appropriate dosage and absorption rate vary among individuals. Many women have no problems with absorption, but those who do need to be patient and willing to experiment, keeping in close contact with their counselor or physician.

6. **When to Begin and End Therapy**
Therapy is very individual. Your physician and counselor will give you instructions on the best regimen for you. It is important to start progesterone early enough in your

cycle to build up the blood levels of progesterone prior to the time when symptoms would begin. Women often ignore this advice, taking progesterone only when they feel symptoms. Treatment is never as successful if begun too late. If the pattern of symptoms regularly occurs in the last few days or week of the cycle (pattern A; see chart on PMS symptoms), a woman should start taking her progesterone five days ahead of the time when she expects her symptoms. If her symptoms occur at ovulation (patterns B and C), she should begin two days ahead.

Women are often told to stop taking their progesterone a couple of days before menstruation in order to bring on their period. This is not advisable because the period often doesn't start within the two days, and there may be a return and worsening of symptoms during menstruation. To prevent this, stay on the progesterone until bleeding occurs, even if the period is delayed each cycle for the first two or three cycles. Generally, women should not take progesterone after bleeding ends because it may cause breakthrough bleeding or irregular periods.

But there are exceptions to this rule. For instance, if a woman has very severe, long-standing problems, some physicians prescribe continual progesterone therapy for two or three months to settle down their symptoms and then cycle the progesterone treatments. If you did well for the first week after ovulation, but not so well around menstruation, you probably took too little progesterone, too late to help. You should take a high enough dose of progesterone, early enough (around the time of ovulation) to help you feel better just before your period occurs.

The Necessity of Keeping a Calendar and Journal   You are largely responsible for monitoring your own therapy, and your subsequent well-being depends to a great extent on doing it properly. When you begin progesterone therapy, use a calendar to calculate ahead when you need to start taking your progesterone. Buy a small pocket calendar which you can carry around with you. Write an "M" on each day when you bleed. Write down "1" on the first day of bleeding. Count forward from the first day until the day when you expect to ovulate (this only works if you are fairly regular). Then mark two days earlier, and that is when you should begin your treatment. If symptoms begin earlier than expected, you may start taking the progesterone then.

You should mark your calendar ahead every time your period begins. Having PMS often makes it hard to be disciplined, but discipline is needed to begin the therapy early enough and to make sure that you take the progesterone regularly. If you can't do this, you need to enlist someone else, perhaps your husband or a close friend, to help you remember. It is also very helpful to keep a journal noting how you feel day by day, which will help gauge your progress.

How Long Will I Have to Take Progesterone?   Some young women with PMS may be able to stop using progesterone after taking it for six to nine months. This is because taking progesterone for a while sometimes stimulates the pituitary to produce its own progesterone, and the PMS condition corrects itself. This ability of the pituitary gland to start functioning properly on its own seems to decrease as women age, and the symptoms may return later in life. Women over 30 who have had PMS since puberty usually have to take progesterone at least until menopause.

When you have taken progesterone successfully for some months, you may try to lower the dosage or shorten the time during which you take it. Both should be done gradually; your symptoms will indicate whether you can manage with less. Some women can go off of it for a few cycles and then use it when necessary. But remember, women over 35 with severe symptoms should expect to stay on progesterone for a portion of every month until they begin menopause. Many can then discontinue treatment, but if a woman still has her uterus and starts taking estrogen at menopause, she will need to keep taking progesterone to counteract the effect of estrogen. A few women taking progesterone only will need to stay on progesterone into their sixties, because they still experience recurring PMS-like symptoms despite the fact that menstruation has ceased.

Taking Progesterone—A Summary　　While these instructions may seem complex, taking progesterone is simple in actual experience. Remember the following points:

- **Faithfully fill in your calendar.** Determine, based on the previous month, when you can expect to ovulate this month. Mark your calendar to start the progesterone therapy two days ahead of ovulation (if that is when you start symptoms) or five days ahead of symptoms (if you have pattern A PMS; see chart on PMS symptoms).
- **Start the treatment early enough.** If you get symptoms a few days before they are expected, start the treatment then.
- Once you figure out your individual dosage, **take the progesterone consistently** through the second part of the cycle when you need it. Maintain the dose as needed at an even rate on a daily basis. Don't skip doses or days. Once you increase the dosage, keep it at the same level until you stop taking it.
- **Reorder progesterone early enough** that you always have at least one month's supply on hand.
- **Stop taking the progesterone at the right time, and don't stop it suddenly.** Taper off the dosage (by cutting it in half for one or two days, and then stopping it) at the time when you would normally cease having symptoms.
- Make appointments with your counselor or physician for follow-up treatment until you feel better. It's worth it.
- Seek to become symptom-free, not just a little better.

OTHER TREATMENTS FOR PMS

I have listed guidelines for treatment that will help the majority of women with PMS, but not everyone responds to the same therapy. In fact, women whose symptoms and histories appear similar may respond to quite different therapies. Following are some suggestions for alternative treatments:

Treating Coexisting Conditions

Women with PMS caused by infections, or coexisting with other conditions such as endometriosis or polycystic ovaries, will require treatment for the other conditions, and this will sometimes stop their PMS symptoms. This is also true when a woman has endocrine problems such as a swollen pituitary, a hypothalamic or pituitary tumor, or thyroid problems. The specific problem causing PMS or worsening PMS needs to be dealt with.

Estrogen for PMS

Dr. John Studd of St. Thomas' Hospital in London has used the surgical implantation of estrogen pellets as a treatment for PMS; he has performed thousands of these minor surgeries with great success. He is against the use of natural progesterone to treat PMS, which I feel is unfortunate because it works for many women.

Dr. Studd used to say that women who do not ovulate do not get PMS; the estrogen pellet with its continuous output of estrogen into the bloodstream prevents ovulation. However, I have worked with physicians who have seen many women who don't ovulate and who have PMS-like symptoms (though not in a definite pattern). One of these doctors says that once he can produce ovulation in these women, he can treat their PMS. Dr. Studd now says that estrogen lessens depression directly.[30] There is no doubt that some women with PMS do respond to estrogen therapy, and should read Chapter 11 on estrogen and depression.

It is now known that taking estrogen increases the number of progesterone receptors and primes them. Also, progesterone can both switch on and switch off estrogen receptors, possibly a reason why some women who have been on progesterone for a while find that it "no longer works." I believe these facts make the case for sometimes using a combination of both hormones for PMS.

As I said earlier, it seems to me that there are "progesterone types" and "estrogen types." Women respond to one hormone or the other, and often their initial response will stay the same for decades. I have always responded positively to estrogen; natural progesterone is a downer for me. But I have long-time friends who took progesterone and had a positive response within five or ten minutes, and that positive response has continued for 15 years. They don't feel any improvement if they take estrogen.

If you try natural progesterone and it doesn't work, you might need to add a little estrogen. Young women with PMS may only need a little estrogen, and I would suggest beginning with $1/4$ mg of Estrace taken twice daily, morning and night.

The Thyroid Connection

Thyroid disorders cause menstrual irregularities (heavy bleeding, cramps, infertility, or irregular periods), and in some cases may be the direct cause of PMS. Many women with PMS have a family history of thyroid disorders.

See Chapter 8, on thyroid problems.

The Adrenals May Be Involved

Very little has been written about the possibility of adrenal involvement in PMS, despite the fact that many women with PMS have allergy problems, terrible chronic fatigue, and recurrent infections—all symptoms of adrenal deficiency. The stresses of life—caused by outer factors as well as physiology—can lead to a high output of adrenaline and cortisol. Sometimes this overfunction gets stuck in high gear. These women will have the symptoms of too much adrenaline production—rapid heart rate, heart palpitations, inability to sleep, panic attacks, and feeling nervous—but, in fact, end up adrenal depleted. Some women's hot flashes are due to low adrenal function not just low estrogen.

Prednisone, the usual form of cortisone used for treating adrenal deficiency diseases, has understandably come into disfavor because of the very serious side effects of high doses. However, some alternative physicians give women small physiologic doses of hydrocortisone, a type of cortisone that is several times weaker than prednisone. This is a controversial treatment, but I mention it because sometimes it's an important factor for some women.

As with thyroid, women should not try to medicate themselves or adjust dosage with cortisone, because the side effects are much more serious than with progesterone or estrogen, and overmedication can be fatal.

Treating Yeast Infections and Allergies

Many women with hormonal problems suffer from systemic yeast infections, allergy problems, or both. In fact, some researchers believe that candida (yeast) is the primary cause of PMS. However, when the immune system is not functioning properly, adrenal function is low, and PMS, infections, and allergies often occur together. Sometimes hormone therapy alleviates candida and allergies because it helps the immune system. This is particularly true if allergies only appear premenstrually. Sometimes candida worsens with progesterone therapy because progesterone increases the metabolism of sugar.

Treatment for candida ranges from dietary changes to prescription treatment for either local yeast manifestations or systemic yeast problems. A blood test is available to test systemic yeast.

Changes in lifestyle include eliminating all types of sugars, grains, foods that mold easily, and anything else in the diet that encourages the growth of the yeast. Some researchers think that fruit should be largely eliminated, at least for a while. Others think grains are more of a problem. Health food stores sell various antifungal agents, such as pau d'arco (a South American herb), and Caprystatin (caprylic acid).

Vaginal infections can be treated locally—for instance, with Monistat, Gyne-Lotrimin, or other, stronger medications. Yeast in the digestive tract may respond to oral tablets of Nystatin. Systemic treatment includes Nizoral, which is potent and expensive. Women on Nizoral need frequent tests of their liver enzyme levels. There is a newer drug available, called Diflucan (generic: fluconazole), that is even stronger, and it is very expensive. A single dose of Diflucan has been recently approved by the FDA as treatment for vaginal yeast infections. For more information, I suggest that you read *The Yeast Syndrome*, by John Parks Trowbridge, M.D.

Chronic Fatigue Syndrome

My son had chronic fatigue syndrome (CFS; also called chronic fatigue immune disorder syndrome, or CFIDS) for eight years, so I know how debilitating this disease can be. Every so often, I see women who are unfortunate enough to have CFS in combination with hormonal problems, and I feel terribly sorry for them. It's enough to have either problem; it's terrible to have both.

CFS is an immune system disease in which, it is believed, a person's killer cells multiply and start attacking their immune system. At present, researchers think it is the hyperactivity of these killer cells that is responsible for the miserable symptoms this disease produces.

In the past, CFS has been blamed on various viruses, such as Epstein-Barr, Herpes VI, or Cytomegalovirus, but now these are seen as opportunistic infections that can occur because the immune system is damaged.

Those with CFS have extraordinarily incapacitating fatigue, which strikes them in varying degrees. Some sufferers are fairly functional, but others cannot even lift their heads off the pillow.

There is presently no known cure for CFS. The body must mend itself. But certain remedies have been helpful for a few, such as Acyclovir and Zovirax, which attack the herpes virus. A combination of gamma globulin and sex hormones may help others. As with PMS, there are many supplements touted to cure CFS. They probably all help some people, and there is little to lose by trying them. Rest and nutrition are extremely important, and counseling may help, since those with CFS are usually very driven people. Antidepressants also have a role.

Treatment for Chronic Depression

Women with severe hormonal depression are often sent to psychiatrists for treatment with antidepressants. I have talked to women who have received tremendous benefits from taking antidepressants and tranquilizers, and others who try the whole gamut of available treatments and are treatment failures. Sometimes women with these problems are even given shock therapy, which is coming back into favor as a treatment choice. (Most of the women I have talked to experienced no benefit from it.)

Among my case histories, you have read of Sandra; she had the worst hormonal problems I have seen to date, and was not stabilized emotionally until she went on lithium along with hormones. You will also read of Jeannie who was made worse by Parnate. The reader needs to study these medications, read about their possible benefits and side effects, and make an informed choice.

Women who are taking antidepressants, or contemplating taking them, would benefit from reading Harvard psychiatrist Peter Breggins' book *Toxic Psychiatry*. He is opposed to antidepressants and shock therapy and, while some may think his view is too narrow, his book is very thorough. It is a viewpoint that must be heard, and I feel that his emphasis on the possible side effects from various antidepressants is correct. However, I still acknowledge the fact that some women have miraculous results from taking antidepressants.

Women with PMS are often put on Prozac. It does seem to help some women dramatically, while others don't respond at all, even to higher doses. A female psychiatrist friend says that a quarter dose of liquid Prozac (5 mg) may be all that is needed to treat PMS.

Dr. Breggins says that people will feel better on Prozac because it is an upper. He worries that its basic action—making serotonin more available in the brain—will backfire one day because people taking it will eventually need more and more serotonin and will end up worse off than when they began the therapy. He also worries that Prozac is similar in chemical makeup to the neuroleptics, such as Stelazine, and may eventually produce similar side effects: a 30 to 40 percent chance of developing tardive dyskinesia (involuntary muscle jerking) and other similar problems that can be permanent. He says there is already some evidence in the literature that this is so. Also, the serious side effects of Prozac prompting some people to violence and suicide have already been well publicized.

One of Prozac's common side effects (in possibly 30 to 40 percent of women taking it) is the disappearance of the ability to have orgasms. This may be a lesser problem in the beginning if the depression goes away, but it is a real problem if it continues.

For more information about the side effects of Prozac and other SSRIs (selective serotonin re-uptake inhibitors), see information about the Prozac Survivor's Support Group, Inc. in the Recommended Reading at the back of the book. Also read Robin's story in Chapter 9 on thyroid and depression.

As mentioned earlier in this book, studies on estrogen and natural progesterone show that there is positive action by both on the central nervous system and the neurotransmitters in the brain. These hormones, particularly estrogen, have an antidepressant action and a catalyst action which enhances the use of antidepressants. What this means is that some women with hormonal depression may respond to hormone therapy alone, and others may need a combination of hormones and an antidepressant. There are also a few women who appear to have a hormonal depression but do not respond to hormone therapy.

QUICK TIPS FOR PMS

This is a summary of the preceding Treatment section.

Dietary Recommendations
General suggestions:

- Eat a diet that is largely vegetarian, with an abundance of fresh, unprocessed foods.
- Eat mainly fruits, vegetables, whole grains, and legumes.
- Avoid refined sugars, refined carbohydrates, and processed fats.
- Limit concentrated foods—foods high in fat, protein, sugar, or salt—including animal products (meat, milk, butter, cream, etc.). Use concentrated foods as a garnish, not a main dish.
- Restrict intake of both animal fat and highly processed vegetable fats such as cooking oil, margarine, and so on.

- Cut down on caffeine (coffee, cola drinks).
- Cut out smoking, alcohol, and illegal drugs.

Hypoglycemia diet:

A woman with PMS almost always has fluctuating blood sugar levels with a tendency toward functional low blood sugar. This can bring on headaches and sudden mood changes. She should eat more frequently when symptomatic—some carbohydrate such as bread, crackers, potatoes, corn, or oats every three or four hours.

She should eat six meals a day, but needs only to eat small portions, including some carbohydrate with each meal to help maintain the blood sugar level (a half slice of bread, a few crackers, half a potato, etc.).

Keeping the blood sugar level elevated and stable may help alleviate the mood swings, headaches, irritability, and violent outbursts that characterize PMS.

Some women need stick only to the diet to keep PMS under control (about 60 percent of women, according to Dr. Dalton). Women taking hormone treatments should also follow this diet; treatment may fail if these suggestions are not carried out.

Helpful Supplements:

There are a number of multi-vitamin and mineral supplements specifically made for women who have PMS or who are going through menopause. As examples, Dr. Guy Abrahams formulated a PMS supplement called Optovite, and Dr. Susan Lark formulated another marketed by Schiff Products. These products contain all the supplemental nutrients you need.

Vitamin B_6   The level of vitamin B_6 in the recommended daily dose of six tablets of Optovite is 300 mg, considered high by some researchers. Dr. Katherina Dalton says that more than 50 mg of B_6 can cause peripheral neuritis (pain and tingling in the extremities), but not everyone agrees with this statement.

Vitamin E   400 mg twice a day.

Magnesium and potassium   Taken in a trace mineral supplement. This may be particularly helpful for women with migraines and muscle and joint pain. Occasionally, a potassium supplement such as Klorvess (or K-Lyte) might be prescribed to help women with persistent muscle problems.

Evening Primrose Oil (Efamol)   You can also use borage, black currant, flaxseed, or linseed oil. These all contain an essential fatty acid helpful in the production of hormones. It is also said to reduce prolactin levels (prolactin may cause excessive bloating and breast tenderness). The recommended dose of evening primrose oil is six capsules per day, taken daily until symptoms diminish; then three capsules a day. In my experience, women with sore breasts, bloating, and acne do best on evening primrose oil.

Herbs   There are several fine herbal supplements available; I recommend that you consult an expert. Vitex (agnus castus) is often recommended as a good hormone balancer. Others commonly mentioned are: astragalus, burdock root, comfrey, dong quai, fo-ti, ginger, horsetail, licorice root, motherwort, nettle, oatstraw, pau d'arco, raspberry leaf, red clover, squawvine, wild yam root, and yellow dock.

L-Tyrosine and L-Phenylalanine   These amino acids are said to be particularly helpful for depression, though I suggest that you read the label on the bottle to avoid taking them in excess. L-Tryptophan used to be on the market and was withdrawn after a polluted batch caused bad side effects. It's a shame that this is only available by prescription from some alternative physicians, because it really helped a lot of women.

Pro-Gest®   This is a natural progesterone cream, available without prescription. It can generally be purchased through a health professional (chiropractor, naturopath, etc.). One eighth to one quarter of a teaspoon is a general daily dosage. It is rubbed onto the fatty parts of the body (the inside of the upper arm, thighs, belly, etc.) during days 10–26 of the menstrual cycle for PMS, or during days 1–25 for postmenopausal women. See Appendix 2 for sources of Pro-Gest®.

Natural Hormones by Prescription

Pharmacies that compound natural hormones have their own protocols for taking them; ask each pharmacist for details. The following are only guidelines:

Natural Progesterone   As a treatment for PMS that lasts from ovulation until menstrual bleeding, you could take 100-mg oral capsules of micronized[30] progesterone in oil (to be swallowed) or 100-to-200-mg sublingual (under the tongue) tablets, two or three times a day from day 12 of the menstrual cycle (two days ahead of expected symptoms if they begin at ovulation), counting the first day of the previous flow as day one. Be consistent when taking progesterone; taking it haphazardly can lead to breakthrough bleeding and a return of symptoms. I think it's best to take the progesterone until day one of bleeding, because stopping it early can bring the symptoms back. Some women need to take progesterone until the end of each menstrual period if they still have symptoms. More details about this later!

After menopause, after a hysterectomy, or when continual treatment with progesterone is advised, you could take a 100-mg oral capsule of micronized progesterone in oil once a day, or a 100-mg sublingual tablet every night before sleeping.

When a woman has had a hysterectomy and is taking estrogen, some think that it is advisable for her to have some progesterone to counteract the effect of estrogen on the breasts, though generally doctors prescribe estrogen without progesterone. A small proportion of women actually find progesterone more helpful than estrogen after menopause or hysterectomy. If you decide to take progesterone, how much you should take depends on your reaction to it. You could take 100 mg each night for a week or ten days. If it makes you feel better, you could take progesterone every day and increase the dosage. If taking the amount suggested makes you sleepy, take less. If you react negatively to natural progesterone, you can discard it.

Estrogen   Some women who are hormone-sensitive feel better and have fewer side effects on Estrace than on

Premarin because estradiol is more physiologic (i.e., it matches what the body naturally produces). Estradiol is the main type of estrogen in the body, and the key that opens the cell receptors. However, some women do feel better on Premarin or Ogen, and you need freedom to try alternatives.

If you take Estrace and want to begin with a low dose, you might start with 0.25 to 0.5 mg, taken sublingually (under the tongue). You can swallow the tablet, but Dr. Katherine Morris says that it is more potent when taken sublingually or vaginally, and so you should be able to use less this way. The tablet can be cut with scissors or crushed and divided with a razor blade. Absorption is very good because these routes bypass the digestive system. Alternatively, you could use one of the estrogen patches. The old Estraderm patch was changed every three to four days. The new Climara patch lasts five to seven days. The new Vivelle patch is available in four doses, rather than just two. For more details, contact your pharmacist.

Sometimes you can just take estrogen in relation to when you have symptoms. For headaches around the time of menstrual bleeding, you might only need to use estrogen for a few days. For PMS, you might need it for part or all of the last two weeks of your cycle. But at menopause, you probably need to take it every day, particularly if you have symptoms many days of the month. The dosage can be increased according to your symptoms.

Thyroid If family or personal history suggests subclinical (meaning mild enough to not show up in blood tests) hypothyroidism, some physicians will give low replacement doses of thyroid. There is a difference of opinion on whether to prescribe Armour thyroid or Westhroid (both brands of animal thyroid) or Synthroid (synthetic T4). Most pharmacists feel more comfortable with Synthroid because the concentration is more reliable, and it better matches human thyroid. However, many women do better on Armour, and others feel better on a combination of Synthroid and a low dose of Cytomel (T3). Cytomel seems to be particularly helpful for depression and extreme fatigue because it provides instant energy. It is also helpful for women who build up high T4 levels on Synthroid alone. But it is more active, and women are more likely to have symptoms of excess from taking Cytomel.

A low starting dose of Synthroid (such as 0.25 mg to 0.05 mg) is suggested. Thyroid should be taken every day, and sometimes taken for life. Watch your pulse rate and temperature to avoid "thyroid storm" (medication-induced overdose).

Testosterone   It is better to use natural testosterone than methyl testosterone, which is a synthetic. Natural testosterone is available from most of the pharmacies that make natural progesterone. Testosterone is often the first hormone to take a nose-dive in the late thirties or early forties. The dosage is usually 1.25 to 5.0 mg once a day, probably best taken in the morning to avoid sleep disturbances at night.

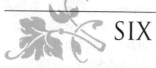

SIX

THE BIRTH CONTROL PILL

Gina came to see me on the advice of her mother, a counselor who had heard me speak on the radio.

Gina was depressed and very hostile, and the hostility was directed specifically toward the mother who had been so concerned about her. Gina spent most of the interview telling me about this terrible woman who had brought her into the world, but the conversation didn't seem quite rational. The mother seemed very nice.

The only factor I could see was that Gina was taking the birth control pill, and when I talked to her about the effect the pill sometimes has on the mind, she decided to go off of it and see if she felt less depressed.

A couple of months later, I met Gina's mother again, and asked her diplomatically how her daughter was doing. She didn't know what Gina had said to me, but she told me that Gina was a different person now that she was off the birth control pill, and that they were getting along much better.

Gina didn't need hormone treatment after stopping the pill. Her body came back to normal just by stopping it. Unfortunately, some women don't return to normal after taking the birth control pill. Their pituitary doesn't seem to function properly again, and they only find relief from their symptoms by taking hormone replacement therapy.

Treatment and Cause

The birth control pill has been widely prescribed in this country, not only as an oral contraceptive, but as a successful treatment for PMS, hormone-related mental depression, heavy menstrual bleeding and cramps, and perimenopausal symptoms. Many women feel better when taking the pill, and they are very thankful for it.

There are also women who are particularly sensitive to the synthetic progestin component of the birth control pill. These women are likely to become more depressed on the pill, and it may trigger or worsen their hormonal symptoms. Such women should either avoid taking birth control pills or switch to a pill that contains lower doses of progestin (accompanied by somewhat higher doses of ethinyl estradiol), such as Ovcon 35, Brevicon, or Modicon. These brands are less likely to cause depression, according to Dr. Elizabeth Lee Vliet, who has prescribed them extensively in her practice for younger women who need estrogen. If women do not do well on these particular oral contraceptives, they will probably not do well on any type.

Fascinating History of the Birth Control Pill

The history of the birth control pill's creation, as told by Paul Vaughan in *The Pill on Trial*,[1] makes for fascinating reading. Vaughan was at one time the chief press officer for the British Medical Association. His was the first book I read in the early seventies that pointed out that the synthetic progestin portion of the pill caused depression.

A more recent book on this subject, by Carl Djerassi, is called *The Pill, Pygmy Chimps, and Degas' Horse*.[2] This is the autobiography of the scientist who synthesized the birth control pill, and includes chapters called "The Birth of the Pill," "The Pill at Twenty," and "The Pill at Forty: What Now?"

The Pill Intended for Birth Control

The pill, of course, was produced in a concerted effort to find a new form of birth control, not for purposes of relieving the hormonal symptoms of PMS or menopause. The history Vaughan recites shows that the reason the pill causes and often worsens PMS is the fact that it is made from synthetic hormones that do not match the body's own hormones.

Margaret Sanger played a leading role in the history of the pill, urging research biologist Dr. Gregory Pincus, in the 1950s, to find a new approach to contraception—not so much for Western women, but to control the population in third-world countries. Mrs. Stanley McCormick, a wealthy widow, provided funds for the research.

Progesterone had been synthesized from a sow's ovaries, about a decade before this, by a chemist named Russell Marker. Estrogen had also been isolated around that time, and was being used to treat women who had painful menstruation. It was already known that either estrogen or progesterone could prevent women from ovulating. Professor Fuller Albright of Harvard had talked about the possibility of birth control by the use of hormones as early as 1945.

Hormones were still being manufactured from animal sources, and what was needed was a cheap and convenient way of manufacturing them in bulk. Russell Marker was an extremely clever professor of organic chemistry. He had a touchy personality, had difficulty maintaining personal relationships, and had stormed out of several jobs. With backing from the drug company Parke, Davis & Co., Marker produced a steady flow of research material about the chemistry of steroids, which included the sex hormones.

Marker wanted to find a new source for the commercial manufacture of sex hormones, and he began this search in 1939. The best source he found was a substance called sapogenin, a form of which—sarsapogenin—was found in the sarsaparilla plant. But the yield was too small to have any commercial value, so he set about finding other plants of the sarsaparilla family. He felt that the most likely place to find them was in the subtropical southwest of the U.S. and in Mexico. In 1940, Marker spent his summer vacation searching for the plant, and enlisted other botanists to help him. He apparently sifted through five tons of tropical greenery, and found a plant that yielded the most sapogenin in the form of diosgenin. Its name was *cabeza de negro*, a species of wild yam.

When Marker tried to find someone to provide the capital to produce progesterone from diosgenin, he got a lukewarm response, because Mexico was so far away and there was a war going on. He left his teaching job and went to Mexico City to synthesize progesterone from the wild yam plant. When he had a considerable amount, he went to a small pharmaceutical company in Mexico City called Laboratorios Hormona, run by two immigrants from Europe, and offered them four-and-a-half pounds of progesterone, worth tens of thousands of dollars at the time. Marker and the two pharmacists went into business partnership and incorporated as Syntex, SA. Subsequent production of progesterone was slow, and tension grew among the three partners until Marker walked out yet again, taking the notes on his laboratory process with him.

A Hungarian, Dr. George Rosenkranz, continued the work Marker had begun at Syntex, and produced progesterone, testosterone, and desoxycorticosterone, an adrenal hormone. Another chemist at Syntex, Carl Djerassi, produced the estrogens estrone and estradiol. By the early fifties, Syntex had become the major supplier of synthetic hormones to drug houses in Europe and America.

However, there was a serious problem to overcome: progesterone, whether from an animal or a plant source, was ineffective when taken by mouth. At the time, it had to be given by injection. To make a birth control pill, an oral form of progesterone was needed. A chemistry professor at the University of Pennsylvania, Professor Max Ehrenstein, felt that one could change the structure of progesterone and yet not change its effects.

In 1950, Carl Djerassi tackled the problem of creating synthetic progesterone, the step that would lead directly to the production of the pill. The first synthetic progestin he produced was norethisterone, a powerful testosterone derivative. At the same time, G. D. Searle & Co., in Chicago, produced a similar progestin called norethynodrel.

The Basic Problem with the Pill

At this point in the story, Vaughan points out that the progestins and the estrogenic compounds that were in the classic
birth control pill are not natural products, but synthetic adap-
tations with subtle variations. He says that, though the differences may seem trivial on paper, they may produce gross
differences in effect in the body, where the machinery is too
intricate and too sensitive to be misled.

Though the pills have changed over the years, using lower
doses of hormones, and, in some cases, synthetic progestin
only, they still have the same problem that Paul Vaughan described in 1970. They have molecular variations that may
cause side effects in the body, including lowering of mood.

This thesis fits with the suggestions of Drs. Katherina and
Maureen Dalton in England: that while synthetic progestins
prevent ovulation and cause sloughing off of the lining of the
uterus, they do not function properly in the progesterone receptors in the cells. Synthetic progestins are like a "key" that
fits into the progesterone receptor "lock" but will not "open" it.
While the synthetic progestin is in the "lock," there is no room
for the progesterone molecule to enter, and the overall effect is
to decrease progesterone levels. Also, the synthetic progestins
are very potent and may overpower the pituitary function either temporarily or permanently. This is similar to taking thyroid medication, wherein, above a certain dose, the pituitary
may shut down and become lazy; when a person goes off the
thyroid medication, the pituitary function may not return.

Therefore, at one level or another, the pill may inhibit production of the body's own sex hormones, leading to a lowering of mood and the side effects of irritability, anger, and other
emotional and physical symptoms.

A Caveat

Having said all this against the birth control pill, I should add
that some women do lose their PMS symptoms while taking
the pill, which is why some doctors automatically put women

on it. Some women also find the pill wonderful if they have painful, heavy periods and wildly irregular cycles. However, most of the women I have seen with hormonal problems have had adverse reactions to the pill; I advise women that if they are subject to PMS, they probably would be better to avoid the pill and other synthetic progestins.

CHAPTER

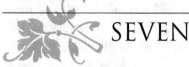

SEVEN

POSTPARTUM DEPRESSION

 Denise didn't know what depression was until her new baby was about four months old. She was sitting in her chair one night, watching television, when she felt a total body change come over her, and she soon went into a deep depression.

Nobody in her family could understand it. She and her husband had wanted the baby. The pregnancy had been fine. There seemed to be no reason why Denise should be so depressed.

It was very hard for Denise to tell anyone, even her husband, how dreadful she felt. At times, she was so angry with him and the baby that the idea of harming them kept entering her mind. It seemed impossible to control her thoughts, and because these evil thoughts kept coming back, she felt that she was going insane. It was as though she was floating outside her body watching herself—a spectator, alienated, and out of touch with reality. She felt spaced out, exhausted, and anxious; she was beginning to lose hope of ever returning to normal.

Denise found a sympathetic ear with her physician, who had just had a baby herself and knew from experience that some mothers go through a hormonal imbalance for a while. She told Denise that she had postpartum depression (PPD).

The doctor put Denise on natural progesterone and checked her thyroid levels. Sure enough, Denise had border-line low thyroid, a temporary result of the dramatic changes that occur during pregnancy and delivery. The doctor said that Denise might also need a little estrogen and proges-terone, as well as thyroid, and, perhaps, an antidepressant. She could keep breastfeeding while on progesterone, be-cause it was metabolized so fast that it didn't reach the milk. But if she went on estrogen or the antidepressant, she would probably have to stop breastfeeding. Fortunately, taking progesterone and thyroid were sufficient in Denise's case to effect a big change in her outlook. Within a couple of months, the worst was over and she was able to stop taking the hormones.

Hard to Find Help with PPD

It's even harder to find enlightened treatment for postpartum depression than it is for premenstrual syndrome. The subject of PPD is barely dealt with in most baby-care books. Unlike PMS, which only occurs during part of the month and allows a woman to function normally for most of the time, PPD can be continuous. It sometimes affects a woman almost 24 hours a day, especially if she has insomnia.

If a woman has never had PMS, and suddenly finds herself with severe PPD, the unexpected mood swings can be terrify-ing. She may feel as though she is living on another planet and has lost contact with the real world. Coupled with a loss of feeling, numbness, and an inability to reach out in love to her husband and baby, this can be an incredibly painful and lonely experience.

Women with PPD frequently find themselves unable to feel anything emotionally, and it is common for them to think they don't love their husbands and that they want a divorce. The husband is often hurt and bewildered when he becomes the target of the woman's irritability and anger.

VARYING TYPES AND DEPTHS OF PPD

According to Dr. Katherina Dalton, there are varying stages of depression after childbirth.

The Baby Blues

About half of all women who give birth suffer from this mild form of PPD, which occurs shortly after delivery and only lasts a few hours, a few days, or a couple of weeks. It is a short-lived condition that goes away relatively quickly and is soon forgotten.

Other women suffer from extreme fatigue for the first few months of their baby's life. With a new baby, this makes life especially hard for a while. A woman may feel as though she is walking through wet concrete, but this feeling usually goes away with time. It is not accompanied by the terrifying emotional problems of serious PPD. Along with this deadening fatigue, some women also have drying of the vagina and low sex drive due to the low estrogen levels that occur after delivery.

Postpartum Depression

Ten to twenty percent of women who give birth experience this form of PPD, with its exhaustion, irritability, depression, mood swings, and anger. It generally ends some time during the first year after the baby is born. It is frequently triggered by the return of menstruation or when the mother stops breastfeeding. The intensity and length of PPD varies with individuals. While it is usually self-limiting (which means that it will go away, whether treated or not, within a few months or a year), there are cases in which women have unresolved postpartum depression for many years and never fully return to health. Many women say that their health broke down after a certain pregnancy.

PPD occasionally happens a long time after the delivery. I saw a woman who had no problems with her hormones until her baby was 21 months old. She had been breastfeeding her child, and menstruation had not returned. At twenty-one months, she weaned the child and her periods returned, bringing severe PPD and a breakdown of her immune system.

Postpartum Psychosis

One in 500 to one in 3,000 women who give birth undergo this relatively rare but extremely severe condition. Such women are obviously mentally ill and may have delusions, hallucinations, mania, agitation, and deep depression. They may be suicidal or murderous. The life and safety of their babies or other members of the family may be at risk, and appeals for help should be taken seriously. These women are often unconscious of what is happening and may return abruptly to normalcy as suddenly as they left it.

THE PICTURE PUZZLE OF PPD

Dr. James Alexander Hamilton, a San Francisco physician, divides PPD into two general levels, which he calls the lesser and major syndromes.

The Lesser Syndromes

These syndromes are very common and will be experienced by one third to one half of all new mothers, and one tenth of all women having their second child.

1. **Maternity Blues**—occurring day three to day ten after delivery. Symptoms include weeping episodes, insomnia, and exhaustion.
2. **Postpartum Depression**—mild to moderate depression, apparent three or more weeks after delivery. Incidence is one in ten births. Symptoms include gradual personality change, feelings of alienation, wishing to divorce, and problems with rearing children.

The Major Syndromes

Each of the major syndromes is characterized by inability to handle stress, apprehensiveness, sensitivity, anxiety, and fear.

1. **The Early Agitated Syndrome or Puerperal Psychosis**
   Onset postpartum 4 to 20 days. The symptoms include confusion, delirium, hallucinations, delusions, extreme bipolar mood swings, sudden mercurial changes, and potential violence. Possible cause: temporary low adrenal function because of sluggish pituitary function following childbirth.

2. **The Late Depressive Syndrome or Severe Postpartum Depression**
   Onset three weeks after delivery. The symptoms include insidious, slowly increasing depression accompanied by many physical symptoms, and suicidal tendencies. Possible cause: low thyroid production because of low pituitary function following childbirth.

3. **The Late Mercurial Syndrome or Postpartum Psychotic Depression**
   Onset three to four weeks after delivery; may evolve from the other two syndromes. Moderate to severe symptoms include confusion, dullness, and slow thinking, punctuated by unpredictable, explosive episodes of psychosis, with extreme agitation, hallucinations, auditory hallucinations which seem like commands, bizarre thinking and behavior, and frequent amnesia about behavior. Violence, suicide, and infanticide are serious concerns.

Symptoms of PPD

Agitation	Alienation	Anger
Anxiety	Crying jags	Confusion
Delusions	Depression	Dizziness
Drying of vagina	Euphoria	Fatigue
Fear	Forgetfulness	Futility
Guilt	Hair loss	Hallucinations
Headaches	Hopelessness	Inability to concentrate
Insomnia	Irritability	Lack of energy
Lack of motivation	Loneliness	Low self-esteem
Low sex drive	Marital conflict	Mood swings
Obsession	Panic attacks	Paranoia

Sadness	Shame	Strange thoughts
Suicidal tendencies	Swollen feet	Trance
Violent thoughts	Vomiting	Weakness
Weight gain	Weight loss	Worry

What Happens Hormonally After Delivery

Dr. Hamilton describes the precipitous drop in serum levels of estrogen and progesterone soon after delivery, from the very high levels of pregnancy to being almost absent by the end of the first week postpartum. There is a latent period, the three-day interval after birth, when symptoms are rare.

Around day three, levels of bound and free cortisol and β-endorphins drop dramatically to about a third of the predelivery levels. Levels of thyroxine also typically drop below normal, reaching a low about three weeks after delivery. These drops in hormone levels vary with the individual, though they are fairly common to all women.

Dr. Hamilton treats PPD as an endocrine problem, not just as a typical depression, and designs the treatment according to the timing, type, and severity of the symptoms.

Unpredictable Incidence in Individuals

Women often wonder, "If I had PPD once, will I get it again?" One client of mine had such a terrible time after giving birth to her first child that she decided against having any more.

Actually, unless there is a strong familial history of PPD, the incidence is unpredictable. A woman could have several pregnancies without PPD, and then suddenly have it with the next child. Another woman might have PPD with her first child and dread the second, but find, with great relief, that it doesn't recur.

But overall, women who have a family and personal history of PPD are more likely to have it again. And women who have postpartum psychosis are 300 times more likely to experience it with a subsequent pregnancy.[1] There are some women who have severe PPD after each child that worsens as they get older, never becoming fully resolved.

Those Horrible Feelings

The hardest thing for women to cope with is the emotional impact of PPD. They feel "spaced out" and alienated from those around them. They are sure that no one really understands what they are going through, and they are sometimes too ashamed to discuss their real feelings with their husbands.

Panic attacks, frequently occurring at night, along with inability to sleep, create a high level of fear and anxiety. Women may find themselves incomprehensibly sad and inexplicably angry with their husbands—alternately weeping uncontrollably, then hostile and angry. Hostility toward their baby may sweep over these women, and the urge to do the child bodily harm makes women extremely fearful and guilt-ridden. Sometimes, they become preoccupied with thoughts of gloom and death. They feel powerless to control these feelings.

Complicating the problem, most of these women are quite aware that these emotions are abnormal, but they still blame themselves. Their rational mind can acknowledge that they have everything going for them—a loving husband, a beautiful new child—but they are unable to pull themselves out of the morass of depression. Sometimes they even see the PPD as a judgment on something they've done in their past. This can happen particularly if the PPD is a result of a terminated pregnancy.

Women feel that if only they had a little more self-control, they could overcome this hostility and pull themselves out of the depression, but trying to control it rationally just doesn't work.

They are "out of control," and they need sympathy, understanding, and medical help.

It Can Happen to Anyone

There is no particular type of woman who is predisposed to having PPD. While family history is a factor, it can happen to any woman, regardless of age, race, social standing, religious affiliation, or previous psychiatric good health. It happens whether the child is wanted or unwanted. It is a physiologically-based problem that occurs as a result of extreme hormonal changes during pregnancy; it is not "just in her head."

Two Types of Pregnancy

In general, there are two distinct types of pregnancy that precede PPD. In the first type, women may feel great during the second or third trimester. If they have previously suffered from PMS, they may find that, once morning sickness passes, they feel the best they've ever felt in their lives during the rest of the pregnancy. It is normal for women to feel wonderful during pregnancy, with a characteristic glow of contentment. It's a time when, ideally, they should have fewer physical and psychological problems, and fewer allergies and infections than normal.

In the second type of pregnancy, women may feel sick all the way through and be troubled with depression or physical symptoms, such as breakthrough bleeding, nausea, and premature labor pains. Their physicians may be concerned about their high blood pressure because of possible pre-eclampsia (borderline toxemia).

Both extremes of pregnancies—good and bad—may lead to PPD.

MASSIVE PHYSICAL CHANGES DURING PREGNANCY

During pregnancy, the uterus changes from the size of a small pear to the size of a large watermelon, including baby, placenta, and fluid. The skeleton and body cavities are pulled out of shape, and the amount of blood that circulates is doubled. Consequently the heart, liver, and kidneys have to work much harder.

Hormone Levels Rise During Pregnancy

When a woman becomes pregnant, her hormone levels rise dramatically. For the first 12 to 16 weeks, estrogen and progesterone are produced in her ovaries at much higher levels than normal. Then, the placenta produces 170 times[2] the pre-pregnancy amount of progesterone by full-term, and hundreds of times the pre-pregnancy amount of estradiol. Prolactin levels, which prepare the breasts for lactation, also rise, and so does production of cortisol and thyroid. Four other hormones are produced only during pregnancy, the primary one being human chorionic gonadotropin (HCG). HCG is made by the placenta and acts very much like LH (luteinizing hormone) does in the non-pregnant woman. It controls and stimulates the excess hormone production that occurs during pregnancy. As mentioned before, if all goes well, women will blossom with the increased hormonal activity. But if hormone levels don't rise properly, women can be miserable during pregnancy.

It has recently been discovered in Japan that progesterone has an MAO-inhibiting effect during pregnancy, which means that progesterone inhibits monoamine oxidase production in the brain, countering depression the way the antidepressants Nardil and Parnate do. Dr. Maureen Dalton believes that this is why progesterone plays a role in lowering high blood pressure and preventing toxemia later in pregnancy.

Hormone Levels Drop After Delivery

As mentioned earlier, after the baby and placenta are delivered, the levels of estrogen and progesterone suddenly plummet—estrogen to about 1/200th of the pregnancy levels within 24 hours, progesterone to zero within a week. The four unique pregnancy hormones disappear completely, and cortisol levels also plummet. Prolactin is still produced at high levels while the woman breastfeeds, and these high levels help inhibit the pituitary stimulation and ovarian production of estrogen and progesterone. Prolactin not only inhibits the pituitary precursor of progesterone—luteinizing hormone (LH)—but thyroid stimulating hormone (TSH) levels may also drop, because LH is chemically similar to part of TSH (TSH-α). Changes in TSH levels may result in temporary thyroid problems.

Autoimmune Rebound

During pregnancy, the high levels of hormones have produced a cortisone-like effect, and many women with joint pain find that it disappears with pregnancy. But after delivery, the drastic drop in hormone levels produces an autoimmune rebound. Consequently, postpartum thyroiditis is a very common phenomenon, with onset occurring after 11 percent of pregnancies.[3]

All of the changes that take place throughout pregnancy are supposed to return to normal levels within six weeks. It is no wonder that some women don't pull out of these massive changes in their body's chemistry without problems.

Sheehan's Syndrome

In fact, some women, who have severe trauma with labor (hemorrhaging, sudden loss of the placenta, or prolonged retention of the placenta) actually suffer partial death of their pituitary gland. This is called Sheehan's syndrome, and it occurs as a result of internal chemical injury to the pituitary. The shock from the loss of blood causes a prolonged spasm of the small blood vessels to the anterior pituitary,[4] resulting in clotting, blockage, and death of these small arteries. Women who have this problem may have permanent multiple endocrine deficiencies. Note that one of the symptoms of Sheehan's syndrome is psychosis; some specialists believe that postpartum depression is a mild version of Sheehan's syndrome.

The Woman with PPD Needs Support

A woman's husband and family need to realize that PPD is a real problem, and that it can be a terrifying experience for the new mother. She needs to be able to talk about what she is experiencing in a nonjudgmental environment. She already feels alienated, confused, estranged, and even insane. It is hard for her to make decisions, and her family may need to help her get medical attention and follow through with it.

CASE HISTORIES

Terrie's Story

Terrie has never known what it is to have mood swings, even though she had a hysterectomy and oophorectomy in her thirties. However, she was put on estrogen after the surgery because she had developed osteoporosis, partly due to having a benign tumor on her parathyroid gland.

Several months after Terrie first met her husband, he asked her if she ever had menstrual periods, because she was the only woman he knew who didn't have mood swings. She laughed and told him that of course she had periods, but that she had never had PMS. In her twenties, she delivered her only children—twin boys. The delivery was very difficult, and for about two years afterward she had a terrible problem with insomnia. Even with medication, she would not sleep for more than three hours a night.

At a party one day, Terrie overheard a psychiatrist talking about someone who sounded as though she had a similar problem to hers. She made an appointment for the whole family to see this psychiatrist, and he told her that the rest of the family was fine, but that she was depressed. In her case, it had nothing to do with mood swings; it was a sleep disorder. He gave her Elavil at a fairly low dose and told her that if this was her problem, she would sleep for a long time. After taking the first dose, she slept continuously for three days. She continued taking the Elavil for six months and then went off of it and had no more problems with sleeping.

Despite having had her ovaries removed in her thirties, Terrie still does not get depressed whether she takes estrogen or not, but, as mentioned, she takes estrogen for osteoporosis.

Terrie's problem is an example of a non-hormonal sleep disturbance occurring after pregnancy that responded not to hormones but to a short-term antidepressant.

Jeannie's Story

I was sitting in my office one day when a man knocked at the door and asked if he could speak with me about his wife. He was a Christian minister, had heard me speak about PMS on my husband's radio program, and wondered if I could help her. She had been put on a series of antidepressants and was presently taking Parnate, a fairly heavy-duty medication that required certain food restrictions. So far, she had not improved, and the next step was shock therapy. Jeannie's husband was vague about her problems, so I didn't know if I could help her.

When Jeannie came with her husband to see me, she looked like a zombie—stricken, pale, and deeply shaken by her experience. She told me that her problems began when she had toxemia during her second pregnancy. Afterward, she had severe postpartum depression, became anorexic, and had no menstrual periods for three years. Her doctors tried the birth control pill and Provera, but she did not feel good when taking them, so they decided to leave her without treatment. She did not go on antidepressants at that time.

She struggled with depression ever since, and it worsened in her early thirties. Along with the depression, she was having strong hot flashes, night sweats, panic attacks, and very heavy menstrual periods. One physician told her that if she weren't so young, he would have thought she was going through menopause. She was put on a series of antidepressants—Tofranil, Prozac, Xanax, Pamelor, and finally Parnate. She actually felt a little better on Prozac, but her doctor was reluctant to keep her on it because of the controversy surrounding it, and took her off it. Jeannie was given a little Cytomel (thyroid medication) to boost the Pamelor, but the Pamelor never rose to a therapeutic level, so her psychiatrist put her in the hospital and did a "wash out," taking her off of all medication. He told Jeannie that it would take three to four days for the medication to leave her system, but she became very ill with chronic fatigue, flu-like symptoms, forgetfulness, and weepiness. Her doctor put her back on Xanax and Restoril, and added Parnate at that time.

When Jeannie's mother was the same age, she suffered from hormonal problems with severe mood swings and outbursts of anger. She had been put on Valium, and her uterus was removed when she was 37. Later, her ovaries were removed, and she was very sick afterward. Jeannie's mother, now age 70, told me that she had osteoporosis and arthritis, and that her vagina was "raw." But the doctors had told her that she could never go on estrogen because she had a history of strokes. I tried to tell Jeannie's mother that she might be able to go on the post-menopausal doses now. The strong stroke warnings had been related to high doses of synthetic estrogens such as those in the birth control pill and the older forms of estrogen-replacement therapy. Now, a woman could have a blood test for her antithrombin levels, which indicates whether she is at high risk for a stroke. But, because she was frightened by what her doctor had told her years ago, the advice fell on deaf ears.

I believed that Jeannie was indeed going through pre-menopausal changes when she started having the night sweats and panic attacks, and that these probably were initiated by the postpartum depression and amenorrhea following the birth of her second child. I sent her to a female OB/GYN who would put her on hormones.

But Jeannie had to wait a month to get an appointment with this doctor and, during that time, she inadvertently ate the wrong food and had a violent reaction to the Parnate she was taking. She went to the emergency room with a terrible headache. Jeannie had been warned by her psychiatrist what to expect if she had an adverse reaction, and her symptoms were classic. But, amazingly, the doctors at the emergency room did not know what Parnate was! Nor did they consult with the pharmacist. When Jeannie tried to explain, the nurse who was attending her rudely told her to shut up. It wasn't that Jeannie was aggressive; by nature she was quite the opposite.

She was sent home without treatment, her headache worsening. When she called her psychiatrist, he told her that the problem was related to the medication and that she should go to another emergency room. While there, because she had a fever, they thought she might have spinal meningitis and performed a spinal tap. Unfortunately, the procedure was done too low in her spine, and she became temporarily paralyzed. The staff further worsened her headache by making her stand up and walk around too soon. She was given several strong medications for her headache, including morphine, but nothing worked. At the same time, Jeannie was bleeding very heavily, and her doctors felt that they could do nothing about that until they relieved her headache.

She was taken off all medication and sent home. Gradually, over about 10 days, the headache subsided. She kept her appointment with the OB/GYN, who was horrified at Jeannie's story. The doctor planned a D&C (scraping and removal of the lining of the uterus) and a hysteroscope examination (insertion of a scope through the cervix in order to view the uterine wall) to find out what was causing the bleeding. Because of Jeannie's experience with the Parnate, both these procedures had to be performed without an anesthetic, which was excruciatingly painful.

Afterward, having determined that there was no major problem, the doctor put her on natural progesterone and, later, on estrogen. The progesterone helped stopped the bleeding, and the combination of hormones alleviated the other symptoms she had been experiencing. Jeannie had gone cold turkey off the Parnate, and was on no other medication. Despite the severity of her problems and the hair-raising experience she had just been through, when I spoke to her a few weeks later, I couldn't believe the improvement in her physical and emotional health. Nor could her husband.

I don't want to convey the idea that Jeannie's terrible reaction to Parnate is typical. On the other hand, I had a similar reaction when I was on it, and I nearly died. I think it is unfortunate when women like Jeannie and myself, who both had hormonal problems, are automatically sent to a psychiatrist for treatment with potentially lethal psychotropic medication that is not appropriate for this type of problem. How much better it would be to treat a woman who has obvious hormonal symptoms with estrogen and progesterone first, than to give them a heavy-duty drug like Parnate.

I try to keep an open mind on this issue, since some women do seem to need psychotropic medication and definitely benefit from antidepressants. Others I see have no response to this type of medication, and still others have major problems after taking them. Jeannie's story is a good example of what can happen when antidepressant medication makes a bad situation much worse.

What's Happening Now?   Jeannie is doing much better now than when we first met. Shortly after I first wrote this chapter, she was given a hysterectomy because she was hemorrhaging so badly. Subsequently, she took 2 mg of Estrace daily with sublingual natural progesterone. The estrogen helped her, but the progesterone made no difference so she stopped taking it. Jeannie says she has done very well, apart from severe hot flashes. Her physician told her that 2 mg of Estrace daily was the upper limit, and that she couldn't prescribe any more. Because of this, Jeannie was put back on Paxil, and it does lessen the hot flashes. They are intolerable when she goes off Paxil.

Jeannie's OB/GYN sent her to an immunologist, who diagnosed her as having chronic fatigue syndrome. Her Epstein-Barr titer was very high. The immunologist felt that the excessive hemorrhaging, the hysterectomy, and the adverse reaction to Parnate had caused Jeannie such trauma that it resulted in chronic fatigue. But, even before the hysterectomy, she was suffering from terrible exhaustion.

I called Jeannie to update her case history, and asked about her sex drive and muscle strength. Both were very low. I asked her if her physician had suggested testosterone. When the ovaries are removed, most women need added testosterone. Jeannie said that she had recently read an article about it, and was going to ask her OB/GYN to consider prescribing testosterone for her.

I suggested to Jeannie what I had suggested three years before, after her hysterectomy—that she probably would do better with an estrogen and testosterone pellet implant—and referred her to a local doctor who does them. I recommended that she first ask her OB/GYN to try her for a short time on the same amount of Estrace, but taken under the tongue in divided doses, and to add the low-dose Estraderm patch. Even if she only tried it for a few weeks, she would be able to see if more estrogen helped. I also suggested that she try testosterone, beginning with 1.25 mg of natural testosterone (not methyl testosterone) twice a day. I think these changes will make a big difference to her.

Trauma from hemorrhage and other causes, as in Jeannie's case, often requires a long, long recovery. While there are other forms of treatment that can also be helpful, if someone needs particular hormones, nothing else will help in quite the same way.

TREATMENT FOR POSTPARTUM DEPRESSION

Postpartum Depression manifests itself in different ways. For some women, it will go away by itself in a few days or weeks. Others may have it for a few months and then it will lift. Some have it for a year, and then it fades away. A few have it forever.

There are also different levels of severity. One woman will feel sad for a short time. Another woman might become psychotic and hallucinate.

Treatment depends on severity. Most women can take comfort from the fact that PPD often goes away by itself when it has run its course, and may not recur with another pregnancy.

When women feel alienated, depressed, and anxious, they need the reassurance of knowing they are not alone in having this problem. They are not going insane, and the depression in most cases will not last forever. For some women, that reassurance is enough to get them through.

However, if PPD is interfering seriously with a woman's life, there are options for treatment. As with Terrie, a short course of the right antidepressant may take care of the problem. Other women will need one or more hormones, and possibly an antidepressant as well.

It is extremely important for all women with PPD to get as much emotional and practical support as possible while having these problems. They need plenty of rest and lots of sympathy.

Dr. Dalton's Treatment

The treatment recommended by Dr. Katherina Dalton for women who have delivered their babies, but have not yet

resumed menstruation, is daily administration of 100-mg intramuscular shots of natural progesterone[5] (in alternate buttocks to avoid scarring). Dr. Dalton prefers injections into the
outer lower buttock where fat and muscle combine. Her past
work has recently been validated by a well-researched study
from the University of Cardiff in Wales.[6]

For women with milder problems, Dr. Dalton recommends 400-mg vaginal or anal suppositories of natural progesterone one to three times a day, depending on symptoms.
This regimen is then varied according to the response of the
individual woman.

Dr. Dalton has written a book on PPD called *Depression
After Childbirth*. It is available from PMS Access in Madison,
Wisconsin (1-800-222-4PMS). Dr. Dalton has also written a
brochure called *Guide to Progesterone for Postnatal Depression*. It is
available from PMS Help, P.O. Box 100, St. Albans, Hertfordshire, AL1 4UQ, England.

Other Suggestions

Physicians in the U.S. frequently use natural progesterone
(not synthetic progestins) in oral form—micronized powder
made into capsules or tablets. Tablets and capsules in oil may
be swallowed. Powder capsules are frequently used under the
tongue. (See progesterone treatment section in Chapter 5 on
PMS for details.)

According to Dr. Dalton, you may keep breastfeeding
while taking progesterone, because progesterone is quickly
metabolized and does not migrate into the milk. Dr. Dalton
says that using progesterone may actually help to increase
milk flow.

Once menstruation resumes, progesterone is usually given
during the last half of the cycle, as with PMS.

Some women may need estrogen, but they should not
breastfeed their babies if they decide to take it. Other women
may need a little thyroid temporarily, and some may need it
permanently. Sometimes it is the onset of hypothyroidism or
the appearance of a goiter that causes PPD. Some women
treated with thyroid will lose their depression.

Some women who do not respond to hormones alone may need treatment with an antidepressant or antipsychotic medication. If the mental disorder is obviously very severe, it is not wise to use hormones alone because of the risk of suicide.

Women with severe PPD could try ceasing breastfeeding to see if it helps the hormone levels return to normal. When prolactin is high, the ovarian hormones may remain subnormal. Other women are fine while they breastfeed, and have problems when they stop.

Preventive Treatment

Having low levels of progesterone often causes premature births and also causes repeated miscarriages in some women. Women with a history of repeated miscarriages or toxemia are sometimes given natural progesterone during pregnancy, particularly during the first trimester. Women with depression during pregnancy may also be given natural progesterone.

Women who have PPD after each pregnancy may be given preventive injections of progesterone immediately after delivery.

Dr. Hamilton's Treatment

Dr. James Alexander Hamilton, M.D., of San Francisco, sees PPD as a polyendocrine disorder caused by the sudden drop in estrogen levels immediately after delivery; this can cause pituitary shock, which primarily affects the levels of cortisol, β-endorphins, and thyroxine.[7] Anyone seriously interested in treatment for postpartum problems should read Dr. Hamilton's book (co-edited with Patricia Neal Harberger), *Postpartum Psychiatric Illness: A Picture Puzzle*. This book outlines preventive treatment for women who have had previous bouts of severe PPD, and reflects the cutting edge of research in postpartum depression, and many of the suggestions made in it are available only under research conditions.

Dr. Hamilton has given women injections of estrogen at delivery, followed by oral estrogen during days one through fourteen after delivery. There is some need for caution in giving women estrogen soon after delivery (particularly high doses of synthetic estrogens) because of the possibility of increasing the clotting factor and causing thrombosis. But many physicians believe that this is not a problem if normal doses of natural estradiol are used.

Dr. Hamilton has also given injections of intramuscular natural progesterone at delivery and for the following seven days, followed by progesterone suppositories twice a day for two months or until the onset of menstruation. However, having seen a serious problem occur in a woman given natural progesterone alone, Dr. Hamilton is opposed to using it as a sole treatment for severe postpartum depression.

Dr. Hamilton also mentions giving 50 mg of vitamin B_6 during days one to thirty after delivery, because he believes that this substance may prevent a drop in the level of serotonin, a neurotransmitter.

Dr. Hamilton theorizes that, for extreme cases, taking a little cortisone twice a day for three weeks may help alleviate postpartum psychosis (experienced from day three or four), and that a low dose of thyroid, starting three weeks after delivery, may help lighten a late depressive syndrome. The thyroid dose should be closely monitored.

FOR FURTHER HELP:

Contact Depression After Delivery, P.O. Box 1282, Morrisville, Pennsylvania 19067, USA.

Read *Depression After Childbirth*, by Katharina Dalton, M.D., Oxford University Press, New York, 1980, 1989, available from Madison Pharmacy and Associates in Madison, Wisconsin (1-800-588-7046).

Read *Postpartum Psychiatric Illness: A Picture Puzzle*, edited by Dr. James Alexander Hamilton and Patricia Neal Harberger, University of Pennsylvania Press, 1992.

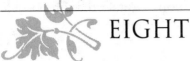

CHAPTER

EIGHT

THE THYROID LINK

 Doreen's family includes several women with thyroid problems. Her grandmother had a goiter, and her mother, one sister, and a cousin are taking thyroid medication. Doreen started menstruating late, at about age 16, with severe cramps. Sometimes she would go three or four months without a period and then have an extremely heavy one. Because of her family history, she had often been tested for low thyroid, but the tests always came back within the normal range, though borderline low.

She had trouble becoming pregnant and, like her mother, had two miscarriages. When I saw her, she had a six-month-old baby and was suffering from severe postpartum depression after having borderline toxemia during her pregnancy.

Doreen's thyroid seemed to be the main culprit. She was suffering from extreme exhaustion. Her hair was very dry and fell out easily. She was highly susceptible to cold air temperatures, and her basal temperature was low.

When she went to the doctor again, her thyroid test results were low, but she probably had been suffering from a subclinical hypothyroid condition all her life. After only a few days of being on thyroid medication, she said that, impossible though it seemed, she was already feeling better.

Thyroid Affects Many of the Body's Functions

Many of the women I see have a family history of thyroid disease, particularly on their maternal side, and they have the signs and symptoms themselves. This is not surprising; if glands were cities, the thyroid might be Rome, because it is linked to so many places.

Researchers have always found strong links between thyroid problems and menstrual difficulties, pregnancy problems, difficulties at menopause, autoimmune problems, and emotional disorders.

It's important for women to know about these links, because thyroid disorders are prevalent and frequently overlooked. Not all women, even those with major thyroid disorders, will show a lot of symptoms. Some women find out by accident that they are low thyroid and have few or no symptoms. Others, even with subclinical conditions, have many symptoms. "Subclinical" means that the condition is mild and may not show up in routine blood tests.

Menstrual Problems Are Common Among Low-Thyroid Patients   The thyroid gland varies in size during the normal menstrual cycle,[1] and women who have thyroid disorders frequently have associated menstrual problems,[2] including one or more of the following:[3] irregular cycles, painful cramps, heavy bleeding, premenstrual syndrome, endometriosis, infertility, infrequent or abnormal ovulation, ovarian cysts and polycystic ovaries, habitual miscarriage, difficult pregnancies, toxemia in pregnancy, lactation failure, postpartum depression, and premature menopause.

Sometimes Thyroid Is the Main Culprit   A study by Brayshaw suggested that PMS itself might be a form of thyroid dysfunction, but this was a small study and not widely accepted.[4]

Probably the women with thyroid disorders as the sole cause of their PMS are a subgroup.

The same could be said of women with postpartum depression. Postpartum thyroiditis is a very common phenomenon. Again, how much it contributes to postpartum depression is a controversial subject.

Some women may lose their hormonal symptoms just by treating their thyroid problem. Other women will find that they need other treatment.

Abnormal Thyroid, Normal Tests

Sometimes a woman's thyroid test results show up as normal despite suspicious symptoms or a family history of thyroid problems. Even if her thyroid levels are borderline low, they are often not considered low enough to treat.

Sometimes a woman is resistant to her own thyroid. This means that she apparently produces enough thyroid hormone, but her body can't use it. Or she may have thyroiditis, in which antibodies turn against her body and begin to destroy her thyroid gland. These antibodies can block thyroid function in the gland itself, in the bloodstream, or in the cell receptor.

Hereditary Thyroid Problems

It is well known that thyroid problems can be inherited. Over half the women I see with hormonal problems have at least one close relative (frequently their maternal grandmother, mother, or sister) who have a diagnosed thyroid condition. For many of these women, several or all of their female family members have thyroid problems.[5] Thyroid trouble is the first thing a woman should suspect, if her mother has a diagnosed thyroid problem.

Typical Low Thyroid Symptoms

The following list of symptoms may help you to determine if you have a thyroid problem:

Allergies

Arthritis

Asthma

Brittle and ridged nails

Cold extremities

Colitis or constipation

Confusion, inability to think clearly, lack of concentration, poor memory

Decreased sweating

Depression and other emotional problems, including paranoid thoughts and even psychosis

Diabetes or hypoglycemia

Dry, coarse, rough, scaly skin

Dry, brittle hair; fine hair; hair that falls out easily

Energy pattern: a tendency to wake up slowly, be fatigued in the afternoon, and feel best after 8:00 P.M.

Excessively high or low blood pressure

Fatigue, listlessness, languor, indolence, lack of endurance, muscle weakness

Flat, puffy look to the face

Formication (crawling feelings on skin)

Headaches and migraines

Heart irregularities—(rapid or slow pulse rate, palpitations, murmur, mitral valve prolapse, family history of stroke or heart attack)

High cholesterol

Hoarseness

Inability to tolerate extremes of temperature

Insomnia

Irritability

Loss of the outer portion of the eyebrows

Low sex drive

Menstrual cramps, excessive flow, irregular menstruation, infertility, habitual miscarriage, toxemia in pregnancy, endometriosis

Peripheral neuritis, symptoms similar to carpal tunnel syndrome

Recurrent colds

Respiratory problems—tonsillitis, sinusitis, ear and mastoid infections

Skin problems such as boils, eczema, psoriasis, and acne
Slowness in speech or movements, slurred speech
Slowing down of the circulation, which may cause fluid re-
    tention and edema of the eyes, abdomen, and ankles

Some of these symptoms are the symptoms of myxedema,
which is an extreme thyroid disease. Nobody has every symptom in the list, and some have only a few.

Six Common Symptoms of Hypothyroidism

Dr. Broda Barnes was a well-known American physician who
used to be called "Mr. Thyroid." He died in the 1980s, after
spending most of his life researching the thyroid gland. Dr.
Barnes completed a Ph.D. in physiology, specializing in thyroid, and later taught endocrinology at the University of
Chicago. Subsequently, he added an M.D. degree. In his medical practice, he found that thyroid problems were extremely
common and caused many different symptoms. Dr. Barnes'
work is now being carried on by the Broda Barnes Foundation in Trumble, Connecticut.

Dr. Barnes found six common denominators among mild
cases of hypothyroidism:

1. Subnormal body temperature (below 97.8°F)—sufferers
   feel the cold deep inside, especially in their hands and feet;
2. Fatigue, particularly upon rising and in the afternoon;
   more energy at night;
3. Drowsiness;
4. Depression;
5. "Female" problems;
6. Recurrent infections.

Dr. Barnes developed the basal temperature and basal metabolism tests for low thyroid (but found the latter to be less
reliable). Because of his influence, the basal temperature test
was reported in JAMA in 1942 and featured in the *Physician's
Desk Reference*. It was used for years to detect low thyroid problems. When blood tests came into prominence, the basal temperature test went out of fashion. Some, including Dr. Barnes,

thought this unfortunate because antibodies and other factors often cause the thyroid blood tests to be as much as 40 percent in error. Many physicians use both the thyroid blood tests and the basal temperature test, the combination giving more accuracy than either one.

Thyroid and Body Temperature

The reason temperature is important is that it is a true measure of your metabolic heat. When there is a marked discrepancy between your basal temperature and the norm, it means that your metabolism may not be working efficiently. This would affect many body systems, including the production of enzymes.

Stress, anxiety, allergies, low pituitary or low adrenal function, the presence of a virus, and slower heart rate from athletic exercise can also be associated with lower body temperature. Nevertheless, the basal temperature test is helpful in pointing out the likelihood of a subclinical thyroid problem.

How to Take Your Basal Temperature Dr. Barnes felt that the best time for performing this test is immediately upon awakening in the morning. Shake down a basal thermometer and put it on the bedside table the night before. As soon as you awaken, put the thermometer under your armpit for ten minutes. Oral temperatures are often misleading, because any sinus or respiratory infection will elevate the temperature of the mouth.

The normal temperature under the armpit should be above 97.2°F. If your temperature taken this way is consistently well below 97.2°F, you may have low thyroid activity.

Which Days to Take Your Temperature Menstruating women can use the basal thermometer test only during the first two days of their period, when ovulation does not affect the results. However, you may take your temperature for longer than two days. When women are postmenopausal or post-hysterectomy, the temperature may be taken any day.

Unless you are running a fever from an infection or inflammation, a 10- to 15-day average of your basal temperatures will give you the most natural and accurate measurements. Or you can take your temperature for a whole month.

If you have temperature readings that are obviously very low as a result of a viral infection, or if you are running a fever due to a bacterial infection, ignore those readings.

The Thyroid Hormones

The thyroid gland produces two main thyroid hormones, produced by the interaction of thyroid stimulating hormone (TSH), from the pituitary gland, with dietary iodine. The primary hormone made in the thyroid gland is called thyroxine, or T4. It makes up 83% of the thyroid gland's total production. The other hormone is called triiodothyronine, or T3. It represents 17 percent of the thyroid gland's total production. T4 is bound by protein and stored in the body to be broken down as needed by an enzyme (5-deiodinase) into T3. T3 is the active form of thyroid hormone. It is four times more active at the cell level than T4. Besides its many other physical functions in the body, T3 is the hormone that targets the brain and interacts with brain neurotransmitters to influence mood and emotion.

Thyroid Blood Tests

Hormones measured in the bloodstream consist of a "free" and a "bound" portion. The free portion represents the part that is available to be used. The bound portion represents the part that is bound by protein and not usable until broken down. One of the problems with blood tests for hormone levels is that it is not easy to accurately measure the free, usable part.

In the case of thyroid, physicians usually order a thyroid panel—a group of blood tests used to calculate the level of free T4. These include: a total T4 by radioimmune assay (normal range 5–13 mg/dl); a radioactive T3 resin uptake (normal range between 25 and 30 percent, varies with the method);

and a free thyroxine index (FTI) (normal range varies with different labs). Currently, a TSH test is usually included. Note that the T3 uptake is not a measurement of free T3. Rather it is used to help calculate the amount of free T4. Doctors use an equation:

$$\frac{\text{Total T4} \times \text{T3 uptake}}{\text{Average FTI} = 30} = \text{Approximate level of free T4}$$

The most reliable test for free T4 is called the T7 test. It is a more expensive test and cumbersome to perform, and therefore not included in the thyroid panel and rarely done. A free T3 test is available, but it is usually only used to determine if a patient has hyperthyroidism, not hypothyroidism.

If the TSH level is high, even if the thyroid panel is normal, the patient is considered hypothyroid (low). It means that the pituitary gland is producing high levels in an attempt to stimulate the thyroid gland to produce more thyroxine. If the TSH level is low, the patient is considered hyperthyroid (high). The newer TSH tests are called ultrasensitive, and they are considered much more accurate than previous methods of measuring TSH. The TSH measurement is considered to be the gold standard of thyroid tests.

Thyroid test results need to be read carefully by a physician, because there are many nonthyroidal factors that complicate the interpretation of the results.

Blood Tests Are Not Always Reliable   Many physicians are unwilling to treat a thyroid problem unless it clearly shows up in blood tests, despite the fact that research has shown that blood tests are not always conclusive.[6]

For instance, the Center for Disease Control regularly sends out blood samples to 7 percent of all laboratories in the U.S. Between 8 and 25 percent of tests yield erroneous results.[7]

Niels Lauersen says:

> The results of the T3 and T4 tests might vary from laboratory to laboratory, so a doctor should carefully scrutinize all lab reports. If he sees a low, or what is called a "low-normal,"

reading for thyroid function, he should prescribe a minimal dose of thyroid medication.[8]

Rule Out Thyroiditis

Thyroiditis is a general word describing a number of auto-immune thyroid disorders.[9] Hashimoto's thyroiditis (named after the Japanese researcher who discovered it) is the most common cause of low thyroid function; some think that it is one of the most common thyroid diseases that exists.[10] It affects up to 1 in 8 people[11] and is up to 25 to 50 times more common in women than men.[12] It is not uncommon in children, adolescents, or women over 45.[13] A number of researchers believe that the incidence of thyroiditis is on the increase.[14]

In the women's center where I work, we routinely check for thyroid antibodies because thyroiditis is so common. We do this, because the other blood test results can be normal while the antibody test result is abnormal. Thyroiditis can take years to show up on the other thyroid tests. Meanwhile, thyroid destruction is gradually taking its course.

Thyroiditis can be hereditary—passed through the placenta from mother to child—or it can be due to antigen defects. It can also begin with an infection.

How Thyroiditis Occurs

In thyroiditis, the immune system mistakes the person's own thyroid tissue for an enemy, and makes thyroid autoantibodies. These attack the thyroid gland, affect the production of thyroid hormones in the bloodstream and in the cells, and frequently result in chronic inflammation of the thyroid gland.

The onset of Hashimoto's thyroiditis is often slow.[15] In the early stages, thyroid levels may be alternately high and low; this fluctuation is characteristic of the disease. However, the test results can also remain normal (euthyroid) for a long time in the early years. The thyroid gland may be swollen or have nodules on it, or it may feel normal.

Testing for Hashimoto's Thyroiditis   A test for thyroid antibodies (antithyroglobulin and antimicrosomal) will usually

Female/Male Ratio of Autoimmune Disease[16]

Hashimoto's Thyroiditis	25 to 50:1
SLE (Lupus)	9:1
Sjøgren's	9:1
Thyrotoxicosis	4 to 8:1
Hypothyroidism	6:1
Type 1 diabetes	5:1
Rheumatoid arthritis	5:1
Myasthenia gravis	2:1
Multiple sclerosis	1 to 5:1

—*Richard Bronson*

show positive for thyroiditis, though the level of antibodies may fluctuate from test to test, and the intensity of the symptoms may not correspond with how high or low the antibodies are. Hashimoto's can also be diagnosed by aspiration needle biopsy.

Graves' Disease and Hyperthyroidism

Graves' disease causes the thyroid gland to overproduce thyroxine. It is also an autoimmune disease and is four to eight times as common in women as in men (much less common than Hashimoto's thyroiditis). In Graves' disease, antibodies are produced against thyroid stimulating hormone (TSH) at the pituitary level.

Sometimes Graves' disease is a triggering factor in women with PMS whose main symptoms are racing heart, agitation, and exhaustion. In the onset of the disease, or in borderline cases, symptoms may sometimes show up only premenstrually.

Thyroid Is a Major Hinge

There is a great sympathy between the endocrine and immune systems, and the thyroid plays a central role in this. The combinations and variations of possible problems seem endless. A woman with chronic fatigue syndrome might also have thyroid problems and PMS. Or a woman with postpartum depression might have autoimmune thyroiditis. Or a woman with lupus might develop Graves' disease around the same time and be having trouble at menopause. Or a woman might have a multiple autoimmune/endocrine disease in which she has diabetes, adrenal failure, thyroid failure, and ovarian failure in a slow progression. For more information and references on autoimmune links with thyroid, see Appendix 3.

AUTOIMMUNE DISEASES

Autoimmune disease can be triggered when the immune system is fighting chemical toxins or viruses that enter the body from outside. These invaders can have components that are similar to human tissue. When the immune system sets out to fight these invaders, if it finds similar tissue in the body, it may produce "autoantibodies" (meaning that they begin to attack the self). There are numerous diseases involving different types of antibodies that occur because the immune system mistakes the person's own body for an enemy.

These diseases are much more common in women. Their immune system is more sophisticated because of maintaining pregnancy, and so more subject to failure. Different immune system diseases, such as lupus, thyroiditis, and myasthenia gravis, involve different autoantibodies. But these different autoantibodies can coexist, and thyroiditis is a central factor in autoimmune disease.

Classification of Polyendocrine Autoimmune Disease

I   Candidiasis, hypoparathyroidism, Addison disease
II Addison disease and thyroid autoimmune disease and/or insulin-diabetes mellitus

   III a. Thyroid autoimmune disease and insulin-dependent diabetes mellitus
       b. Thyroid autoimmune disease and pernicious anemia
       c. Thyroid autoimmune disease and vitiligo and/or alopecia and/or other organ-specific autoimmune diseases not falling into the previous categories.

The APICH Syndrome

The name APICH (involving **a**utoimmune disease, **p**olyendocrinopathy, **i**mmune dysregulation, **c**andidiasis, and **h**ypersensitivity) was coined by Nathan Becker, M.D., and Phyllis Saifer, M.D., physicians in the Bay Area in California. The APICH syndrome represents one form of polyglandular autoimmune syndrome, also called candidiasis endocrinopathy. It comprises a variety of symptoms, but Hashimoto's thyroiditis, yeast problems, respiratory problems, and allergies are involved.

Polyendocrine means, as we have said, that more than one endocrine gland is affected, and the autoimmune factor binds all these disorders together. The cause of these disorders may be genetic, and therefore strongly hereditary, but it may also be brought on by other factors, such as trauma, shock, or virus.

According to Drs. Becker and Saifer's article, "Allergy and Autoimmune Endocrinopathy: APICH Syndrome,"[17] ten times more women than men suffer from the APICH syndrome. Many women with hormonal problems to whom I have given Becker and Saifer's article identify closely with the description of this disease.

For instance, Sandra's case history in Chapter 5 is an example of someone with an obvious autoimmune polyendocrine problem. Robin's case history in Chapter 9 reveals a family history in which thyroid problems and collagen disease are interlinked. According to Dr. Gio Morino, a family physician who works with Chapa-De Indian Health in Auburn, California, the North American Indian population commonly has thyroiditis, diabetes mellitus, pernicious anemia, and other autoimmune diseases (maybe 50 percent of the North American Indian population has diabetes).

Though considered rare, I wonder if these autoimmune problems are more common than we think.

Symptoms of the APICH Syndrome

Women with the APICH syndrome may have multiple and divergent symptoms, including:

Afternoon fatigue	Allergies	Autoimmune disease
Black under-eyes	Blurred vision	Candida (yeast)
Coarse skin	Colds	Depression
Difficulty swallowing	Edema or swelling	Eye sensitivity
Fatigue	Frequent urination	Headaches
Irritability	Low blood pressure	Low temperature
Memory loss	Menstrual problems	Mood swings
Morning fatigue	Nasal congestion	Need to sleep a lot
Night alertness	Pallor	Photophobia
PMS	Poor concentration	Prematurely gray
Respiratory problems	Ridged nails	Ringing in ears
Sleep disturbances	Sore throat	Suicidal tendencies
Thin, brittle hair	Weight fluctuation	

Intolerance to temperature change—chills easily, wilts in hot weather

History of the APICH Patient   Women with these symptoms may also show certain tendencies in their history, such as:

- a family history of thyroid disease, goiters, thyroidectomies or irradiation of the thyroid
- acne
- alcoholism
- eczema
- endometriosis
- fibrocystic breasts;
- hypoglycemia;
- irradiation for acne, thymus, birth marks, tumors
- juvenile onset diabetes
- mitral valve prolapse
- mononucleosis

- nervous breakdown
- pernicious anemia
- postpartum depression
- psychiatric problems
- rheumatoid arthritis;
- tonsillitis, tonsillectomy;
- toxemia in pregnancy.

SUMMARY

There is a common link with the thyroid gland among PMS, pregnancy and postpartum difficulties, and problems around menopause.

Though the thyroid connection is not important for all women with hormonal problems, it is often a central or co-existing issue that needs to be addressed. This issue is very important for a large, well-defined group of women who are often overlooked by the medical profession. Women who have a family history and typical symptoms of thyroid disorders should investigate this first, and not be easily discouraged in their search.

Further Information

The Broda O. Barnes, M.D., Research Foundation
P.O. Box 98
Trumbull, Connecticut 06611
203-261-2101.
fax: 203-261-3017

The Barnes Foundation is a nonprofit organization dedicated to continuing research, education, and distribution of information on thyroid and other endocrine dysfunctions. A 24-hour comprehensive urine test is available from the foundation to test thyroid and adrenal hormone levels. The foundation also acts as a networking organization that will provide, upon request, a list of physicians who use Dr. Barnes' clinical and familial techniques.

CASE HISTORY

Dana's Story

Dana, a 36-year-old intensive care nurse and mother of one, had mild PMS and suffered dreadfully from allergies. She came to me because of the difficulty she had carrying her pregnancies to term. She believed that she had thyroid problems but was having difficulty convincing her doctors of this.

Dana's mother had been on thyroid medication since the age of 18. There was a history of Hashimoto's thyroiditis, as well as breast and other hormonal cancer, in her mother's family. Her two oldest aunts received short-term treatment for schizophrenia, which Dana thought might have been a misdiagnosed hormonal problem. At 54, her mother had a hysterectomy because of precancerous lesions on her cervix. She was presently having monthly estrogen injections and bimonthly testosterone injections. Whenever her hormone levels dropped, she became angry and paranoid.

As a child, Dana was very healthy and rarely sick, except for occasional earaches and a bout of bronchitis at age eight. Secondary changes occurred with dramatic weight gain at age ten, but Dana did not have menstrual periods until age 16. She had no other health problems until she was about 19 years old, when she had painful tonsillitis with a fever of 104°F. This lasted for about six months, and she was on penicillin for most of that time. She has since been told that this was a classic indicator of Hashimoto's disease, which was not diagnosed then. She had a tonsillectomy at age 19, and her headaches, which began at puberty, developed into severe migraines after this surgery.

Dana's menstrual periods were always irregular, and, at age 29, they became even more irregular, and she developed a male body-hair pattern. Polycystic ovaries were suspected; and this was confirmed by tests, but her hormone levels were always within normal limits. Her yearly prolactin levels were usually slightly over high-normal (high prolactin levels are sometimes linked with hypothyroidism).

At age 30, Dana was put on Clomid for infertility. Despite increasing doses, her periods remained 45 to 60 days apart, and her progesterone levels were always low. A year later, on the tenth day of her cycle, she had a laparoscopy and hysterosalpingogram (an X-ray study in which dye is injected into the uterus and tubes), which were both normal, showing no apparent reason for infertility. By day 45, because her period had not started, she was given a shot of progesterone to induce menstrual bleeding. She had no period, but 10 days later she had sharp pains in her left ovary. On examination, the doctor thought that she was pregnant, but a blood test was negative.

When she was given Clomid the following month, she had an extraordinarily severe migraine that day. Dana thinks she conceived at that time; this proved to be her only full-term pregnancy.

For the first three months of her pregnancy, she had severe headaches, and her blood sugar level was erratic. Twenty weeks into the pregnancy, she became very tired; this seemed understandable since she was working for five physicians at the time. At her 30-week checkup, they found that the baby had dropped and her cervix was dilated. Bed rest was advised, and she stayed in bed, on her left side, for about eight weeks. The baby's heart rate was erratic, so labor was induced; this turned out to be due to the umbilical cord being around its neck, but that was not known at the time.

After delivery, the baby developed thrush (an oral candida infection), which lasted eight months. She was colicky, had allergies, and failed to thrive. Dana's health worsened; she became dehydrated and had gastritis, diarrhea, congestion from allergies, one or two migraines a week, bladder problems, and pain on intercourse (which was relieved after treatment for the yeast infection).

When the baby was a year old, Dana was doing better on a yeast-free diet and taking Nystatin, but she still had a lot of diarrhea and stomachaches, and her hair and skin were dry. It was several years before these problems were resolved.

Her second pregnancy was unplanned, and Dana conceived without medical intervention. She had less diarrhea because she continued on a yeast-free diet and so felt better. At 13 weeks, an ultrasound examination revealed that she had a blighted ovum; she had a miscarriage 24 hours later, with heavy bleeding. She became anemic, and her gastritis and allergy symptoms returned. Within two months, she lost another 10 pounds, bringing her total weight loss to 35 pounds in one year.

After the miscarriage, she went to Dr. K., who had been treating her for the yeast problems. He put her on thyroid medication and referred her to an endocrinologist, Dr. B. For a year, Dr. B. managed Dana's thyroid problems. He also gave her low-dose hydrocortisone; because he believed that she had Schmidt's syndrome, an autoimmune disease involving thyroiditis and adrenal failure. During this time, her menstrual cycles ranged from 37 to 55 days in length, and she had mild PMS. She controlled the migraines and the gastritis with the yeast-free diet, though both symptoms were still present. In 1989, Dana saw a gastroenterologist, who determined by a stool sample that she had blastocystis hominis, a type of intestinal parasite. A course of Flagyl cleared the bowel symptoms, but she had migraines during the whole six weeks while she was on medication. For the next six months, Dana felt better than she had since her baby was delivered in 1986. Her periods were 33 to 40 days apart; her PMS was mild, and mainly consisted of sore breasts. She craved alcohol premenstrually, but limited her intake because it brought on migraines.

Early in 1990, Dana's menstrual cycles suddenly lengthened to 80 days, then 60 days. Dr. B. increased her thyroid medication to 0.15 mg of Synthroid. One month later, Dana became pregnant. She went off all alcohol. During this pregnancy, she had severe fatigue, and her blood sugar level dipped precariously low. She had one to three headaches a week. An ultrasound examination was planned at fourteen weeks, as no heartbeat could be found; the ultrasound confirmed that the fetus was dead. All test results were within normal limits.

Dana's blood sugar levels remained low after having a D&C (removal of the uterine lining). She saw another endocrinologist, who told her that she had no business taking thyroid. She told him that she felt healthier on thyroid than she had ever felt before, but he said that her test results did not indicate that she needed it. Dana agreed to lower her dosage gradually, and eventually stopped taking thyroid medication. She then experienced a progressive return of her symptoms and severe PMS. Another physician, who examined her for possible pituitary dysfunction felt that she could not have conceived if she had a pituitary problem. He did not object to her using thyroid and wanted her to go back on Clomid.

From July, 1991, when Dana stopped taking thyroid medication, until I saw her in September, 1991, she had only had one period. Her migraines had returned, and her allergies were much worse. Repeated TSH tests were mainly normal, but one test was borderline high-normal.

Dana went to yet another endocrinologist, who put her back on thyroid and explained that in the case of thyroiditis, blood tests can appear normal. "It's not whether you have thyroid in the bloodstream; it's whether it is available at cell level." Since she had taken thyroid medication before, and was so much healthier when taking it, he knew that she would feel better again once she resumed taking it. She was also a candidate for progesterone therapy because of her PMS, but since her PMS tended to go away when she was taking thyroid medication, he thought that she might not need progesterone.

Dana's story is a good illustration of a woman who is suffering from incapacitating symptoms of a thyroid problem, yet her tests are mainly normal. She is a very intelligent woman and has worked for years in the medical field. She understands how doctors' opinions differ even if they are trained in the same specialty. Her instincts told her that she should be on thyroid medication, but the varying opinions of the specialists she went to confused her.

I find myself sympathetic with both the doctors and patients. The doctor wants to go by the textbook and is understandably cautious about prescribing thyroid medication if it is not absolutely necessary; the side effects of overdose can be serious. However, the doctors I work with generally have not seen any serious side effects from small doses of thyroid medication.

On the other hand, the physician doesn't understand how miserable women feel with their symptoms, which are very real whether the test results are in the normal range or not. When a woman with problems like Dana's takes even a little bit of thyroid medication, the effect can be dramatic, relieving a lot of symptoms. Given the choice, women with long-standing chronic problems often prefer to take the small risk of side effects, because they feel so much better on thyroid medication. In fact, they know that their bodies work better with a little help.

Why is it that physicians so freely hand out antidepressants, which are chemically alien to the human body and can produce toxic side effects, yet are so reluctant to prescribe hormones, which the body produces naturally?

Says Dana, "I used to think there was a large body of information out there that all doctors tapped into. But it's not like that. They all have their own opinions and prejudices. When you work as a nurse, as I do, you realize that doctors are not infallible."

What's Happening Now?   Dana is doing very well. In exploring the possibilities of pregnancy, it was found that she was producing a type of antibody that caused her miscarriages. She talked frankly with her endocrinologist, who advised her against getting pregnant again because of the dangers to her own health. Dana and her husband discussed the situation and decided that pregnancy was not worth putting her own health at risk. She is reconciled to this and feels fortunate that she has one child.

Dana is still taking thyroid medication. Her new endocrinologist has some unconventional ideas about cell metabolism and has her taking a special, expensive calcium- and-vitamin-D supplement twice a week. She says that this supplement makes a tremendous difference in how she feels.

While on this treatment, Dana has no PMS or allergies and seems to be in good health.

NINE

THYROID AND DEPRESSION

Having looked at the links between thyroid problems and other physical health problems, let us look at the connection between thyroid problems and various emotional disorders. This connection has been much more thoroughly researched than the link between estrogen and depression.

The link between the thyroid gland and mental disease has been known for over a century. The term "myxedema madness" was first coined in 1888. (Myxedema is an extreme low thyroid condition.)[1]

According to Victor Reus, M.D., head of the psychiatry department at the University of California at San Francisco, depression is two to three times higher in women than in men, particularly up to age 45.[2] A number of researchers have also pointed out that thyroid problems are more common in women.[3] Therefore, there may be a link between low thyroid and depression in women because of a common incidence. While this might be partly due to the pressures of society, there appears to be a hormonal link.

There have been links made between abnormalities in the hypothalamic-pituitary-thyroid axis and a number of other mental disorders:[4] panic attacks, suicide, agitation, mania (bipolar disorders), paranoia, schizophrenia, psychosis, autism, Down's syndrome, dementia, Alzheimer's disease, attention deficit hyperactivity disorder (ADHD), obsessive-compulsive disorder, and seasonal affective disorder (SAD).[5] There is also a link with bulimia and anorexia nervosa.[6] The reason why thyroid has so many effects on behavior is that it targets the brain and interacts with brain messengers that influence mood and emotions.

Early Stage Thyroiditis Can Cause Emotional Problems

Chapter 8 mentioned that Hashimoto's thyroiditis begins gradually, and that overt hypothyroidism may take years to occur. However, even in the early stages while thyroid function is normal, Hashimoto's thyroiditis has been linked with a number of moderate-to-severe emotional disorders.

According to Hall, Popkin, and others:

> The mental symptoms associated with Hashimoto's thyroiditis may precede the full-blown, classic picture of hypothyroidism. The psychiatric symptoms include various mental aberrations, depression, irritability, and confusion. Indeed, patients may be mislabeled as having psychotic depression, paranoid schizophrenia, or the manic phase of a manic-depressive disorder. The workup must include a thorough evaluation of thyroid function, including tests for autoantibodies. Patients usually respond favorably to thyroid replacement hormone therapy.[7]

Hashimoto's Thyroiditis Not Always Easy to Detect   Only one-fifth of cases of Hashimoto's thyroiditis are clinically low thyroid at the time of diagnosis. But at the onset of the disease, the patient may appear hyperthyroid or hypothyroid or alternate between symptoms of both. (If treatment begins in this early stage, it can be very difficult to regulate the dose of thyroid medication because of the fluctuation between hyper- and hypothyroid symptoms.)

The thyroid gland may typically appear either normal or swollen but pain-free. Rarely, it is enlarged with pain and tenderness. Thyroid destruction is gradual in most cases, and usually takes years to develop. Occasionally, a patient will have a dramatic progression to clinical hypothyroidism.

The Psychiatric Aspects of Hashimoto's Thyroiditis   Accordinging to Hall and others:

> Hashimoto's thyroiditis usually presents either as a chronic insidious change in personality manifested by lability, anxiety, and withdrawal, or as a progressive depression, often so gradual that it seems most compatible with a psychogenic etiology [from a psychological cause]. Alternately the disease may present as classic "myxedema madness." In this case the patient may appear to suffer from paranoid schizophrenia, psychotic depression, or manic depressive disease (manic type). The typical picture includes generalized agitation, disorientation, persecutory delusions, hallucinations, and bouts of extreme restlessness. Patients are often in a hallucinative, irritable, delusional, paranoid state with concomitant auditory and visual hallucinations. Hypersexuality may also occur during these episodes: a marked increase in sexual drive is the most characteristic feature reported.[8]

Physical symptoms also occur:

> In the more gradually progressing cases, patients may report a variety of nondescript complaints, including poorly defined abdominal or peripheral pain, lassitude, weakness, menstrual irregularities, joint aches, weight gain, and changes in hair and skin.[9]

Using Thyroid to Treat Depression

There is a lot of research connecting thyroid and depression, and thyroid medication has been commonly used to treat endogenous depression. Endogenous depression is a term used to describe depression that is biochemically caused and comes from within, not from outside circumstances.

The use of active thyroid to treat depression on its own or as a "helper" for tricyclic antidepressant treatment (e.g. Elavil), has been common for the last 25 years.[10] It has been used even when thyroid function is "normal" according to the TSH standard.

Says Jeri Miller (quoting Irl Extein, M.D., the former medical director of the mood disorders center at Lake Hospital of the Palm Beaches, in Florida):

> Depressed patients who do not respond completely to a tricyclic antidepressant tend to respond when thyroid hormone is used to potentiate or boost the antidepressant. "This is probably the main finding in the area of unipolar depressed patients," Extein said, adding that it is not yet known if thyroid hormone also boosts noncyclic antidepressants.[11]

The article goes on to say that patients without hypothyroidism or elevated TSH can respond to thyroid hormone potentiation. About 50 percent of patients who do not respond to a tricyclic antidepressant will show marked improvement when T3 (brand name Cytomel) is added. Extein says that if the improvement doesn't occur within two weeks, it probably isn't going to occur.

A conclusion could be made that, for some women with hormonal mood swings, thyroid (and possibly estrogen) may be a more appropriate first choice for treating depression than antidepressants. In fact, for many women with hormonal depression, antidepressants just don't work.

Difference of Opinions Between Endocrinologists and Biopsychiatrists Sometimes there are differences of opinion among specialists. Expert endocrinologists emphasize the fact that the TSH test is so sensitive a test that it indicates hypothyroidism very early. Therefore, endocrinologists are generally reluctant to treat subclinical cases—those in which the TSH test result is normal. This is the position most doctors take.

To illustrate this point, I quote a helpful letter that I received from Robert Volpé, M.D., a Canadian endocrinologist in the Division of Endocrinology at the University of Toronto. Dr. Volpé has been an expert on thyroid diseases his whole professional life, and has written extensively on the subject. After reading something I had written, he wrote:

> . . . There is one paragraph in your section on hypothyroidism with which I could not agree. You state that thyroid function tests "do not always reveal marginal or borderline thyroid function problems." While such tests do not always show the early stages of Hashimoto's thyroiditis and do not demonstrate the presence or absence of thyroid nodules, they are completely reflective of thyroid functional disturbance.
>
> If the TSH is normal, that patient is *not* hypothyroid. I make this emphatic since there are practitioners of various types who will insist that patients can be hypothyroid despite having a normal TSH, and that is clearly *not* the case. As you know, the TSH will rise even before thyroid hormones levels start to fall and is an extremely sensitive index of the slightest degree of hypothyroidism. Thus your remarks that "specialist researchers in this area think that the TSH is not the last word for diagnosis" do not reflect the views of main-line endocrinologists or academics in this field.[12]

What can I say? Many women feel intuitively, as I do, that a thyroid disorder is part of their problem. And indeed many, like me, find that taking thyroid medication helps when many others treatments have not. My TSH level has always been normal, whether I'm taking thyroid medication or not.

Too Much Thyroid Medication Can Be Dangerous

There are sound reasons for caution about prescribing thyroid medication; it has serious side effects if given too liberally or inappropriately. As two examples of many side effects, thyroid affects the heart muscle. Too much can increase heart rate and cause a heart attack. Thyroid also affects bone, increasing osteoclast activity (osteoclasts are chewers that eat your bone), so too much thyroid medication can cause osteoporosis in women. However, even this is a controversial subject. Alan Gaby, M.D., who wrote *Preventing and Reversing Osteoporosis,* brings into question the conclusions of two main studies used to show an increase in bone loss in women on thyroid medication.[13] He quotes a *Lancet* study by Franklyn that shows that thyroid hormones in normal amounts do not cause osteoporosis.[14]

TRH Test, a Marker for Depression

As we have mentioned, research psychiatrists say that thyroid tests can be used for more than identifying patients with thyroid dysfunction. They can also be a marker for depression.

Jeri Miller enlarges on this point, again quoting Irl Extein, M.D.:

> The brain is not only the master regulator of the thyroid system but also a target organ. One of the reasons the thyroid is so important in depression and mood disorders is that there has to be normal stimulation of thyroid hormones for certain brain systems to work properly—such as the norepinephrine system.
>
> Thyroid testing is used both to identify patients with thyroid dysfunction—hypothyroidism being much more common in the psychiatric population—and as a diagnostic marker for depressive disorder and mania.
>
> . . . The TSH measure tells the clinician whether the pituitary "thinks" a patient is hypothyroid. . . .
>
> Another commonly used thyroid function test consists of intravenous infusion of TRH followed by measurement of subsequent TSH increases in the bloodstream: this test doubles the sensitivity of TSH in identifying subclinical hypothyroidism. Of eight patients in a study with positive antithyroid antibodies, only half had high TSH, whereas all had high scores on TRH tests. 'This shows you if you are only using TSH, you are still missing about half of your depressed patients who have positive antibodies,' Extein said.[15]

Not a Common Test, Though a Common Problem   The TRH test is not commonly used in general practice; I have seen only two women who have received it. Yet Victor Reus, M.D., says that approximately 25 percent of hospitalized depressed patients have a "reduced" TSH response to TRH infusion.[16] He continues, saying that:

> The . . . significance of "subclinical hypothyroidism" and the role of replacement therapy remain controversial in the endocrinologic literature. . . . In the best controlled study thus far, however, "subclinical" hypothyroid patients were found to be suffering from a variety of nonspecific symptoms of malaise that *did respond* to replacement therapy.[17]

Differences in Opinion   I wrote back to Dr. Volpé and learned that he is very much aware of the psychiatric use of TRH to define endogenous depression. But he maintains that TSH is the standard test for primary hypothyroidism. He says that if you find someone with a borderline high TSH and an increased response to TRH, that person will probably have no symptoms of thyroid disorder.[18]

I think it's important to understand these differences of opinion, because your doctor's approach to your problem will depend on his or her training, experience, and prejudices.

On a practical level, I see many women who are depressed and who have relatives with thyroid problems or who identify with the symptoms of thyroid disorder. Many of them were taking thyroid medication at some previous time but were taken off it later. Their doctor may order a thyroid panel and a TSH test; If the results are normal, the doctor may recommend that no treatment be given.

But if such a woman went to a psychiatrist who was well-read about thyroid, she might be given a trial of low-dose thyroid as an adjunct to treatment. Or if she went to a family physician who thought that she had the profile and symptoms of hypothyroidism, he might try thyroid treatment despite normal test results. But I've seen a number of endocrinologists slap the primary care physician's hand if they find out that thyroid is being prescribed when the TSH test result is normal.

This is one reason why most doctors take a conservative stand and won't prescribe thyroid medication unless the test results are conclusive.

A Physician Uses Thyroid for PMS

Kathryn Morris, M.D, is one of a number of physicians I know who will try a course of low-dose thyroid treatment if the patient's symptoms indicate that it may help. She says:

> Our experience is that many women with significant PMS respond to low-dose thyroid treatment. Since the thyroid function tests may not be accurate, we also evaluate patients by their symptoms. We find that women who have more than ten symptoms of hypothyroidism are very likely to respond to thyroid treatment. Not only does their PMS clear, but many of their other symptoms diminish as well.

> The symptoms of low thyroid include the following: low body temperature, fatigue, cold hands or feet, difficulty losing weight, constipation, difficulty waking in the morning, depression, irritability, headache, poor memory, frequent colds or infections, acne, eczema/dry skin, hair loss, hypoglycemia, asthma, arthritis/arthralgia, hypertension/hypotension, water retention, irregular menses, heavy menses, menstrual cramps, infertility, repeated miscarriages, low libido, and PMS.[19]

My Own Experience with Thyroid

I might add that when a woman with a borderline thyroid problem takes thyroid medication, sometimes it will help and sometimes it won't. In my case, it helps. I first felt the sudden descent of devastating lassitude (with no viral symptoms), as I describe in my own story, at the age of 11. I had the symptoms of hypothyroidism from then on, including depression and fatigue. My mother and sister both had goiters. Both had surgery to remove part of their thyroid but were never treated with medication. They had lots of symptoms and both had hysterectomies. We all had severe PMS.

My thyroid blood tests were always normal until I was age 44, when a doctor checked my thyroid antibodies and found them high. My basal temperature was about 95°F. Since I began taking thyroid daily, the tiredness I struggled with all my life has been lessened. I have tried enough "solutions" over the years to know what works for me, and this isn't a placebo! Taking estrogen relieves my depression, but thyroid is the medication that helps with the fatigue.

Finding Help for Thyroid Problems

If you are convinced that you have a thyroid problem and you can't find anyone to prescribe it for you, you may have to look to alternative healers, such as chiropractors, herbalists, or naturopaths who believe in subclinical hypothyroidism and often use glandular preparations to treat it

Or, if Drs. Ray Peat and John Lee are correct, you may find that Pro-Gest® cream helps stimulate thyroid function.[20]

CASE HISTORIES

Laura's Story

Laura was about 27 years old when I first met her. She was married and had two small children. Laura had problems beginning in puberty, which were compounded by repeated surgeries and her pregnancies.

Her mother and maternal aunt had goiters, and the maternal aunt and a cousin had dermoid cysts,[21] but nobody in the family had the severe problems that Laura had.

Her periods were irregular, two months apart, and long and heavy, and they lasted two or three weeks. The excessive bleeding caused her to become very anemic. She was diagnosed as being hypothyroid at age 16 and was put on thyroid medication and the birth control pill. The thyroid medication made her feel better and gave her more energy, but after a year the family moved, and she stopped taking it. Some time during her teens, she was anorexic and bulimic, and her weight went down to 85 pounds. She drank heavily and describes herself as a borderline alcoholic.

Laura took the birth control pill until she was 23, when she was diagnosed with cancer of the cervix. She was having a lot of pain and bleeding with her periods; at that time, she discovered that she was sterile. Her uterus was tipped, and her fallopian tubes were blocked with endometriosis, so she had surgery to clear out the tubes in 1978.

She had many medical problems after she was married in her early twenties, including a disease in the glands in her groin, resulting in six or seven surgeries. She went on Clomid to help her ovulate, but didn't become pregnant while taking it. Later, in 1980, she was able to conceive and become pregnant. She described herself as very emotional during this pregnancy, but not enough to keep her from enjoying the pregnancy. She had toxemia toward the end, and the pregnancy lasted three weeks past her due date. She didn't dilate, and, because of this and the fact that she had a small pelvis, she had a Cesarean birth (C-section). After the surgery, she lost a lot of blood, was very anemic, and had very low blood pressure. She felt as though she was dying, and was extremely weak.

In 1982, Laura became pregnant again, and became exhausted and emotional. She did not have toxemia this time, but did have another C-section. She has RH-negative blood, but that caused no problems. Initially, she felt better after this pregnancy than the first, but within a short time, postpartum depression crept up on her and she had great difficulty maintaining control.

Shortly afterward, Laura thinks she had a miscarriage. She hemorrhaged for a week just like she did during her second labor. Afterward, she had pain in her right ovary, and her gynecologist thought that she had either a swollen ovary or a tubal pregnancy, and put her on the birth control pill because her condition was not clear. She saw another doctor who did an emergency laparoscopy and, unfortunately, punctured her ovary.

The ovary remained swollen, and Laura was told that she had postpartum depression, since she was hysterical and seemed to be on the verge of a nervous breakdown. In 1983, a doctor put her on 400 mg of natural progesterone, three to four times a day. This apparently did not help; he wanted to put her on the pill, which she refused because of her previous bad experience with it. Instead, she took Librium and sleeping pills, worked on her diet, and took vitamins.

Her doctor told her that her ovary was larger than a golf ball (a healthy ovary is about the size of an almond). At the time everything hurt, and she couldn't have intercourse because of the pain. Her uterus felt as though it was falling out, and it even hurt her to walk. Later, her ovary and uterus swelled again and became excruciatingly painful. She also had severe pain at the site of her C-section surgery. She had no periods for three months, and her uterus was growing larger. A doctor said that she needed a hysterectomy, and that he would also examine her ovaries. He removed her uterus and fallopian tubes, but left the swollen ovary alone even though it was bigger than the other one. He found she had lacerations of the bladder which were causing internal bleeding, so he patched the bladder and repaired adhesions from previous surgery.

When I subsequently met Laura, she had extreme PMS. She would cry, scream, become violent, and throw things. She described herself as nervous, jumpy, and irritable. She suffered from insomnia, and was having night sweats and hot flashes every day.

I sent Laura to a doctor, who put her on a combination of estrogen, progesterone, and thyroid treatment. It was the estrogen that helped her most significantly. Eventually, it became necessary to have her second ovary removed. Some time later, her husband called me because she was having a return of her symptoms. She had lost a lot of weight, weighed under 100 pounds, and felt as though she was dying. They had moved from California, and were living in Tennessee at the time.

I suggested that she go to a clinic in Atlanta, Georgia, to get an estrogen implant. Like me, she had an immediate response to the implant and found that it worked better than any other method of taking estrogen. The physician implanted five 25-mg estradiol pellets and one testosterone pellet, and she felt immediate and dramatic relief.

Laura now lives in California again, and does well as long as she has a new implant every three months. She and I have a similar need for estrogen. The implant only lasts us a relatively short time, but while it works it is wonderful. She also takes thyroid medication, but says she gets no obvious benefit from progesterone so doesn't take it (when you've had a hysterectomy, taking progesterone is optional). Laura also takes Prozac, which she says has been a lifesaver; it helps a lot with her depression.

Laura looks fine and is able to work full time. It is sad to see a woman in her early thirties who has had to go through such terrible problems most of her adult life. But Laura is grateful that eventually she found some help, and her family is glad that she is back to being relatively normal.

Robin's Story

I first saw Robin 13 years ago, when she was 28 years old. She is now 41. Her family history consisted of health issues associated with thyroid (goiter) and autoimmune diseases (lupus erythematosus and Felty's syndrome).

Robin began her periods at age 13. They were always irregular. At age 16, she was prescribed a low dose of thyroid to combat low energy levels, irregular periods, and moodiness. At age 18, she went off the thyroid medication, feeling that she probably didn't need it. She took the birth control pill for approximately eight years, off and on. This seemed to aggravate her ongoing symptoms of PMS.

At age 26, she gave birth to her first child, and did not have postpartum depression. But after her second child was born, a year later, she did have postpartum depression. It was around that time that she came to see me. One of the doctors I work with prescribed natural progesterone. It helped stabilize her moods and control the food cravings associated with PMS and postpartum depression. She felt very well on it for a number of years.

About age 33, the progesterone wasn't working anymore. She was having severe PMS beginning at ovulation, with food cravings and insomnia the week before her period. The week after ovulation was the worst; then, a day or so before her period, she felt a sudden calm, and her depression lifted. However, only one or two days into the flow, her symptoms returned, and she felt as though she were on a roller coaster. She was having symptoms most of the month, but they were at their worst before her period. I suggested that she try estrogen because of the symptoms at the end of her period. She did try it, and it did help.

Robin became pregnant again at age 34 and discontinued the hormones. Her pregnancy was normal, but she was extremely tired. This baby was large—10 lbs 2 oz—and, subsequently, Robin slid into postpartum depression. She was extremely fatigued and feeling depressed. At that time, she began taking a combination of estrogen, natural progesterone, and Armour thyroid. She felt considerably better until her thyroid dose was increased to 2 grains, which gave her heart palpitations. She suspected that this was due to the thyroid, but nobody was listening. One day, she and I were sitting in a restaurant, and Robin described her symptoms to me again. I took her pulse and found that it was 120! Meanwhile, she had been to the emergency room with heart palpitations. She was suffering from thyroid storm (too much thyroid medication).

At that point, Robin stopped taking thyroid, though she probably would have been fine taking a lower dose after her body settled down again. At that time, the doctor who had prescribed her thyroid medication died in an accident, and subsequently no one would prescribe thyroid for her. She was only fiddling with taking estrogen, not really trying it seriously. She was on natural progesterone for fourteen days a month, but it was not helping much.

At age 38, Robin went to her internist. She felt terrible and told him about her hormone problems. The internist sat back in his chair and said that her problem wasn't hormonal at all—that she was clinically depressed. He gave her samples of Prozac, and told her that she would be feeling fine in a few weeks.

After four days on Prozac, her husband rushed her to the emergency room; this happened twice, and she was found to have an elevated white blood cell count. She felt that the problem was the Prozac, but the doctors at the hospital wrote it off as a virus, and she was sent home. Her doctor said that she was just anxious, and that she needed Prozac, along with Xanax to calm her down and enable her to sleep. She followed this regimen for about two-and-a-half weeks, until the toxic reaction became unbearable. She had a 15-pound rapid weight loss from diarrhea (she was already thin), found herself unable to eat, and had seizures, a skin rash, insomnia, agitation, and total fatigue. At this point, she was diagnosed with chronic fatigue syndrome, and her cytomegalovirus titers were extremely elevated. Robin is convinced that Prozac adversely affected her immune and endocrine systems. She was told by a psychiatrist that she should stop taking the drug as all her symptoms indicated a toxic reaction.

She was sick for nearly a year and was passed from one specialist to another, having every medical test imaginable run to determine the cause of her problems. At that point, she went to another doctor, Dr. M., who worked in two very different practices—one regular medicine and the other alternative and nutritional. Dr. M. told her that she was severely hypothyroid. She was pasty, thin, and her blood pressure was only 90/50. She had no reflexes and was extremely fatigued. Her menstrual cycle was erratic with bleeding every 15 to 17 days.

Dr. M. described a course of action that would bring her back to health. Robin sought out new doctors, including an OB/GYN and an endocrinologist who were willing to work on her delicate health issues. Their first step was to put her back on a combination of estrogen and natural progesterone. The endocrinologist prescribed 0.05 mg of Synthroid. Dr. M. prescribed a one-week course of Diflucan to treat her yeast problems, which helped with several body processes. Along with this, she took numerous vitamin supplements.

Robin has been doing very well for the last couple of years but has to watch out for her health in the early spring—a time when may hypothyroid people feel extra low, maybe due to the colder weather. She is very grateful to have doctors who have diligently worked with her to safely regain her health.

About a month after her reaction to Prozac, Robin discovered Dr. Peter Breggin, the author of *Talking Back to Prozac* (see Recommended Reading). He gave her the telephone number of the Prozac Survivor's Support Group. Guy McConnell, the national director of this group, told her that her immune reaction was not an uncommon side effect with Prozac, which can potentially affect every body system.

In February of 1994, Robin accepted the Northern California directorship of the Prozac Survivor's Support Group. This is a nonprofit group formed to distribute information to people who are thinking of taking the drug, those who are taking it, and friends and relatives of those taking it. While many physicians have been told that this group is linked to The Church of Scientology, this is not true. The organization is made up of people who have either had a bad personal experience with Prozac-like drugs, or who have a close family member or friend who did.

While many people are grateful for the positive changes they have experienced while taking Prozac (see Laura's story), not everyone who has used it or the other SSRIs (selective serotonin re-uptake inhibitors), such as Zoloft, Paxil, and Effexor, have had a positive experience. Because so many people are being given these drugs for a wide variety of problems (they are being distributed like candy by many practitioners), the small proportion of people who have a drastic adverse reaction to them is growing.[22] Many would like to see the side effects of suicidal ideation and violent tendencies more prominently displayed on the package inserts.

I am particularly concerned because there have been quite a number of research papers written that recommend Prozac for women with PMS. Many women who are given Prozac are in their mid-thirties to mid-forties—the very women who are going through perimenopausal anxiety and depression. Some of the former leading advocates of natural progesterone are enthusiastically recommending this class of drug. While not denying the obvious help that taking Prozac has given to many people, I would like to add a cautionary note.

Prozac Survivor's Support Group, Inc.

The Prozac Survivor's Support Group, Inc., is a national non-profit organization. If you have questions about adverse events associated with taking Prozac, this group is available to answer them.

The Prozac Survivor's Support Group, Inc. has directors across the United States, in Canada, and in Europe. They have brochures available upon request, as well as an extensive packet available for $20.00. This includes scientific research, FDA studies, psychiatric reports, personal accounts, newspaper articles, and more.

To learn more about the Prozac Survivor's Support Group, Inc., please call 1-800-392-0640, or write:

Robin Berkley
P.O. Box 891
Folsom, CA 95763
or
Guy E. McConnell
96 14th Ave. N.E., Apt #C
Birmingham, AL 35215

TREATMENT FOR THYROID PROBLEMS

Experts differ in their opinions about early treatment of thyroid problems. Patients can show symptoms in the early stages of thyroiditis, even though their test results may be normal. Some doctors say that it is better to treat such patients early in order to prevent further destruction of the thyroid gland. Other doctors choose not to treat what may be a transient problem; not all people with Hashimoto's thyroiditis go on to develop full-blown hypothyroidism.

Nutritional Thyroid Boosters

In his book, *Nutrition and Vitamin Therapy,* Dr. Michael Lesser says that he prescribes organic iodine, extra vitamin B 1 (thiamine), B-complex, and vitamin E for people who have sluggish thyroid glands. He recommends kelp, seafood, and iodized salt as sources of iodine. Dr. Lesser also mentions avoiding foods that contain goitrin, an antithyroid factor: beans, beets, cabbage, carrots, lettuce, peaches, spinach, and strawberries.

It may be possible to consume too much iodine, however. While people who live in areas where iodine is deficient in the diet tend to develop goiters (swelling of the thyroid), a number of studies point out that there are higher levels of Hashimoto's thyroiditis in countries where iodine levels in the diet are high (for example, Japan, where a lot of seafood is consumed).

There are over-the-counter formulations available that contain animal thyroid hormones. Some of these may have very low levels of T3,[23] the active portion of thyroid, in them.

Drs. John Lee and Ray Peat say that using Pro-Gest® skin cream can improve the function of a sluggish thyroid,[24] but this needs the support of further studies.

When Thyroid Medication Is Needed

When there is obvious thyroid deficiency, as determined by blood tests, family and personal history, symptoms, and basal temperature, thyroid supplementation may be needed. As mentioned, some physicians (for example, Dr. Boris Catz), will treat a patient with symptoms of thyroiditis before the blood tests show a problem.[25]

Thyroid medication must be taken under the supervision of a physician. In general, however, women with symptoms of subclinical thyroid function may be started on 0.025 to 0.1 mg of Synthroid daily; and 5 mcg of Cytomel may be added if afternoon fatigue does not go away.

Different Types of Thyroid Medication   There are several forms of thyroid treatment; finding the most suitable form for each individual is important.

Some physicians prefer to prescribe animal thyroid for the same reason that they like to use conjugated animal estrogens; they are more "natural" than synthetic thyroid, and they contain all the types of thyroid hormone that a human produces, along with the hormone calcitonin.

Dr. Broda Barnes, who helped develop Armour thyroid (an animal-based thyroid medication), felt that his patients did much better on Armour than on Synthroid. In fact, the Barnes Foundation has used the 24-hour urine test since 1984, and finds that desiccated animal thyroid is more readily utilized in the body than the synthetic kind. They feel that there is a greater bioequivalency with the natural thyroid.[26]

On the other hand, animal thyroid is only "natural" for the animal that produces it, and humans can produce antibodies to it. This can produce side effects, probably because the hormone cell receptors can detect the difference.

Synthetic thyroid medication usually contains only one type of thyroid hormone, such as T3 or T4. Many pharmacists and physicians prefer synthetic forms of thyroid medication because the dosage is more reliable. They say that animal thyroid tablets vary in strength, depending on which animal they are taken from. They also believe that a synthetic thyroid hormone, such as Synthroid, is a good copy of human thyroid hormone. Animal thyroid works immediately, but Synthroid takes five to six weeks to reach its optimal effect with each dosage change. In this respect, synthetic thyroid more closely resembles the way human thyroid works.

When women take Synthroid (T4) their bodies should normally break it down into T3. In some women, the enzyme that does this (5-deiodinase) is missing, and this breakdown does not take place. They may need to also take Cytomel (synthetic T3).

Precautions in Taking Thyroid Medication

Many physicians are understandably cautious about prescribing thyroid medication. Taking thyroid above certain doses can cause the pituitary gland to cease production of thyroxine and create the need to take thyroid indefinitely—and this "certain dose" is different for every individual. Moreover, overmedication with thyroid can affect the heart and bones adversely. And if a woman who is manic-depressive takes too much thyroid, it can push her into a manic phase. The ideal amount to give is that which normalizes but does not suppress the TSH levels.

Experimenting with different doses and types of thyroid medication may be necessary, but all dose changes should be done with the full knowledge and consent of your physician. While physicians who use progesterone for PMS encourage women to experiment with their dosage, they don't encourage women to change their thyroid dosage at will. The potential side effects of thyroid overdose are much more serious than those from progesterone.

Taking too much thyroid medication can lead to "thyroid storm," characterized by rapid heart rate, potentially leading to a heart attack. Long-term thyroid overdose may cause osteoporosis,[27] though opinions vary on this.[28] Again, adjustment of thyroid doses should never be treated casually, and should be monitored by a physician.

Some women with PMS will benefit immensely from thyroid treatment, but it is critical that they regularly check their pulse and temperature, which both tend to rise if the dosage is too high. Occasional blood tests to monitor thyroid levels are also wise.

Denise Mark, M.D., on Thyroid   Dr. Mark uses thyroid replacement therapy, based on both a patient's blood tests and their symptoms. She says that it is not uncommon to see low-normal T4 and high-normal TSH levels in women with mild hypothyroid symptoms. She finds that a small amount of thyroid replacement can be beneficial to many women.

As a general rule, it is better not to oversuppress the TSH level by using thyroid treatment (taking thyroid tends to lower the TSH). However, Dr. Mark finds that sometimes it's necessary to do this in order for the patient to maintain a good quality of life. In many years of practice, she has had no clinical problems among patients on thyroid treatment who have suppressed TSH levels. She makes sure they have no symptoms of thyroid overdose and regularly monitors their bone density to be sure that osteoporosis is not a problem; so far, it hasn't been.

Dr. Mark also uses natural progesterone and androgens to support the thyroid medication where necessary.

Be Aware of Possible Side Effects   Because the doctors I work with use small doses only, they rarely see serious side effects from thyroid overdose. But they do caution women to watch for signs and symptoms.

When beginning to take thyroid medication, patients may experience more rapid heart rate as the medication stimulates their heart. They may feel nervous, have insomnia, get severe headaches, experience a rise in body temperature and pulse rate, or notice a reddening of their hands and feet as the blood rushes to their extremities. These symptoms may be temporary and due to the sudden stimulation of the heart by the extra thyroid, or they can be ongoing and indicate an overdose.

If a patient initially experiences fatigue, the dosage is increased slowly. Sometimes the thyroid gland becomes sore and tender. If heart palpitations, nervousness, and irritability occur, the patient is advised to stop taking the medication for three days, then try again. If the symptoms recur, the patient should again stop taking the medication for three days and then begin again on a miminal dose.

Treatment for the APICH Syndrome

The APICH syndrome is essentially thyroiditis, oophoritis (ovarian inflammation), and associated immune system problems (see Chapter 8, The Thyroid Link). Drs. Nathan Becker and Phyllis Saifer treat women with symptoms of the APICH syndrome as follows: L-thyroxine (Synthroid, T4) is given in small doses at first (0.025 mg), and the dosage is gradually increased over four to six weeks to 0.15 mg or 0.2 mg daily (approximately 80 percent of body weight). That is, if you weigh 150 pounds, you would take approximately 1.25 mg of Synthroid (the closest easy increment to 1.2 mg, which is 80 percent of 150).

For people who build up excessive levels of T4 (the main thyroid hormone the body produces) and do not convert T4 to T3, a low dose of T3 (Cytomel) may be added to provide instant energy and relieve afternoon fatigue.[29] Rarely, a patient with the APICH syndrome may develop Graves' disease. There are rare patients with the APICH syndrome whose thyroiditis and high antibody levels are not kept under control by L-thyroxine, and who require a total thyroidectomy with subsequent thyroid replacement therapy.

Other Treatments for Women with the APICH Syndrome For women who have severe allergies, immunization therapy has sometimes been helpful.

Women with cyclical, PMS-type symptoms may need treatment with natural progesterone or a combination of estrogen and natural progesterone.

Because of their history of allergy, infection, and menstrual problems, many women with APICH syndrome have been on the birth control pill or on repeated antibiotics. This may have allowed yeast overgrowth (candidiasis), causing numerous problems, including repeated vaginal infections. Where there is evidence of yeast-related problems, a trial of oral Nystatin has been used for three weeks with success. There are many natural antifungal agents available without prescription from health food stores.

Use of Treatments for Autoimmune Problems Various researchers are using cyclosporin, gamma globulin, and Depo-Medrol to treat polyglandular autoimmune problems, but these are considered controversial treatments.[30] Cyclosporin is a chemical compound that acts as an antiviral antibody and is used to inhibit organ-rejection in transplant patients. Gamma globulin is part of the blood that supports immunity.

Norman Beals, Jr., M.D., (now retired) used to give a course of injections of Depo-Medrol (a cousin of cortisone) to women who show evidence of having antibodies. He doesn't try this unless standard therapies fail. He says:

> In adults, chronic diseases often don't respond to standard medical treatment. With those who don't respond to normal hormone replacement, we individualize their treatment with

higher doses of hormones. If that doesn't work, we then attempt to treat their autoimmune problems.

After prescribing six to eight weeks of hormone treatments for a woman patient, he may add Depo-Medrol injections if it seems as though antibodies are attacking the hormone supplements. This is not a commonly accepted practice, but it may be helpful information for some women.

Dr. Beals recommends three to six 0.5-cc injections of Depo-Medrol weekly. He learned this technique years ago from Dr. Robert Greenblatt, a famous U.S. hormone pioneer. He finds that Depo-Medrol works successfully and rapidly by reducing the sensitivity of the antibodies. In most cases, this corrects the problem. On a few occasions, Dr. Beals has had to give a couple of repeat shots.

Thyroid Problems Associated with Other Hormonal Problems

Pat Puglio of the Broda Barnes Foundation agrees that hormonal problems often coexist with other disorders:

> Certain other cases of menstrual disorders may need more than thyroid therapy alone. Some women with PMS, excessive blood flow, or irregular menses may need estrogen and/or progesterone therapy along with thyroid, in which cases we use only the natural forms of estrogen and progesterone. Others may show some degree of adrenal insufficiency, which may need to be treated along with the thyroid and ovarian deficiencies.[31]

CHAPTER

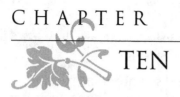

TEN

PERIMENOPAUSE
AND MENOPAUSE

 Paula is a 35-year-old woman who had a sudden
onset of panic attacks two months prior to seeing
me. She had only had one previous attack 14 years
before. The recent panic attacks typically began when she was
driving, and they either occurred premenstrually or on the
first day of her period. These episodes were severe enough to
warrant going to the emergency room.

When the panic attacks occurred, Paula would experience
a sudden physical change, with exhaustion, a fear that she was
dying, heart palpitations, and mental depression. Each time her
menstrual cycle passed, the problem disappeared.

When she went to her doctor, he did extensive bloodwork,
including checking her thyroid. Everything was normal. The
doctor diagnosed her as having panic attacks and depression
due to life stress. Initially, he gave her Trazodone and Librium.
Even after adjusting the dose, these only worked for a short
time. Then he switched her to Zoloft, but she had severe and
immediate side effects. She tried it more than once and gave
up. Then the doctor put her on Tofranil, but she found that the
side effects, mainly drowsiness, were worse than the problem.

232

When we looked at Paula's history, there was no excessive stress, sexual abuse, physical injury, or trauma—all common factors in panic attacks. There were some symptoms of hypothyroidism, and her mother was on thyroid medication at age 20 for a few years. At the age of 18, Paula was diagnosed as having polycystic ovaries, also called Stein Levanthal syndrome. She had a wedge resection done to treat this problem, and her symptoms (weight gain, irregular periods, and body hair) seemed to resolve themselves. She subsequently had normal periods and four fairly normal pregnancies, but the last pregnancy was more difficult because of gestational diabetes in the seventh month.

I asked a specialist if the wedge resection Paula had in her teens could result in early menopause. He said that it was a wonder she didn't have problems much sooner, since often one- to two-thirds of the ovaries are removed in wedge resections. He concluded that she might be borderline hypothyroid, and that she was probably premenopausal because of the surgery.

Women often begin having panic attacks in their mid-thirties. Panic attacks are a multifactorial problem. Sometimes they are related to the revival of memories of early abuse or trauma. Or too much stress and not enough rest can increase the output of adrenaline and cortisol. This can lead to adrenal depletion or burnout, bringing panic attacks and adrenal hot flashes.

But panic is often part of a gestalt of perimenopausal symptoms that occur as hormone levels decline. There is usually some hormonal event in the past that has triggered the present problem. In Paula's case, it was probably her early wedge resection. Women like Paula often respond poorly to antidepressants and tranquilizers, since such treatments can only mask the real problem of hormone deficiency.

Sometimes the presenting symptom in a premenopausal woman will be panic attacks, but yours might be quite different. If you suspect that you are having premenopausal changes, read on and find out about the common symptoms that occur in the years before and during menopause.

THE STAGES OF MENOPAUSE

Menopause is the point of time in a woman's life when her menstrual periods cease. On average, this happens at the age of 51.4 years, but there is a wide range. Some women go through premature natural menopause before the age of 40. Others go through surgical menopause at an early age. At the other end of the spectrum, about 5 percent of women go through menopause between ages 55 and 60.

Diet can affect the age when menstruation begins and ends, because menstruation is not triggered until a woman's body achieves a certain proportion of body fat. Women who eat more animal fat tend to start menstruating earlier and to finish later than those who are on a vegetarian diet.

Premenopause is the phase before menopause actually takes place, when ovarian hormone production is declining. This process can last for as long as 5 to 15 years. Perimenopause is the 3 to 4 year span around the menopause; premenopause is a broader term. Women who are premenopausal and perimenopausal often have more symptoms than postmenopausal women whose hormones have leveled out. These women with early problems are often told that they are too young for menopause, and their hormonal symptoms are often overlooked or ignored.

What You Might Experience During Premenopause

There is a relatively small number of women who hardly notice any changes at menopause. Their periods just stop overnight, and they have few if any symptoms. But many women who haven't previously experienced hormonal problems begin to notice premenopausal changes between the ages of 35 and 45, and occasionally even younger. As a woman's ovaries gradually decrease in function, she can begin having a number of disturbing symptoms. These include mood swings, panic attacks, sleep disturbances with frequent awakenings, depression, changes in tolerance of temperature change, joint pain, fibromyalgia (muscle pain), and onset of allergies, headaches, or migraines. These symptoms of early estrogen deficiency sometimes occur even though the FSH level is still normal and menstrual periods are still regular.

Changes in Cycle and Flow in Pre- and Perimenopause

Women's cycles (counting from day one of a flow to day one of the next flow) can become shorter or longer, or both alternately, as menopause approaches. When estrogen levels begin to drop during the first half of the menstrual cycle, the follicular phase may be shortened from about 14 days to about 10 days. This can shorten the total cycle length from 28–30 days to 24–26 days, resulting in more frequent periods. Sometimes women will start bleeding immediately after an unsuccessful ovulation and have two periods a month. If they also get longer, heavier flow at this time, they may feel that they are always bleeding.

On the other hand, some women begin having longer cycles (over 40 days) because they are not ovulating as frequently. Or their cycles may become very irregular; they may go several months without bleeding. Some women's flow may change, with lighter, more watery bleeding and less clotting due to reduced estrogen levels. These women tend to have breakthrough bleeding, with premenstrual, postmenstrual, or mid-cycle spotting. Or the opposite can happen; about 10 percent of women begin to bleed very heavily, to the point of hemorrhage, with unpleasant clotting for several days. This is due to temporarily high estrogen- levels—the last hurrah as menopause approaches—accompanied by low progesterone levels as ovulation fails.

Though these erratic changes aren't really "normal," they are so common at menopause that they are almost thought of as normal.

When Is Menopause Complete?

When menstrual periods have not occurred for a full year, menopause is considered complete. A blood test of the levels of FSH (follicle-stimulating hormone) can confirm that a woman has passed through menopause. FSH levels are very high before puberty. During the menstrual years, FSH levels vary depending on the time in the cycle, with the highest level at ovulation. After menopause, FSH levels can rise to over 100 mIU/ml. FSH levels often begin to increase once a woman is in her thirties or forties. Once the levels are over 40 mIU/ml, a woman is considered menopausal. But an elevated FSH does not guarantee that a woman could not suddenly ovulate and become pregnant. It is smart to continue using birth control for a year or two after bleeding ceases.

Why is there any risk of ovulation? According to Leon Speroff, M.D., the luteinizing hormone (LH) level also rises at menopause, but it does so about a decade later and only to about one-third of the level that the FSH rises to.[1] Until the LH level is also elevated to about 30 to 40 mIU/ml, a woman might still occasionally ovulate.

The readings for FSH and LH are best done on the first day of the menstrual cycle. At ovulation in a young woman, FSH can rise to 30 mIU/ml, and LH can rise to 100 mIU/ml, so you could easily get a false reading of menopause if blood is drawn mid-cycle.

What Happens After Menopause

When the last menstrual period occurs, the ovaries stop their major production of estradiol, the main female estrogen. Medicine has described typical postmenstrual symptom progression as follows: menstrual periods cease at about age 51; hot flashes begin at about age 52; vaginal dryness occurs at about age 53; bladder problems and incontinence appear at about age 55; and osteoporosis and heart disease begin at about age 58. You should remember that this is a textbook ideal of the average menopause. It is like the textbook pregnancy—doctors remark on it when it happens, because it is relatively rare.

In reality, many women have more symptoms during premenopause, and find that when they finally reach menopause they feel better. This is why there are always two audiences at a talk on menopause: some are premenopausal and have mood swings, assortments of pain, and bleeding concerns; others are postmenopausal, often no longer experience mood swings, and are not interested in "all that hormonal stuff," but are concerned about osteoporosis and heart disease.

It is interesting that the women who seek me out for help with their hormones are usually the ones experiencing symptoms in their thirties and forties. The postmenopausal group is mainly finished with the type of symptoms I commonly see in younger women. These younger women seek help because medicine generally has not yet embraced the hormonal connections among the headaches, mood swings, panic attacks, and joint and muscle pains that women commonly get in their thirties and forties. It's as though premenopausal women are invisible.

Medicine generally views osteoporosis and heart disease as problems confined to older women. At the clinic where I work, we recently did a bone mineral density test on two young women age 27. Both had full-blown osteoporosis, though they were not thin and looked perfectly healthy on the outside. There is an epidemic of bone loss in younger women for a variety of reasons (refer to the sections on osteoporosis later in this chapter for more information). These reasons include an emphasis on thinness that leads to frequent dieting, insufficient calorie consumption, anorexia, bulimia, and overexercise. And remember that heart disease is the leading cause of death in women from age 40 to 65. Age 40 is pretty young!

So it doesn't pay to think about menopause in too narrow a time frame. The issues that are involved really span decades.

What Is Happening?

As menopause approaches, the ovaries begin to fail as the number of eggs decreases. Estrogen levels are dropping. Low levels of circulating estrogen may cause the pituitary gland to compensate by producing high levels of FSH. The high FSH level then overstimulates the few remaining eggs and causes high levels of estrogen. Estrogen dominance at this time of life is a temporary phenomenon. It precedes and heralds the ultimate estrogen low at menopause. But while these changes take place, estrogen levels can swing dramatically from low to high, and back again.

If the estrogen level is too high or too low, ovulation may not occur, and the progesterone level becomes low or nonexistent. Sometimes the corpus luteum (yellow patch left on the ovary after ovulation) will remain on the egg and grow into a large ovarian cyst, producing excessive levels of progesterone. So progesterone levels can also fluctuate.

Menstrual periods will tend to reflect specific hormonal changes. Low estrogen levels will cause menstrual bleeding to become lighter and lighter, sometimes with spotting between periods. High levels of estrogen will cause heavy, clotted bleeding, especially if progesterone levels are low.

Women with heavy menstrual periods, or those who go for months at a time without periods, would both probably benefit from taking progesterone. If they are producing high levels of estrogen and not ovulating, they may develop endometrial hyperplasia (abnormal thickening of the lining of the uterus) and be at risk for developing endometrial cancer.

How Long Does Menopause Last?

The amount of time it takes for a woman to complete the process of menopause varies a great deal. Perimenopause can begin and end quickly; a woman may suddenly cease to have periods and show no other symptoms of menopause. At the other extreme, menopause can last 35 years or more; some women experience hot flashes years before their periods cease and still have them in their seventies.

MENOPAUSE OCCURS IN A VARIETY OF WAYS

The average lifespan of American women has increased dramatically over the last few decades, with the result that a larger number of women are facing the changes associated with menopause and are confronted with its problems. While most women, today, expect to go through menopause, their individual passage through it varies tremendously. The following are examples of the variety of ways in which women experience menopause:

The Fortunate Few

Some women live their whole lives without knowing what hormonal problems are like. They breeze through their periods, don't experience premenstrual syndrome, have little trouble during or after pregnancy, and may go on the pill, have a tubal ligation, or have a hysterectomy—all without side effects. About one women in ten goes through menopause overnight, just ceasing to have periods and having no associated symptoms. They are the fortunate few.

The Average Experience

The typical woman experiences some discomfort through menopause and is aware of hormonal changes in her body, but these changes do not disrupt her life. Her periods may come late or early and they may be short or long, light or heavy; they may stop and start spasmodically, or vanish for months and return. Such a woman may experience some discomfort from hot flashes, and have depression, mood swings, insomnia, and loss of sexual drive. The average woman may complete menopause within a couple of years.

Women with Previous Hormonal Problems

Other women may have had hormonal problems, starting with PMS, since puberty. Their mothers and grandmothers had PMS; their sisters, aunts, and cousins all have the familiar pattern of cyclical symptoms before their periods. Some women who suffer from years of PMS go through the transition of menopause very easily, but for some PMS sufferers, menopause marks a worsening and deepening of the hormonal problems they've battled for many years.

A Drastic Change

Some women have sudden and drastic menopause at a younger age than usual, as a result of one or more of the following events:

1. **Hysterectomy or ovarian surgery** (removal of ovary, uterus, fallopian tubes, or any combination of these).
2. **Tubal ligation** (some methods seem to lead to premature menopause). Other abdominal surgery that affects the ovarian blood supply can also trigger problems.
3. **Ovarian failure** (8 to 10 percent of women experience spontaneous menopause before the age of 40, some for genetic reasons, and others go through it as a consequence of autoimmune disease).
4. **Chemotherapy** (used in treating cancer, including the use of Tamoxifen for breast cancer).
5. **The use of Lupron or Synarel** to treat endometriosis (these induce instant chemical menopause, and the effect is occasionally long-term).

The Late Shocker

Some women who have never experienced PMS or postpartum depression, and who are going through menopause "naturally," are unpleasantly surprised, at about age 50, by strong hot flashes, night sweats, fatigue, muscle aches, and a host of other physical problems. Emotional problems, such as depression, irritability, anxiety, and phobias, may also occur, and the mental anguish can be severe. Menopause can also herald the onset of alcoholism, and a few women may attempt or achieve suicide.

EGG SUPPLY, FROM THE FETUS TO MENOPAUSE

Before a female baby is born, all the eggs she will ever have are already present in her ovaries. Production of oocytes, which will eventually mature into eggs, begins in the female fetus at six to seven weeks gestation. Halfway through the pregnancy, at 20 weeks, the baby has six to seven million eggs. These begin to die off and form scar tissue through a little-understood process called atresia, beginning at 15 weeks gestation.

At birth, the baby girl has already lost 80 percent of her eggs. She may have from 500,000 to 5,000,000 eggs in her ovaries (these figures vary depending on the source of information). Different women are born with different numbers of eggs; the number may depend on a combination of genetic factors and early injuries to the ovary.

The egg supply continues to decline. By puberty another 80 percent have been lost, and the numbers are down to about 200,000 to 300,000 eggs. With each menstrual cycle, between 20 and 1,000 eggs are called to the surface of the ovary. Most of these eggs produce estrogen and die. Only one or two eggs per cycle come to maturity.

Ovulation is a monthly miracle that many women take for granted. Estrogen levels ebb and flow like the tide during the follicular phase of the cycle before ovulation. Androgens in the ovaries battle for supremacy over the estrogen surge. Many factors can tip the balance, including stress and a woman's weight. Estrogen has to be at a certain level (not too high, not too low), for about five hours in order for ovulation to take place. That it does so routinely each month in many women is a miracle. Some women are so regular, and their cycles so predictable during their menstrual years, that if their flow varies at all, they are on the phone to their doctors to see if something is wrong.

More Ovulations This Century

In previous generations, women had more pregnancies and fewer ovulations and menstrual periods than do women today—only about 40 to 50 during their lifetime. Now, because of birth control, women have fewer pregnancies and more periods—about 400 to 500 in their lifetime. Every time women ovulate, they can lose hundreds of eggs. Reason suggests that this can induce estrogen levels to go into an earlier decline. Women still often go through menopause in their late forties or fifties, but more women seem to be going through it earlier. And the gradual decline in their estrogen levels may begin 10 or 15 years before their periods actually stop.

Some Reasons for Early Menopause

As we mentioned earlier, the average age for women going through menopause naturally is about 51.4 years, but a small proportion of women at both ends of the scale stop having their periods earlier or later. I have met women who naturally stopped menstruating as early as ages 27, 28, and 31. Their mothers and grandmothers stopped at a similar age, so there is a genetic factor.

Leon Speroff, M.D., Winnifred Cutler, Ph.D., and Christiane Northrup, M.D., report that less than one percent of all women spontaneously and abruptly stop having menstrual periods before age 40.[2] According to Lila Nachtigall, M.D., about 8 to 11 percent of women stop having their periods before age 40.[3]

These figures probably include some women who have not actually gone through menopause, but whose ovaries are not working because their hypothalamus gland function has been suppressed. (This happens sometimes with overexercise and stress.) Definitive studies would require a thorough endocrine workup with blood tests to find out exactly what was happening. I doubt that this is usually done.

Autoimmunity and Premature Ovarian Failure

Any event that damages the ovary can lead to early menopausal changes. One source of damage is coexisting autoimmune disease. The autoimmune process may not be primarily attacking the ovaries; the process may be happening elsewhere in the body, but it can destroy the ovaries if they contain similar target tissue. You may read more about this in Chapter 8, The Thyroid Link.

New Research on Mitochondrial DNA Damage

Gradual change in the mitochondrial DNA is another factor currently being researched in connection with ovarian failure. Like nuclear DNA, another form of genetic material, mitochondrial DNA is found in every cell of the body, including the cytoplasm of the ovary. However, mitochondrial DNA is only transmitted from mother to child and is not passed on by a son; his children will carry the mitochondrial DNA of their mother.

Research is presently being done on damage to particular organs as a result of genetic deletions (missing information) in the mitochondrial DNA. The tendency to have these deletions in the genetic code is passed from a mother to her children, and the deletions become more apparent with advancing age. Oxidation from chemical processes occurring in the body hastens this damage. And mitochondrial DNA does not have the needed mechanisms to fix the damage.

Deletions in the mitochondrial DNA are being linked to Alzheimer's Disease (three times more common in women than in men), other brain deterioration diseases, and some types of diabetes and heart disease.

Our particular interest here is in the ovary. There is a theory that mitochondrial DNA damage in the cytoplasm of the ovary contributes to infertility and early ovarian failure, but this theory is not yet substantiated.

The autoimmune connection with early menopause and the issue of damage to the mitochondrial DNA are both relatively new areas of study. They are important because they show us that there are complex reasons for perimenopausal change that science is only beginning to explore.

Surgical Menopause

Many women go through "premature menopause" after having a tubal ligation, which may damage the ovarian artery—though this is heavily debated. The resulting reduced blood flow lessens the amount of FSH reaching the ovary, causing a decrease in ovarian estrogen production.[4]

Other women become premenopausal or menopausal after having their uterus removed.[5] Approximately half of all women in the U.S. have a hysterectomy by the age of 60, and the average age for hysterectomy is 35.[6]

Women losing both ovaries will obviously suffer from estrogen deficiency unless they take estrogen replacement therapy. Some women who have a hysterectomy but retain their ovaries will also have estrogen deficiency. Others who even have a fallopian tube or part of the ovary removed may experience premature menopause.

At one time, women were told that if a portion of one ovary was left after a hysterectomy, it would produce adequate estrogen until menopause. This is not usually true. During removal of the uterus, a portion of the uterine/ovarian artery is severed, which means that up to 65 percent of the blood flow to the ovary is diminished. Since hormones travel through the bloodstream from the pituitary to the ovary, this can affect the hormone levels of some women.

The Issue Is Estrogen Deficiency

It may be more helpful to think in terms of estrogen deficiency, which is a process, than to use the term *menopause,* which is a point in time. Estrogen deficiency can occur much earlier than menopause.

SOME TYPICAL PERIMENOPAUSAL SYMPTOMS

- Changes in bleeding (heavy bleeding, irregular cycles, missed cycles, light bleeding, clotting)
- Anxiety, fear, depression, irritability, anger, rebellion, crying jags, panic attacks
- Fatigue, loss of energy
- Low self-esteem
- Suicidal thinking
- Inability to tolerate frustration
- Inappropriate emotional responses
- Low noise tolerance
- Sleep disturbances, insomnia, sleepiness
- Inability to concentrate, confusion, short-term memory loss

- Drying and thinning of the gastrointestinal tract (causing constipation, ulceration, stomach pain, colitis, diarrhea, gas)
- Bladder infections, frequency and urgency of urination, burning, incontinence
- Vaginal dryness
- Low sex drive, painful intercourse, reduction of fantasy, lack of lubrication during sex, diminished orgasms, lessened skin and nipple response
- Hot flashes, night sweats, chills
- Dizziness
- Low blood sugar, trembling
- Numbness, tingling, crawling feelings on skin
- Dry, wrinkling skin; loss of collagen, sagging breasts
- Dry, thinning hair; growth of facial hair, male pattern of hair on body
- Brittle, slow-growing, and grooved nails
- Osteoarthritis, bone thinning and loss, loss of height, shifting joint pains, joint degeneration, backache, mid-bone pains, muscle cramps and spasms, muscle weakness, and loss of strength
- Rapid heart rate, palpitations, heart pain, increased cholesterol levels, high blood pressure, shortness of breath
- Headaches, migraines, nausea
- Dark, gloomy circles under the eyes
- Weight loss or gain

SPECIFIC SYMPTOMS AND PROBLEMS

The Hot Flash

Most women experience hot flashes during menopause. Some authorities say that two out of three perimenopausal and menopausal women have hot flashes; others say three out of four, others say nine out of ten. Half of the women who experience hot flashes stop having them within a year. Another third stop having them in two or three years. Other women may have them for five, ten, fifteen, or even twenty years. Two to three percent have them until the day they die.

Some women may have one flash a month or one a week. Other have flashes three or four times a day. Others have 30, 40, or more a day, one after another. Some women feel the flash mainly in their face, some from their chest up, others from their feet up. Hot flashes last from a few seconds to five minutes. They vary from a mildly warm feeling to a very uncomfortable, "volcanic" heat accompanied by profuse sweating and followed by chills. They are often associated with dizziness and heart palpitations.

Hot flashes are usually worse at night, developing into night sweats. Some women become so badly soaked with sweat that they have to change their nightclothes and bedding more than once each night.

The variation in severity among women explains why some women speak of their hot flashes with fondness, and others find them incapacitating and embarrassing.

Hot flashes may be due more to changes in levels of luteinizing hormone (LH) or norepinephrine than to lack of estrogen. But women born without ovaries, or those with nonfunctioning ovaries, do not experience hot flashes. Taking estrogen usually stops hot flashes, so the theory is of little practical consequence.

Migraines and Fibromyalgia

Dr. Elizabeth Lee Vliet, in her excellent book *Screaming to Be Heard: Hormonal Connections Women Suspect and Doctors Ignore* (see Recommended Reading), has a number of chapters dealing with connections between chronic pain and hormonal issues. She particularly mentions women with hormonal migraines and fibromyalgia.

Dr. Vliet points out that migraines are four times more common in women than in men. Typically, onset is at puberty and they disappear at menopause. The migraines almost always worsen around the two days before and the first two days of menstruation. Yet the connection between hormones, particularly estrogen, and migraines is rarely made, even in books on migraines. There are many triggers of migraines, including stress and food reactions. And estrogen treatment, usually with equine estrogens, can actually bring on migraines in some women. But other women find proper hormone balancing, especially the proper use of the more natural human forms of estrogen, tremendously helpful in treating their migraines and headaches.

Dr. Vliet has had a lot of success in treating women with native human estrogen—17-beta estradiol—and using Imitrex for acute episodes. Many of these women have previously been on four or five medications at a time for migraines, and the improvement is quite dramatic. This approach is also less costly.

Fibromyalgia syndrome (FMS) is the name currently used for chronic, diffuse, aching pain that involves the muscles and the connective (fibrous) tissues of the body (the tendons and ligaments). The symptoms include generalized stiffness, numbness, and soreness, which are often worse in the morning. The pain often radiates from the neck, trunk, and hips, but women may have sharp, tender points in places where the muscles and tendons meet. Fatigue and loss of energy, changes in mood, and loss of concentration often accompany the pain.

Dr. Vliet notes that 80 percent of FMS patients are women, and FMS typically begins in women over age 30 after some hormonal event. She finds that these women are typically low in estradiol and testosterone. Restoring hormonal balance, in addition to other treatments, helps significantly to decrease pain and improve sleep.

I recommend that you read Dr. Vliet's excellent book for more details on these two important subjects; I don't believe you will find the information she offers anywhere else.

Osteoporosis—Holes in the Bones

Osteoporosis is a well-known medical term that describes the loss of bone-mineral density and consequent brittleness of the bones that increases the risk of fracture. Most women are familiar with the word and know that osteoporosis is a common problem, particularly in aging women. Osteoporosis is the most common disease in women past menopause; it is the third greatest killer of women over age 60. Women can die as a result of osteoporosis if their bones don't heal, and they need prolonged bed rest after hip fracture surgery. Lying down and being sedentary reduces breathing capacity and reduces oxygen consumption, making a person more prone to getting pneumonia, heart failure, or strokes. Fifteen to twenty percent of women who have hip surgery due to osteoporosis die within three months. Pneumonia can also occur in women with rib fractures or vertebral collapse because of constriction of the lungs.

While osteoporosis has received a lot of media coverage, the real impact of osteoporosis on health and morbidity is still not fully grasped. This is a complex and important subject, which I am only briefly addressing. If you wish to read about it further, I recommend reading *Menopause: A Guide for Women and the Men Who Love Them,* by Winnifred Cutler, Ph.D., and Celso-Ramón García, M.D., *Screaming to Be Heard: Hormonal Connections Women Suspect and Doctors Ignore,* by Elizabeth Lee Vliet, M.D., and *Reversing Osteoporosis,* by Alan Gaby, M.D. (see Recommended Reading at back of book).

The Importance of Your Bones   Bone is a living, constantly changing tissue. We think of it as being solid, but in fact it is spongy and contains holes like Swiss cheese. Blood vessels and nerves enter and exit the bone, and the bloodstream constantly carries calcium and other nutrients in and out. Bone is continually built up and broken down. It contains osteoblasts (bone-builders) and osteoclasts (bone-chewers). After menopause, when estrogen levels drop and calcium is poorly absorbed, there are more osteoclasts and fewer osteoblasts. The osteoclast (chewing) activity increases and the osteoblast (building) activity decreases. This leads to bone loss.

How much bone loss you experience will depend on many factors, including your heredity, your hormone levels, your early and continuing diet, how much you have exercised, and other lifestyle habits. Peak bone mass occurs before age 35. Some women never attain their optimum level of bone mass and begin losing bone relatively early in life.

Achieving and maintaining optimum bone density is critical. It's obvious if you think about it; your skeleton is the frame that everything else hangs on. If the skeleton shrinks and breaks, the muscles and organs contained inside it become compressed, and the body cannot function efficiently.

What Happens Physically to Women with Osteoporosis A backache in the lower part of the spine may be the first symptom of osteoporosis. A woman in her late fifties might fracture one of her small bones—the wrist, the forearm, or the ankle. About age 60, she might have a break or collapse of one or more vertebrae at the places where the spine naturally curves. Her rib cage then ends up resting on her pelvis, which results in loss of height, deformity, and changes in posture. This compresses her lungs and heart and can make it more difficult to breathe.

The femur is the long bone of the thigh. The femur neck, near where it fits into the hip socket, carries most of the weight of the upper body. It can become so weak that even a slight bump can fracture it. Many women fall after a hip fracture, not the other way around.

A woman with full-blown osteoporosis can break a vertebra while being hugged. She can break a rib taking a casserole out of the oven. She can break her arm zipping up her dress. She can break her foot stepping out of bed. She can develop a dowager's hump and be bent over with her head jutting forward. She may have to walk like a bird with her legs spread, walking on tiptoe because of spinal compression.

Young Women Also at Risk for Osteoporosis The above description is a picture of osteoporosis among the elderly, and most hip fractures occur past age 65. But osteoporosis is not just an aging woman's problem. It can occur among young women under a variety of circumstances: if they have an eating disorder such as anorexia or bulimia; if they overexercise (marathoners are a good example); if they don't ovulate and their periods are very irregular or missing; if they diet frequently and never attain their peak bone mass due to lack of calories; if they are on long-term therapy with cortisone; or if they have poor habits, such as being sedentary, smoking, or using too much alcohol or caffeine. A variety of other factors can also cause osteoporosis in the young, such as long-term use (six months or more) of gonadotropin-releasing hormone analogs for treating endometriosis.

According to Elizabeth Lee Vliet, M.D., and Denise Mark, M.D., who perform routine bone-density tests on pre-menopausal women at risk, there is an epidemic of bone loss among young women.

Osteoporosis Statistics

- 25 million people in the U.S. have osteoporosis.
- 20 million of the people with osteoporosis are women; 5 million are men.
- Osteoporosis afflicts up to one-third of American women over the age of 60.
- Less then 1 percent of the people who have osteoporosis currently receive proper treatment.
- Osteoporosis is the most common health problem in women who have passed menopause.
- Osteoporosis is the number-three killer of women over age 60.
- Osteoporotic hip fractures occur in 30 percent of all women over age 65 who don't receive hormone replacement therapy.
- By age 85, 33 percent of all women will have had a hip fracture.
- After a hip fracture, about 15 percent of women die within three to four months; 15 percent end up in long-term institutional care; 25 to 35 percent become dependent on family or others.
- One in four women over 60 can expect to suffer at least one broken bone as a consequence of osteoporosis.
- Twenty-five percent of women will have periodontal disease (a form of osteoporosis) at age 60. Forty percent of women aged 60 will have lost all their teeth. Periodontal disease is a form of osteoporosis.
- Each year, in the U.S., osteoporosis causes 1.3 million fractures, 250,000 broken hips, over 540,000 vertebral fractures and 240,000 wrist fractures.
- The average woman has lost 30 percent of her hip bone by the time she reaches menopause.

- The incidence of fractures rises dramatically with increasing age.
- The main bone loss occurs in the two or three years after menopause or hysterectomy.
- At least 25 percent of women have marked osteoporosis by age 58. Some sources say 50 percent have osteoporosis by age 50.
- By age seventy, 50 percent of all women will have had vertebral compression fractures (of the spine) due to osteoporosis.
- A woman at age 80 can have lost 40 percent of her bone mass.
- Among women with osteoporosis, 88 percent will experience a fracture at some time, and 98 percent will eventually have hip fractures.
- Over 60,000 women a year die from complications of osteoporosis.
- The cost of treating osteoporosis exceeds $10 million annually in the U.S.

Your Diet and Your Bones   It is important to reach optimal bone mass by age 30, and a major factor is your diet. Diet throughout life is important, but it is particularly important in childhood and the teenage years, because calcium loss is experienced much earlier if the diet is poor. Women who consume large quantities of animal products, particularly in their childhood, teens, and twenties, pave the way for bone problems in later years. When more than 15 percent of the diet consists of protein, the kidneys require seven times as much water as normal to excrete it. As a result, minerals in the bones, including calcium, are flushed out with the urine, and this bone damage from calcium loss is irreversible.

Smoking Affects Your Bones   Smokers have lower estrogen levels than nonsmokers because smoking causes the liver to metabolize estrogen faster; smokers generally go through menopause three or four years earlier than nonsmokers. If women who smoke take hormone replacement therapy, they get little or no benefit from it[7] and will have a high incidence of osteoporosis. (Ninety-four percent of women with spinal collapse are smokers.)

Marathoners and the Sedentary Are at Risk   Women who exercise too little are at a higher risk for osteoporosis than the norm. For proper calcium absorption, the bones need pressure, and women need to be on their feet at least two hours a day, preferably moving. Some women cannot do vigorous exercise because of the exhaustion that accompanies their hormonal problems, and walking with friends would be a good choice for them.

Women who overexercise are also at risk. Studies have found that marathoners have a high incidence of osteoporosis, because exercise reduces the proportion of their body fat. Since some estrogen is produced in the fat cells of the body, their estrogen levels diminish, and menstruation may cease. This can lead to a loss of calcium and brittleness of the bones.

The Pros and Cons of Being Overweight   Obese women have an advantage against osteoporosis since they produce more estrogen in their fatty tissues than do thinner women. However, overweight women also have a higher risk of diabetes and heart disease. And it is the women with android obesity (fat around the middle) who produce excess estrone that is believed to contribute to breast cancer.

What Can I Do to Assess My Risk of Osteoporosis?   Don't wait until age 60 to find out if you have osteoporosis. The more advanced bone loss is, the more difficult it is to treat. It is much better to prevent osteoporosis than to treat it. It is a good idea to have a base-line bone densitometry test done at age 35 to assess your bone status; repeat the test as indicated, especially after menopause. This test can tell you if you need to begin treatment to arrest bone loss.

Facts About Bone Density   The best bone testing to date uses the dual-photon bone densitometry (DEXA) test. This is a low-dose X-ray technique. Lunar and Hologic are two com-

Who Is at Risk for Osteoporosis?

Osteoporosis can occur in women of any size, shape, or color. But the following types of women are particularly at risk:

- Slight, small-boned, fair-skinned women, particularly of Northern European or Asian descent (women of color have the least genetic tendency to osteoporosis);
- Women who have either a natural or artificial menopause before the age of forty;
- Women whose female relatives became shorter in old age (i.e., have a history of osteoporosis);
- Women who were heavy meat-eaters (high protein) in their childhood, teens, and twenties;
- Women who have been on many weight-loss diets, particularly high protein diets;
- Women on low-calcium diets;
- Women who smoke;
- Women who drink a lot of alcohol;
- Women who drink a lot of caffeine;
- Women who drink a lot of cola drinks (due to the phosphate content);
- Women who have a sedentary lifestyle (the bones need the pressure of at least two hours of standing and exercising each day);
- Some women with thyroid or parathyroid disorders;
- Women who use too high a dose of thyroid medication;
- Women who use cortisone long-term;
- Women with hormone imbalances that affect calcium absorption;
- Women who use a lot of aluminum-containing antacids;
- Women with periodontal (gum) disease.

You may not fit into any of these risk categories and still have osteoporosis.

panies that make this equipment. Standard X-ray exams have been designed to test tissue, not bone. Bone loss doesn't show up on such X-rays until you have already lost 25 to 30 percent of your bone mass. Bone densitometry measures the mineral density in the bone by bouncing a dual-photon beam of light off the bone, measuring the difference in density between bone and soft tissue. The amount of radiation is very low—less than you would receive on a coast-to-coast airplane flight. Comparison with other X-ray procedures may help: in a bone densitometry test, you receive approximately one millirem of radiation, compared with 40 for a chest X-ray, and 100 for a mammogram.

It is best to check more than one site, as you can have bone loss in one place and not another. Usually the spine and hip are checked. The results will show whether you have normal bone density for your age, and will compare the results with those of an average young adult. If you have lost between one and two standard deviations of bone, you will be diagnosed as having osteopenia (bone loss). Mild osteopenia is about one standard deviation, moderate is about two standard deviations, and severe is three or more standard deviations. Not all osteopenia is caused by osteoporosis. But if osteoporosis is the cause of your osteopenia, you are considered osteoporotic when you have more than two to two-and-a-half standard deviations in bone loss.

Every loss of a standard deviation doubles or triples your risk of bone fracture.

Uterine and Endometrial Cancer

In the 1970s, many women were given large continuous doses of potent synthetic estrogens over a number of years without countering their effect with progesterone. As a result, incidence of uterine cancer and deaths from it showed a noticeable increase. This is because taking estrogen without progesterone over a period of about 8 years can cause a buildup of the endometrial lining, which may bring on precancerous changes and, eventually, full-blown cancer. So far, this type of cancer has been considered a relatively "good" cancer, because it is rarely fatal and survival rates are high.[8]

Many women who die from uterine cancer have never taken estrogen. Some have a genetic tendency toward endometrial cancer. Others who ovulate infrequently are at higher risk for this type of cancer because they produce high levels of estrogen but no progesterone to oppose the estrogen.

Unopposed estrogen builds up the lining of the uterus and can lead to hyperplasia (abnormal thickening, resulting in organ enlargement) and subsequent precancerous or cancerous lesions. Women who ovulate infrequently should probably take progesterone to counteract the effect of too much estrogen stimulation.

The number of annual deaths from endometrial cancer is usually stated as being around 3,000 to 4,000. There is no doubt that the use of estrogen alone increases the risk of developing endometrial cancer; a woman with an intact uterus should not be on estrogen only, unless she has an annual transvaginal pelvic ultrasound or sampling of her uterine lining.

However, as long as women are given the lower premenopausal doses of natural estrogens, with added progesterone, their likelihood of getting uterine cancer will be less than if they were not on hormones at all.

Heavy Bleeding

Some time during her menopause, it is common for a woman's menstrual bleeding to become lighter and more irregular. However, many women have heavy bleeding, which is also considered normal because it is so common. Physicians like to investigate irregular bleeding because of its association with endometrial cancer. Other reasons for bleeding abnormalities include:

- **High levels of estrogen**. This occurs due to imminent or actual ovarian failure, when the ovary produces insufficient numbers of eggs. When ovarian estrogen levels decrease, the pituitary gland puts out high levels of FSH to compensate. FSH overstimulates the ovaries, leading to high levels of estrogen. This builds up the uterine lining, and heavy bleeding results. While women in this condition still ovulate, they may continue to have regular periods with a very heavy flow full of clots, due to high estrogen levels. This type of bleeding tends to respond to progesterone treatment.
- **Low levels of estrogen**. This can also cause breakthrough bleeding because the endometrium cannot

adhere to the uterine wall, and the lining keeps sloughing off. This type of bleeding tends to be light and watery and responds to estrogen treatment.

- **Low levels of progesterone**. Heavy bleeding also occurs because women tend to ovulate less frequently around menopause. Periods may be relatively regular and normal, but ovulation is irregular. When a woman doesn't ovulate and progesterone levels are low, progesterone's beneficial changes do not occur in the endometrial lining. This can lead to erratic, heavy bleeding and can eventually cause a precancerous condition.
- **Pituitary gland failure**. This is a rare cause of bleeding.

Bleeding Irregularities

Bleeding irregularities around menopause should be investigated. Spotting between periods, heavy bleeding and clotting, or a long time with no periods may all be perfectly normal at that time of life, or they may mask a problem. It's best to be sure.

Postmenopausal bleeding should definitely be looked into, particularly if you are not taking hormones. However, remember that you can have endometrial cancer whether you bleed heavily, spot, or don't bleed at all. The amount of blood is not a significant indicator in itself.

If a woman is not taking hormones and has menstrual bleeding only twice a year, she should see a doctor about the need for some progesterone in order to avoid hyperplasia caused by estrogen overstimulating the uterine lining. But if a woman is on the proper combination of hormones when she is going through menopause or in postmenopause, she may stop bleeding or just bleed occasionally, and this is all right. Progesterone counteracts estrogen, and the uterine lining atrophies, so there is nothing to lose.

If you are concerned, a vaginal sonogram or an endometrial biopsy may put your mind at rest.

Endometrial Sampling May Be Advised   When there are significant bleeding irregularities, physicians like to check the lining of the uterus to ensure that there are no precancerous changes due to estrogen overstimulation. There are a number of types of sampling that can be done.

An ultrasound process, performed with a vaginal wand or probe, is available; this is painless and less invasive than an endometrial biopsy. It can indicate the thickness of the endometrial lining and any abnormalities in the lining. Less than 5 mm of thickness is ideal. More than 8 to 10 mm requires further checking.

Currently, an extension of the Pap smear is done by inserting a tube into the uterus and removing samples of the lining. (This is an office procedure, performed more often these days than a D&C, which usually requires a general anesthetic.) Physicians check for abnormal cells and for signs of ovulation. If the endometrial biopsy results are normal, or if the endometrial changes are in their early stages, a woman will probably be given a course of synthetic progestin or progesterone therapy during the second half of her menstrual cycle. Estrogen may also be prescribed if the problem is due to ovarian failure.

Women at risk may be advised by their physicians to have an annual endometrial biopsy. Some researchers say that an annual biopsy is no longer necessary. A base-line endometrial biopsy may be advised before beginning estrogen and progesterone therapy. Then, a woman may take the Progestin Challenge Test (see below) once a year to assess the condition of her uterine lining.

Endometrial biopsy may not be perfectly reliable, according to Dr. Wulf Utian, because only a small section of the uterus is tested. He believes that anything slightly abnormal should be further investigated.

The Progestin Challenge Test   Dr. Don Gambrell proposed the Progestin Challenge Test, in which a woman takes Provera once a year—10 mg a day for 13 days. If she begins to bleed before the tenth day, her uterus is being overstimulated by estrogen, a condition which is not desirable because too much estrogen can lead to hyperplasia and, eventually, cancer. If the woman begins to bleed after the tenth day, her uterus is probably fine; her progesterone level has been adequate and has been doing its work of opposing estrogen.

If a woman does bleed before the tenth day, she is given a three- or four-month course of cyclical synthetic progestin or natural progesterone, which usually sloughs off the hyperplasia. If she is already taking hormones, the dosage of progesterone is raised for a while.

However, note that the Progestin Challenge Test is not universally accepted as reliable.

You Don't Have to Have Periods After Menopause Many women prefer not to take hormones because they don't want to continue having periods after menopause. They often don't realize that hormones can be taken in a way that eliminates their periods. Today, some doctors tell postmenopausal women to take both estrogen and progesterone daily, instead of cyclically, to discourage monthly bleeding. In theory, the progesterone will oppose the estrogen, and the lining of the uterus will thin out and even disappear. This is an ideal which may not occur without occasional breakthrough bleeding until a woman is a few years past menopause.

Recently, a perimenopausal woman told me that her doctor said she needed to bleed each cycle while taking hormones. He felt that bleeding was the most important indicator that there was no endometrial cancer. However, the important thing in endometrial health is the actual change occurring in the lining of the uterus. If continual progesterone does its work properly, bleeding is not necessary after menopause, though breakthrough bleeding may occur; some doctors say that quite a number of postmenopausal women keep bleeding on continual low doses of progesterone.

Dr. Don Gambrell prefers another method, which he calls the continuous cyclical method. He thinks that a few women will still get endometrial cancer when taking hormones continuously. He prefers to have women take both hormones for the first 25 days of the calendar month, and then go off them both for five to six days. He says the bleeding is very light.

What About Breast Cancer?

The possible connection between estrogen replacement and breast cancer has been voiced so often that many women are afraid to take estrogen. Even the experts are confused; much of the necessary data are not available and will not be ready for a decade or two. If you wish to read the "estrogen causes cancer" position, two recent books on the subject are *Estrogen and Breast Cancer*, by Carol Ann Rinzler, and *Sexual Chemistry: Understanding our Hormones, the Pill, and HRT*, by Ellen Grant.[9] There does seem to be increased risk of breast cancer among women who took the pill for a number of years before their first pregnancy.

But many studies show no causative link between estrogen replacement therapy after menopause and breast cancer.[10] Others say that there is no risk with short-term estrogen therapy, but find some evidence of increased risk in women who have used estrogen for more than 10 to 15 years. Some suggest that estrogen taken in conjunction with progesterone actually helps prevent breast cancer.[11] Others suggest that estrogen acts as a catalyst—not causing breast cancer, but encouraging an already present cancer.

A recent study done in Sweden linked breast cancer with estrogen therapy. But the synthetic estradiol used there is not typically used in the U.S. for postmenopausal women, and the doses were much higher than used here.

Most breast cancers occur in women over 55, yet less than 20 percent of these women are on hormone replacement therapy (HRT), according to Gail Sheehey. Sheehey also reports that the average length of time women stay on estrogen is only nine months.[12]

Better Protected on Estrogen and Progesterone   Dr. Winnifred Cutler believes that women are protected over twice as much against developing breast cancer if they are on the correct estrogen and progesterone combination. Dr. Don Gambrell's extensive research indicates that women on estrogen alone have a lower incidence of breast cancer than women who take no hormones; women on both estrogen and progesterone have an even lower incidence. The present consensus is that estrogen does not cause cancer, but that it may accelerate the progress of estrogen-dependent hormonal cancers.

There is no conclusive data for or against prescribing estrogen replacement therapy for women with past cases of breast cancer, though estrogen has been routinely withheld from these women in the past. This has been done on the presumption that estrogen therapy would cause a return of the cancer, not on the basis of actual studies.

The attitude toward women with estrogen-dependent and other breast cancers is rapidly changing. Some doctors are recognizing the problems these women face at menopause, and are giving women with successfully-treated breast cancer low-dose estrogen replacement therapy. These doctors believe that such women are better off on estrogen, and that it won't encourage a return of the cancer.

At the North American Menopause Society meeting held in September 1992, many experts said that they were waiting one to three years after successful treatment of breast cancer to commence estrogen therapy.

Whether to take hormone replacement therapy after breast cancer may be a difficult choice; in the end, a woman must decide whether she can cope with her menopausal symptoms and their effect on the general quality of her life. (See Chapter 13 on breast cancer for more details on this subject.)

Avoiding Infections

After menopause, estrogen deficiency may be responsible for vaginal and bladder infections. Both the vagina and the bladder are full of estrogen receptors, and these tissues can become quite fragile after menopause. Vaginal estrogen creams help prevent the continual recurrence of vaginal infections. Where there are recurrent bladder infections, but nothing shows up in tests, doctors should not presume that the problem is cystitis; such women should have a urology workup.

Many women (perhaps 45 to 60 percent) have problems with some degree of incontinence after menopause. This is a highly treatable condition, but women rarely seek treatment for it.

How Sexual Response Is Affected by Estrogen

Estrogen contributes to a healthy sex life by keeping the vagina supple. This hormone is responsible for maintaining the size, shape, and flexibility of the vagina, as well as the thickness and lubrication of the lining. When estrogen supplies diminish, the vaginal tissues become dry, narrow, and less pliable. The vagina may shorten, and the entrance to the vagina may become so narrow that intercourse is painful or impossible. Estrogen hastens the blood flow to the pelvic area during sexual arousal; blood surges through the tissues, causing the release of fluid into the vaginal passage. Estrogen also makes the skin, the nipples, and other sensual areas respond more pleasurably to stimulation. It also increases sexual response and the quality of a woman's orgasm.

Some women naturally produce estrogen in their adrenal glands in sufficient quantities to enjoy sex after menopause. Others, whose adrenals have been depleted by stress, may notice estrogen levels diminishing soon after menopause or within the next five to ten years. Women who have had a hysterectomy may notice dryness of the vagina almost immediately. To counteract these symptoms, Dr. Lila Nachtigall advises that most women will need to take estrogen if they want to continue having sexual intercourse after age 60 to 65.

Estrogen, progesterone, thyroid, and testosterone all have their role in a woman's sex life. Women who do not fantasize and who have a low libido may need some testosterone to increase their sex drive. Some women with subnormal or low thyroid levels also have a low sex drive.

I have read that high levels of progesterone can reduce the sex drive, and I've also read that it does the opposite.[13] It probably does either in different women. My observation is that women with PMS often have a very high sex drive, and that natural progesterone normalizes it. I have not heard many complaints from women who take progesterone for PMS that it affects their sex drive adversely. Some pregnant women have a low libido (progesterone levels are high during pregnancy). And I have heard complaints from women receiving natural progesterone injections that it blunted their orgasms.

GOING THROUGH MENOPAUSE NATURALLY

Many women would like "to go through menopause naturally." It sounds like a good idea, and it's a possibility for a significant number. But those who do it should know why they

are doing it, and whether they are making the correct decision. Sometimes the cards are stacked against a woman going
through menopause easily, for various reasons—genes, hormonal makeup, early diet, physical habits over the years, and
past sicknesses.

It's true that, in countries such as Japan, women seem to
have far fewer menopausal problems. Research has linked this
phenomenon—in Japan's case—to the prevalence of soy products in the diet. There is an estrogen-like substance called genestein in soy beans, and women in Japan generally eat soy
products several times a day.[14]

The problem is that many of us have not eaten the right
diet or had the right habits for a long time, and we are reaping
the effects.

Making an Informed Decision

Every woman needs to be able to make an informed decision
about whether she should take estrogen after a certain age.
She needs to find out what will happen to her if she requires
estrogen and doesn't take it. What are the benefits and risks?
Does taking estrogen really cause cancer? Are nutrition,
herbs, and exercise adequate?

Don't Close Your Mind to Estrogen Replacement Therapy Too Early

Estrogen has had a lot of bad press and has been treated as an
enemy rather than a friend. But think for a while on those at-
tributes of spirit and body that make a young woman healthy
and beautiful: energy and joy, soft skin, lustrous hair, clear
eyes, good muscle tone, strong bones, and healthy teeth.
Estrogen, with its 300 functions in the female body, is largely
responsible for these qualities. It is the most important hormone for a woman, just as testosterone is for a man. It makes
sense that when estrogen levels start to decline, a woman can
be profoundly affected in many ways.

Dr. Norman Beals likes the metaphor that his physician father taught him. In 1628, a group of physicians met at a con-

ference in Paris to discuss the female disease in which "the wellspring dried up." These physicians noted that some women's bodies began to crumble from the inside out, affecting their skin, their bones, their mucous membranes—in fact, all their tissues. The symbolism of a wellspring drying up is a good description of the aging process. The Bible, similarly, describes a woman's reproductive system as a fountain. At menopause, the fountain often begins to run dry.

If you think of a woman as a biological organism, it's as though, once she has had her children, nature loses interest in her. Her estrogen production drops, other hormone levels decline, and she gradually begins to age. Her skin and hair become dry; her mucous membranes—the linings of her nose and mouth, esophagus, intestinal tract, bladder, and vagina—can become thin and irritated; her bones begin to crumble. Her cardiovascular system loses its elasticity, and her cholesterol level rises. Muscles become stringy. Joints become swollen. Men go through this, too, but generally they don't have the same abrupt decline in hormones that women do at menopause.

The process is gradual. No one ends up a pile of dust, and it doesn't happen in six months. But, while the picture is exaggerated, the direction is accurate.

Nature's Provision Doesn't Always Work

Nature provides for the production of lower levels of weaker estrogens after menopause through the breakdown of ovarian and adrenal androgens; ideally these should be adequate for the nonmenstruating woman. But this is only successful in women with superior genes who have had good dietary and health habits throughout their lives, particularly in childhood. According to Barbara Sherwin, Ph.D., the ovaries of 50 percent of women stop producing testosterone at menopause.[15]

Another factor that is frequently out of a woman's control is the amount of stress in her life. Grief over the loss of a spouse, involvement in a collision, being the victim of violent crime, or other emotionally draining experiences around menopause may exhaust the adrenal glands, which are not meant to handle stress for long periods of time.

The ovaries are made to last for about 50 years at the most. The adrenal glands may function optimally for another 20 years if you are lucky, says Australian physician Sandra Cabot. This is not so bad if you only live a short while. At the height of the Roman Empire, women only lived an average of 23 years. At the turn of this century, women only lived to an average age of about fifty. Now the average age is over 80. Dr. Cabot says that, in the year 2050, the world will be full of little old ladies; under present conditions, half of them will have broken hips.

Whether to Take Estrogen— an Important Decision

A woman who grits her teeth through night sweats and joint pains, determined never to go on hormones, may be making a great mistake. Also, perimenopausal women can have severe, hidden physical conditions, such as heart disease or osteoporosis, without obvious symptoms until a fairly late stage.

Studies show that the majority of women would be better off taking long-term hormone replacement therapy. Unfortunately, women are not always told why this is so; some doctors don't have the time to spend with them individually. Many women stop taking estrogen because they are tired of having menstrual periods after menopause or because they have side effects, but these problems can be dealt with by adjusting the dosage. Some women think that they are through the worst of menopause and no longer need estrogen; they do not know that when they go off estrogen, it's not long before the benefits disappear.

Facing the Reality of Aging

Sometimes ignoring the issues of menopause comes from a reluctance to face the fact that we're getting older. For many women, aging and losing their attractiveness makes them feel that they are losing their identity and therefore their power. The idea of being dependent on hormones also makes them feel that they are giving up control.

The change of life is a fact of life, and there's no point in sweeping it under the carpet because you don't like the idea of getting older. The big question is not "Will you age?" but "How will you age?"

There are many things about menopause that can make it a positive change—a time to look forward to, not a time to dread. Many women in their forties and fifties start a new, happy phase of their lives after menopause. They no longer have to spend all their energy on their families, and are able to spend time developing their own individuality and talents. They often flourish physically and have high levels of energy. It's often the age of poise.

FURTHER INFORMATION

For information on treatment, see the next section of this chapter. Also see Recommended Reading at the end of the book. For a physician in your area, you may wish to contact:

> The North American Menopause Society
> 11100 Euclid Ave
> Cleveland, OH 44106
> (216) 844-3334,
> (fax) 216/844-3348
> (They request that you write to them).

NAMS offers consumers a helpful reading list and a list of health-care providers in their area who are expert in menopause medicine.

CASE HISTORY

Cassandra's Story

Cassandra, at 51 years old, took hormones because she was having hot flashes and was almost through menopause. She had been put on a typical protocol of 0.625 mg of Premarin and 10 mg of Provera daily. She took the estrogen from day one of the calendar month until day 25 and took the progestin from day 15 to day 25. Then she would have a "pseudo," or induced, menstrual period, after which she would begin taking the hormones again on the first day of the calendar month.

Doctors are comfortable using this protocol for hormone replacement because it has been widely studied for effectiveness at menopause. Researchers have determined exactly how much synthetic progestin is required to ensure that women don't produce excessive buildup of the lining of the uterus, which can result from taking estrogen. They know that women who took high doses of synthetic estrogens without any progestin in the 1970s had a slightly higher incidence of endometrial cancer. Taking low postmenopausal doses of natural estrogens with adequate progestin almost completely eliminates the problem of endometrial cancer.

However, Cassandra felt sluggish and slightly depressed on this Premarin/Provera combination. Her friend, Katie, suggested that she switch to another estrogen, such as Estrace, with natural progesterone. Katie also told her that since she was now probably through menopause, she could take both hormones every day. Soon, the progesterone would "cancel out" the effect of the estrogen, and Cassandra would probably cease menstruating. Katie even gave her a sample of both hormones to try. Cassandra took the hormones and immediately felt better. She found that she had more energy, and her sense of well-being returned.

When she asked her physician to give her a prescription for this combination, he said that he would give her the Estrace, but balked at trying natural progesterone. "We just don't know how much to give to make the beneficial changes in the lining of the uterus. There aren't any studies published on using natural progesterone after menopause."

In fact, some study has been done on natural progesterone for hormone replacement therapy after menopause. It has been determined that 150 mg taken twice a day for 13 days a month, or 150 mg taken every day, is sufficient to make beneficial changes in the uterine lining. Dr. Don Gambrell, a noted hormone researcher, says that using 25-mg suppositories of natural progesterone twice a day for 13 days each cycle is adequate.[16] Not only do many women feel better on natural progesterone than on synthetic progestin, but natural progesterone is better for them physically in a number of ways.

Instead, Cassandra's doctor put her on another synthetic progestin, which made her very irritable. Cassandra didn't feel that she could fight her doctor and ended up going back on Provera.

Cassandra's case is an example of a very mild hormonal problem, one that most women wouldn't even recognize. All such women know is that they are slightly depressed and dissatisfied with their lives. One could hardly say that they are sick, but their lives are definitely affected and the consequences can be significant. Such women may think that the only reason for their dissatisfaction is their marriage or job, when it may be partly fueled by a hormone-related problem. If needed, the right combination of natural hormones can improve a woman's moods and change her outlook on life.

What's Happening Now   Cassandra and I are good friends, so we have a hormone consultation every so often. She is finding herself more and more sensitive to Provera and is tempted to go off it altogether. Her current doctor is not used to prescribing natural progesterone, so I suggested that Cassandra take her the results of the recently published PEPI tests (Postmenopausal Estrogen and Progestin Intervention), to show her that natural progesterone is better for cardiovascular health. That issue is one that most physicians understand.

TREATMENT FOR MENOPAUSE

Many women with estrogen-deficiency symptoms may be able to control their symptoms with simple lifestyle changes and natural remedies—at least for a while. The lifestyle changes recommended for women with PMS are also appropriate for women with estrogen-deficiency symptoms (read Chapters 5 and 17, on PMS and diet).

Treatment for Hot Flashes

During menopause, if the only symptom you experience is hot flashes, treatments other than hormone therapy can be effective. Using the herb vitex (also called agnus castus) can help balance your hormones. Taking Korean ginseng capsules, vitamin E, and hormones such as black cohosh can also be helpful. Women are advised to avoid caffeine and alcohol, which tend to worsen hot flashes, and to avoid large doses of niacin (vitamin B_3), as it also affects vasomotor stability (which causes constriction or dilation of blood vessels).

Herbal Preparations

Hormones were first isolated in the early decades of this century. By contrast, women have used herbs for thousands of years to help balance their endocrine systems and menstrual cycles. Many herbs contain estrogen, and others help to produce progesterone. But, since it may be dangerous to take herbs haphazardly, try to find a well-informed herbalist who uses only fresh organically grown herbs.

Some helpful herbal preparations for menopause include black and blue cohosh, licorice, wild yam, sassafras, sarsaparilla, vitex, kelp, valerian root, ginger, motherwort, licorice, yellow dock, dong quai, false unicorn, sage, dandelion, gingko, gotu kola, and ginseng. Bee pollen and spirulina are also helpful.

Herbs that produce high calcium levels include comfrey, oatstraw, horsetail, borage, and nettle. Some herbs that alleviate hot flashes are sage, blue vervain, motherwort, blessed thistle, and rosemary. Rosemary Gladstar's *Herbs for Menopause* gives very practical and helpful guidance. See Recommended Reading at the end of this book for information.

A Caution Against Herbs   Dr. Lila Nachtigall points out that ginseng is a natural plant estrogen and has the same effects on the body as taking prescribed estrogen. She warns against using it excessively because of the risk of hyperplasia (excessive buildup of the lining of the uterus), and because ginseng is usually taken alone and not countered with progesterone.

She also warns against overdosing on herbs because, while many are used as the basis of our modern pharmacology, they have not been subjected to controlled studies. If you find a well-informed herbalist, taking herbs should not be a problem.

Calcium Supplements

Medical opinion on taking calcium for bone protection varies. Some physicians strongly recommend calcium, along with estrogen. Others believe that calcium has little effect in restoring bone, particularly during the two or three years following menopause, when the highest proportion of bone loss occurs.

If you decide to take calcium, remember that, although milk has a high calcium content, it is a poor source because of its high protein content. Better sources of calcium are green vegetables, oranges, almonds, and other calcium-rich foods (refer to a food chart). The recommended dose of calcium is 1,000 mg per day. Some doctors feel that this is too much, and recommend only about 300 mg (native Chinese and Russian people consume about this much in their diet and have little osteoporosis).

Natural Estrogen and Progesterone Creams

If you have menopausal symptoms but are still ovulating and having a regular menstrual cycle, you may use Pro-Gest® cream (use 1/4 tsp twice per day from day 7 of your menstrual cycle until day 21, then raise the dose to 1/2 tsp twice per day through day 28). Do not use cream during your menstrual period unless you have cramps.[17]

If you are not menstruating any longer, you can use the cream by the calendar month: no cream days 1 to 7; 1/4 tsp twice a day from day 8 to day 21; 1/2 tsp twice a day from day 22 to day 31.

For mild osteoporosis, use 1/8 to 1/4 tsp of Pro-Gest® twice a day from day 8 of the calendar month to the last day of the calendar month (use half of a two-ounce jar per month). Break for 7 days from the first to the seventh. For severe osteoporosis or past fractures, use at least one two-ounce jar—at least 1/4 to 1/2 tsp per day—skipping the first seven days of the calendar month.

Professional and Technical Services, Inc., the company that makes Pro-Gest® cream, also makes an estrogen cream. Their phone number is 1-800-888-6814.

Triple Estrogens

Some compounding pharmacies (for instance Bajamar Women's Healthcare and Women's International Pharmacy), have been making up a combination triple estrogen product called Tri-Est. It contains the three main human estrogens in the ratio of estradiol: 1; estrone: 1; and estriol: 8. This recipe is based on the idea that estriol, a weaker estrogen found in its greatest quantity in pregnancy, is the least carcinogenic form of estrogen and therefore the safest. This is not well researched and is based mainly on research done 25 years ago. But, despite this, the idea has found a lot of acceptance. The use of estriol or triple estrogens may be helpful for women with mild problems and those who have had breast cancer and are afraid of stronger forms of estrogen. Women with severe problems don't find triple estrogens very helpful, in my experience.

ESTROGEN THERAPY

Estrogen Is Back in Favor   Research in the 1970s seemed to show that estrogen was linked with an increase in endometrial cancer, because estrogen promotes the growth of the lining of the uterus. This led physicians to stop prescribing it, and women became afraid to use it.

However, estrogen doses have been substantially lowered, and progestins have been added to the estrogen therapy. Progestins inhibit endometrial growth by reducing the number of cell receptors for estrogen and increasing the level of an enzyme that converts estradiol to estrone sulfate, which is easily excreted. Studies have shown that, among women who take progestin for ten or more days, hyperplasia rarely develops. Actually, correct use of lower doses of estrogen with progesterone is more likely to protect against endometrial cancer than to cause it. While the statistics are less clear regarding breast cancer, reliable studies have been done showing that there is no increased risk for breast cancer associated with current postmenopausal doses of estrogen taken for up to five years.[18]

Medical concern is now focused on osteoporosis and heart disease in postmenopausal women; these are more prevalent than breast cancer and are among the leading causes of death in older women. The benefits of estrogen therapy in treating these diseases far outweigh any danger from cancer; for this reason, estrogen replacement therapy has come back into favor.

Do You Need Estrogen?   How do you decide whether you need estrogen? The level of symptoms you are experiencing is an important indicator, as are your blood test results. Whether you have had surgical menopause is, of course, significant. Your family history is important; you should look for osteoporosis and heart disease (particularly in the women in your family, under age 65). Important tests include: an ovarian serum profile, including estradiol, testosterone, and progesterone levels, and FSH and LH levels. According to Elizabeth Lee Vliet, M.D., these hormone tests should be performed on day one of the menstrual cycle and the estrogen and progesterone level tests repeated on day twenty.

Lipid profiles are also useful, as your HDL cholesterol levels often dip as your estrogen levels decline.

It is important to have a base-line dual photon bone densitometry exam performed at age 35 (earlier if the risk warrants it). DEXA is a good choice.

Your doctor may decide that you need estrogen if your estrogen levels are low or if you have a high follicle-stimulating hormone (FSH) blood level on day one of the cycle. Over 40 mIU/ml is a fairly definite indicator that you are menopausal, but even over 20 mIU/ml is a sign that you are on the way. When LH also reaches a high level, it means that you are no longer ovulating, and taking both hormone tests on day one of the cycle is a better indication of menopause than an FSH-level test alone.

A diagnosed premenopausal or menopausal Pap smear is also helpful. It tells you that the estrogen level is low in the tissues of your cervix.

Sometimes a baseline endometrial biopsy is helpful to rule out adverse changes in the lining of the uterus before beginning to take estrogen, especially where there are bleeding problems. A vaginal probe (ultrasound) is a less invasive procedure that shows the condition and thickness of the endometrial lining.

Common Problems with Taking Estrogen   There are several reasons why some women stop taking hormones: they do not want to continue having menstrual periods; they have side effects such as headaches, bloating, weight gain, or nausea; they don't like taking medication all the time; they put on weight when taking hormones; they are afraid of getting cancer.

There are options to try before making the decision to stop taking hormones:

• Most postmenopausal women will stop having menstrual periods if they take their hormones continually, though this process may take six months;
• Changing medication to other types of estrogen and natural progesterone may dissipate side effects;
• Women tend to put on weight at menopause whether they are taking hormones or not—approximately 10 to 12 pounds, according to a recent study; this is not always directly related to taking estrogen, but reflects a general change in metabolism at mid-life.

Estrogen's Benefits to the Heart   According to Dr. Leon Speroff, a review of the current literature shows overwhelming support for a reduced risk of cardiovascular disease in estrogen users, especially among nonsmokers.[19]

Unfortunately, in 1978 and 1985, the Framingham Study suggested that there was a 50 percent increase in cardiovascular disease among estrogen users. While this study was highly respected, it is now believed that the conclusion about estrogen increasing the chance of heart disease was incorrect. In fact, the study was re-evaluated in 1991, and the conclusion was reversed.

The Nurse's Health Study, which monitored 121,964 nurses who were taking estrogen replacement therapy, has been running for about 20 years. It concludes that there is a 50-percent reduction in heart disease among women who have taken estrogen at some time. Current users showed a 70-percent reduction.

One reason estrogen is so helpful in preventing heart disease is that it dilates the blood vessels and acts as an antioxidant in the body. It also elevates the levels of HDL-cholesterol by retarding its metabolism in the liver. This mainly occurs when estrogen is taken orally. Dr. Speroff says that, while the estrogen patch, the implant, and the topical cream may have profound impact on hot flashes, vaginal dryness, and moods, estrogen taken by these routes has only a limited impact on HDLs. Others differ in their opinion on this matter, as we will see later.

Dr. Speroff comments that the public health importance of the impact of estrogen on cardiovascular disease is even more significant than estrogen's effect on osteoporosis.

Estrogen's Effect on Osteoporosis   Dr. Speroff mentions that three-quarters of the bone loss that occurs in women during the first 20 years after menopause can be attributed to hormone loss, rather than to the process of aging itself. Vertebral bone (the spine) is particularly vulnerable and can begin to decline from the age of 20 onward.

There are two important factors controlling the risk of fracture:

1. Bone mass achieved at maturity (about age 30);
2. Subsequent rate of bone loss.

Exercise and diet (both early and continuing) are important in preventing osteoporosis, but neither will stop bone loss if estrogen levels are below normal.

Taking estrogen will lead to a 50-to-60 percent decrease in the likelihood of arm and hip fractures. When calcium is added to the estrogen, an 80-percent reduction in fractures of the vertebrae is seen. Natural progesterone is also helpful in causing an increase in bone density.

The beneficial effect of estrogen on the bones is seen only in current users. Present recommendations are to take estrogen close to menopause and to take it long-term.

What Else Can I Do to Prevent and Treat Osteoporosis?
Improvements can be made and further bone loss can be prevented, but the earlier osteoporosis is treated, the better. Simple treatments include calcium and other supplementation and moderate exercise. But estrogen therapy is considered the

main treatment for osteoporosis because calcium absorption is poor when estrogen levels are low. Progesterone (see the section on John Lee, M.D., in Chapter 16), and testosterone can also be helpful. For premenopausal women, taking a birth control pill with a higher estrogen and lower progestin content, such as Ovcon 35, Modicon, or Brevicon, may help.

Fluoride compounds have been used, in research trials only, to treat osteoporosis, but they ultimately make the outer bone more brittle and more liable to splinter.

Salmon calcitonin has been found helpful in treating osteoporosis. It is very expensive and has some side effects (nausea, stomach disturbances, vomiting) in about 10 percent of the women who take it. It can also cause the body to produce antibodies that stifle its beneficial effects. It appears to particularly help women experiencing acute pain from osteoporosic fractures, so it is often used on a short-term basis to treat pain. It is now available in a less expensive nasal spray.

A number of biphosphonates have been developed. Etidronate Disodium is one of these. It appears to reduce fractures and increase bone mass. However, John Lee, M.D., says that it only strengthens old bones; new bone is not formed. He says that, over several years, results are less impressive and the likelihood of fractures increases.

Alendronate (brand name Fosamax) is a newly released biphosphonate with supposedly few side effects and a longer beneficial effect than Etidronate.

For women with serious bone loss, or for those who cannot take estrogen, other treatments are being developed.

Estrogen for Migraines   When estrogen levels drop suddenly before and during menstruation, this causes spasms in the blood vessels at the base of the neck and can be responsible for severe headaches. Estrogen (and natural progesterone) frequently help relieve severe hormone-related headaches. But sometimes taking estrogen causes headaches. When this happens, women should try lowering their dosage or taking estrogen more frequently. Or they could try estrogen in a form that bypasses the liver.

Some individuals may find they may have to stop using estrogen because it causes or worsens headaches.

Sumotriptin (brand name Imitrex) is a relatively new "wonder" migraine drug. Until recently, it was only available in this country in a very expensive injectable form. Now it is available in relatively less expensive 25 mg and 50 mg tablets. If you are a woman with incapacitating hormonal migraines that respond to estrogen, you may find the combination of estrogen and Imitrex (as needed) much more effective than other heavy-duty headache medications.

Estrogen for Depression, Dementia, and Panic Attacks In the past, when women have complained about the emotional symptoms connected with menopause, many physicians have not taken them seriously. Even now, books on menopause say that depression at menopause is a side effect of poor sleep patterns or hot flashes or low self-esteem. However, many women know that the depression and anxiety they experience at menopause are valid symptoms and find that their emotional health improves when they are treated with estrogen.

I have already mentioned the impact of estrogen on the mind and the mood. Estrogen functions somewhat like an antidepressant and has MAO-inhibitory and antidopaminergic properties. It increases serotonin levels and the number of serotonin receptors; it increases norepinephrine levels in the hypothalamus; and it raises the level of endorphins in the bloodstream.

Studies show that estrogen increases the ability to do abstract reasoning. It improves short-term verbal memory; it increases paragraph recall; it improves the condition of older patients with dementia, for instance in Alzheimer's disease; it improves intelligence, performance of tasks, psychosocial function, interpersonal relations, care of the self, and memory.[20]

Many women with hormonal problems experience an onset of panic attacks in their thirties and forties. These panic attacks, and the associated heart palpitations are the most common symptoms we see in premenopausal women.

Simply put, the changes in estrogen level cause fluctuations in the output of adrenaline. This can destabilize the blood sugar level and alter the heartbeat. Symptoms of panic attack may include rapid, erratic heartrate, hyperventilation, local pain in the chest and right arm, nausea, and debilitation. These frightening symptoms bring on the fear of heart attack and death, which produces anxiety.

Stress definitely worsens such panic attacks, but this type of attack is often premenstrual and often responds well to hormone therapy.

Estrogen Therapy and Arthritis The word arthritis is made up of "arthro" and "itis." "Arthro" means joint; "itis" means inflammation. So the word *arthritis* describes the joint manifestations of a number of different diseases, including the main forms of arthritis: rheumatoid arthritis (RA), osteoarthritis (OA), and gouty arthritis.

RA, OA, and gout are different diseases, and the way the symptoms manifest themselves varies. Sometimes they are acute and episodic, meaning that they flare up only occasionally, and sometimes they are chronic, meaning that they last for a long period of time. The episodes may be a minor nuisance and short-term, or very severe and long-term. Yet most people's visual picture of arthritis is unfortunately the extreme one—a chronic, worsening, constantly painful, and crippling disease.

It may help to distinguish the characteristics of these three types of arthritis, even though they are sometimes found in combination in the same person.

Rheumatoid arthritis is a systemic autoimmune disease, possibly virally caused. It can be manifested in any joint, but it is characteristically found in the extremities (the outer joints in the fingers and toes, for instance).

Osteoarthritis is a disease of degeneration, and occurs when the bones wear out, so it is more common in weight-bearing bones. It is not an inflammatory disease like rheumatoid arthritis, but it can cause local inflammation when the joints degenerate.

Gouty arthritis is more common in men, but it can occur in women after menopause. Gout takes a long time to develop and is usually a local problem, found in one joint. Only after many years does it affect multiple joints. Gout is a metabolic disease, which causes an increase in sodium urate crystal formation in the synovial fluid (the lubrication found between the body's joints). Gout sufferers typically have been on long-term diuretics, but the problem is also linked to hereditary factors, eating certain foods, and alcohol consumption. Flare-ups are excruciating but short-lived.

Estrogen levels are important, especially 17 beta-estradiol. Because there are many estradiol receptors in the cells in the synovial fluid, it stands to reason that the lubrication process is adversely affected when estrogen levels are low. So estrogen has a general role in helping to moderate the discomfort, and perhaps delay the progress, of arthritis—even though it doesn't cure the basic disease.

Elizabeth Lee Vliet, M.D., medical director and founder of HER Place, Inc., in Tucson, Arizona, and Fort Worth, Texas, says:

> Most women take conjugated equine estrogens which, in
> my clinical experience, appear to worsen these various forms
> of arthritis. When I change women over to an optimal level
> of 17-beta estradiol (the specific estrogen that is lost after
> menopause), I consistently find improvements in pain and
> other symptoms of arthritis.

Estrogen may also be helpful in treating rheumatoid arthritis because osteoporosis often accompanies it, both as a result of the disease (increased lack of activity) and from treatment with cortisone (which encourages bone loss). Hormone replacement therapy can help prevent this bone loss, even when cortisone therapy is used.

It is becoming routine to prescribe hormone replacement therapy to prevent heart disease and osteoporosis in women with a strong family history. Some doctors also think that hormone replacement therapy (HRT) should be considered routine for women with a strong family history of rheumatoid arthritis (HRT at menopause; the better types of birth control pill in younger women). But Dr. Vliet recommends that women with arthritis of all types use natural forms of estradiol, progesterone, and testosterone for hormone therapy.

Summary of Benefits from Estrogen There are many physical and emotional benefits of estrogen therapy. Estrogen can help relieve hot flashes. It can keep the skin toned and moist. It can restore the vagina to a more youthful state—thicker, more moist, more flexible, and with added lubrication.

Estrogen can help prevent vaginal and bladder infections caused by estrogen deficiency. It can prevent further bone loss and accompanying symptoms. By improving the cardiovascular system and lowering cholesterol levels, estrogen can protect women from heart disease. Because estrogen dilates the blood vessels, it can reduce the incidence of headaches and migraines (though it can also initiate headaches).

A recent study has shown that estrogen may also help some women avoid rheumatoid arthritis later in life. But for many women, the emotional benefits of taking estrogen are most important.

Who Should Take Estrogen?

- Women who have severe menopausal symptoms: severe hot flashes, vaginal atrophy, recurrent bladder infections from thinning of the vaginal tissues;
- Women with hormonal depression and anxiety, sometimes before menopause;
- Women at high risk for osteoporosis;
- Possibly, women with a high risk of heart disease (though this is not used as a medical reason yet);
- Possibly, women with a history of rheumatoid arthritis (though this is not used as a medical reason yet);
- Women who wish to enjoy sex past the age of 60;
- Women with Alzheimer's disease and other forms of dementia.

Who Shouldn't Take Estrogen? A woman with any of the following should not use estrogen:

- Known or suspected cancer of the breast, particularly those breast cancers with estrogen receptors;
- Known or suspected cancer of the endometrium;
- Known or suspected estrogen-dependent cancers;

- Undiagnosed vaginal bleeding, especially sudden onset after menopause;
- Active clotting disorders;
- Past history of clotting disorders caused by estrogen (be certain of the cause);
- Fibroids that enlarge when taking estrogen;
- Epilepsy, asthma, migraine, heart disease, or kidney disease, in which fluid retention might worsen the disease;
- Some women with severe liver disease or jaundice.

Treating Women for Heavy Bleeding   Irregular bleeding can occur because of too much estrogen, too little estrogen, or too little progesterone.

Dr. Lila Nachtigall feels that women who have very heavy bleeding during premenopause should not be on estrogen therapy. She says that, at this time when the ovaries are running out of eggs, the pituitary tries to compensate by producing large doses of follicle-stimulating hormone (FSH). This can produce high levels of estrogen; hence the heavy bleeding. These women, she believes, need more progesterone to help slough off the excess endometrial lining, rather than estrogen which adds to it.

But if a woman has continual light spotting, taking estrogen can sometimes stop the bleeding immediately, because it helps stabilize the endometrial lining of the uterus.

Sometimes, women have symptoms of estrogen deficiency for only part of the month. They may produce excessive estrogen in the first half of their menstrual cycle, which leads to heavy periods, but still have very low levels in the second half of the cycle. Dr. Winnifred Cutler mentions that some women may need a little estrogen only in the second half of their cycle.

Sometimes the bleeding results from a woman not ovulating or because progesterone levels are low. Such women benefit from treatment with progesterone for several cycles.

Changes in Thought Concerning Estrogen Use   In the past, FDA warnings about estrogens listed many medical conditions which were either caused or aggravated by the estrogen therapy then in use. Because of this, certain groups of women, predisposed to these medical conditions, were advised against taking estrogens. For instance, if a woman had a personal or family history of hormonal cancer, high blood pressure, thrombosis (blood clotting), stroke, heart disease, or diabetes, estrogen was contraindicated in her case.

Recommendations against the use of estrogens were made for several reasons, including:

1. The use of synthetic DES during pregnancy that led to birth defects in male and female offspring to the second generation, and side effects such as vaginal cancer in female daughters.
2. The much higher doses of synthetic ethinyl estradiol that were formerly for hormone replacement. (Ethinyl estradiol is still used in the oral contraceptive pill, but in much lower doses.)
3. The practice of taking ethinyl estradiol continually for years, without the countering effect of progesterone. This increased the incidence of endometrial hyperplasia and cancer.

These warnings were given, even though these issues had not been widely studied at the time. Today, research has shown that natural forms of estrogen are generally benign when taken in smaller doses along with progesterone. Therefore, many women who were previously advised against using estrogen are now free to use it.

- **Endometrial cancer**—This no longer a major concern because prescribed doses are now smaller, and progesterone or progestin is added to counter the effects of estrogen on the uterus. Three-quarters of the cases of endometrial cancer occur in those who have never been on estrogen. Also, compared to the large numbers of women who die from osteoporosis and heart disease, endometrial cancer is less of a life threat (2,900 a year die of endometrial cancer and only a quarter of them have been on estrogen therapy). Women are actually less likely to get endometrial cancer on the correct hormonal protocol. Although estrogen does not cause endometrial cancer, those women who presently have endometrial cancer should not use it.

- **Breast cancer**—Since estrogen influences breast tissue, there has always been concern about its causing or acting as a catalyst for breast cancer. Many studies show no link between estrogen therapy and breast cancer. Other studies indicate that estrogen therapy helps to prevent breast cancer. Currently it is believed that estrogen therapy does not cause breast cancer, and that low levels of estrogen combined with progesterone or progestin decrease one's chances of developing this cancer. Estrogen is often not given to someone who has had breast cancer or who has a strong history of estrogen-dependent breast cancer, but medical opinion is changing. As mentioned earlier, some experts on breast cancer are now giving estrogen and progestin therapy within a year of a simple lumpectomy; others are waiting two or three years. This advice is totally different than that given just a few years ago.

  Another favorable advantage of hormone replacement therapy for the breasts is that correcting hormonal balance may lessen the chances of getting fibrocystic breast disease.

- **Fibroids**—In the past, it was thought that estrogen therapy would cause these benign uterine growths to increase in size. Generally, the estrogen doses given postmenopausally are too small to affect fibroids but, occasionally, even low doses of estrogen will accelerate the growth of fibroids.
- **High blood pressure**—In the past, estrogen elevated levels of the enzymes renin and angiotensin in the kidneys and caused high blood pressure in some predisposed women. Taking estrogen by a method that bypasses the liver usually counters this problem.
- **Gallbladder disease and liver disease**—Women with these problems should take estrogen in cream or patch form, which bypasses the liver.
- **Diabetes**—Some doctors feel that estrogen replacement therapy is important for diabetics because of their high incidence of death from heart attacks. Others note that blood sugar is often more difficult to control in postmenopausal women than in men of a similar age. They feel that hormone

replacement therapy helps to stabilize blood sugar levels in older female diabetics.

- **Blood clotting**—Women on the high-estrogen contraceptive pill were once considered at risk for thrombosis. But the low postmenopausal doses of estrogen are not considered dangerous. Some women are at higher risk for thrombosis than others, but this is relatively rare and can be detected by testing a woman's blood levels of antithrombin, which will show high if the woman is in the high-risk group. She can have regular blood tests to screen these levels.[21]

Side Effects from Taking Estrogen   Most women respond favorably to estrogen therapy, but some experience various difficulties with it. A woman who doesn't receive immediate results from HRT (hormone replacement therapy) should not be discouraged, since there is a wide range of options. HRT is very individual; every woman needs to find, through experimentation, the HRT that suits her best.

Some of the side effects experienced when first taking estrogen may include depression, nausea, vomiting, bloating, increased weight, cramps, swollen or tender breasts, headaches, vertigo, increased susceptibility to vaginal yeast infections, and breakthrough vaginal bleeding.

The body may take a couple of months to adjust to estrogen, in which case these symptoms often quickly disappear. If they don't disappear spontaneously, you may need to adjust your dose, try a different type of estrogen, or vary the method of taking it. About 25 percent of women may have some abnormal uterine bleeding and may need an occasional endometrial biopsy. This should not be required more than once a year. But, if progesterone is taken properly, an annual biopsy should not be necessary.

There Are Different Types of Estrogen   There are three main types of estrogen produced in the female body: estradiol, estrone, and estriol, given in order of potency. Conjugated (mixed) equine estrogens contain them all. Other brands of estrogen may contain only one. Here is a list of some natural and synthetic forms of estrogen available by prescription.

Natural Estrogens
- Estradiol: Tablets (Estrace), patches (Estraderm, Climara), surgically implanted pellets, injections, capsules, and tablets produced by compounding pharmacies.
- Estrone: Tablets (Premarin, Ogen).
- Estriol: Made up by compounding pharmacies such as Bajamar Women's Healthcare and Women's International Pharmacy, usually as a triestrogen with eight parts estriol and one part each of estradiol and estrone.

Synthetic Estrogens
- Ethinyl estradiol, (Estinyl), the estrogen also found in the contraceptive pill.
- Quinestrol, (Estrovis), broken down by the body into ethinyl estradiol.

Hormone Therapy Is an Art and a Science   Hormone therapy is usually simple, but can sometimes be complex. When women seek hormone therapy, it is typical for their physicians to prescribe a standard regimen for all women. The problem is that women aren't all the same, and their needs and responses vary tremendously.

A standard procedure is for a physician to give every woman with menopausal problems the standard regimen of Premarin from day one to twenty-five in the calendar month, then Provera from day sixteen to twenty-five, and then a break.

Because women vary in the extent and severity of their hormonal problems and their sensitivity and reaction to medication, standardized treatments don't always work effectively for all, and women may experience side effects. So treatment needs individual tailoring and fine-tuning.

But don't make it more complicated than it is. For many women, just switching to Estrace or the Climara or Estraderm patch with natural progesterone is a successful first choice.

Estrogen Is Not for Everybody   Remember that there seem to be women who are estrogen types and others who are progesterone types. If you have an adverse reaction to estrogen despite trying different types and doses, you may not be able to take it. Listen to your hormones. You might be able to take natural progesterone or testosterone instead.

The Correct Estrogen for You   Estrogen is prepared in several forms: oral tablets, injections, patches, pellets, and creams. Some consider oral (taken by mouth) estrogens to be more beneficial because they pass through the liver, causing an increase in high-density lipids (HDLs, the good cholesterol); this effect is not as pronounced when women use other methods of taking estrogen. However, some doctors say that the hormones pass through the liver a second time, and so the pellet and higher-dose patch do increase the HDLs.

Not everyone responds equally well to all forms of estrogen. Some women find that certain forms of estrogen give them cramps or sore breasts while other forms do not. Some estrogens take away hot flashes for one individual, and others don't. Some estrogens leave women depressed, while others won't. Some cause headaches for some women; others don't. Women may need to try various types and doses of estrogen therapy before their menopausal symptoms successfully disappear, and before they decide that estrogen is not for them.

Conjugated Oral Estrogens   Conjugated equine estrogens (Premarin) are the most commonly prescribed estrogen, having been on the market since 1941. They are the most thoroughly tested and the most advertised, and they are considered reliable and trustworthy. Some physicians promote the use of these estrogens (made from pregnant mare's urine), because they are "natural" and contain all the forms of estrogen. Others disagree, saying that the quantities and proportions that are natural for horses are not natural for humans.

There are many different estrogenic chemicals in conjugated estrogens, including equilin equine sulfate, an estrogen specific to horses. Some women find this horse estrogen difficult to metabolize or excrete, and it can remain for long periods of time in the human system. The so-called "horse factor" is believed to be a major reason for increased side effects from conjugated estrogens. Some women may also be allergic to the coloring in the tablets. Some women with a tendency toward PMS find that conjugated estrogens cause depression or headaches. Also, conjugated estrogens can have a slightly adverse effect on liver functioning.

Nevertheless, many women feel better on conjugated estrogens than on other forms. That's why you should be prepared to try more than one estrogen to find the best one for you.

Dr. Phillip Warner   Dr. Phillip Warner, an OB/GYN in Los Gatos, California, and director of the Menopause Institute of Northern California, feels strongly that women should be given hormones that are identical with those produced by the human ovary. This means using plant-derived estradiol, estrone, and progesterone, rather than conjugated equine estrogens (Premarin) and medroxyprogesterone acetate (Provera). He says that this is a simple and obvious concept when you think about it.[22]

Premarin has had first position in the market for 50 years. Along with Provera, it has been widely prescribed and used in most research studies in the U.S.

Dr. Warner has been informed by PETA (People for the Ethical Treatment of Animals), a 500,000-member organization that battles cruelty to animals, that they consider the collection of urine from mares sequestered in stalls during the whole of their pregnancy to be cruel. They would prefer to see Premarin made in the laboratory (this product is now undergoing FDA approval).

Dr. Warner's concern is over the issue of physiology (matching human estrogen), not animal abuse. He thinks that women should be given the best estrogen available to match their own. He is not saying that Premarin is a bad product or that it won't work. Rather, he says that plant-derived estradiol and estrone are better products.

In Europe, the main estrogen used is estradiol valerate. This product is comparable to 17-beta estradiol which is available here as a tablet (Estrace), the Estraderm and Climara patches, and the estradiol pellet.

Side Effects of Premarin

- Estrogen may increase the level of antithrombin III, which increases the risk of clotting. Women at risk should have their antithrombin levels tested.

- Estrogen may increase production of the enzymes renin and angiotensin in the kidneys (in approximately one out of twenty women). This causes an increase in blood pressure.
- Estrogen may thicken and concentrate the bile produced by the liver, which can aggravate gallstones. When estrogen is taken by another route, this problem can be avoided.
- Estrogen should not be taken orally by women with damaged livers, but can be taken by other methods.
- About one in twenty women may experience an increase in blood pressure when taking estrogen.
- Another problem with taking either oral tablets or injectable estrogen may be the subsequent peaking and dipping of hormone levels, which may cause mood swings.

Women who are troubled by some of these side effects may wish to use the estrogen transdermal patch or vaginal cream, or estrogen gel that can be rubbed on the arm. These methods bypass the liver.

But note that Elizabeth Lee Vliet, M.D., says that these warnings are based on studies that used conjugated equine estrogens.

Other Oral Estrogens If a woman experiences side effects from taking conjugated estrogens, she may feel better on either Estrace or Ogen. Estrace contains mainly 17-beta estradiol, the most potent estrogen in the female body. Ogen contains mainly estrone, a weaker human estrogen. These hormones are chemically different, and women may do better on one or the other. My experience has been that many women feel better and significantly less depressed on Estrace.[23] Other women find Estrace too strong. It may make them feel hyperactive, tense, or nauseated. They can cut the dose or switch to Ogen.

Oral tablets work well for some women and can help to increase the level of beneficial HDLs. But tablets may not be effective for others, because the liver screens incoming chemicals from the stomach via the bloodstream. In its effort to prevent "foreign invasion," the liver may destroy incoming oral estrogen and also cause side effects.

Taking More Than One Form of Estrogen Some women don't fully lose their symptoms after switching to oral estrogens, but want to continue receiving the beneficial effects on the lipids provided by tablets. If their physician is willing, they may need to take estrogen by both the oral and another route. For instance, some may opt to take a low dose of the patch and a low oral dose.

Estrogen Injections   Monthly injections of long-lasting estrogen are a reliable source of estrogen. Some women with high metabolism may need shots several times a month. This is especially applicable to women who exercise vigorously.

There are several advantages to injectable estrogen. Some women prefer the convenience of having an injection once a month instead of taking tablets every day. Others find that injections work more consistently than tablets or the patch. The dose of estrogen can be adjusted by varying how much is taken up in the syringe.

Some physicians give women with extreme symptoms more frequent injections at a lower dosage (even as many as two or three a week), adding progesterone and testosterone to the shot. They decrease the number of shots as the woman improves.

But many women find it a disadvantage to make regular visits to the doctor's office for an injection. Another disadvantage is that some women who have shots may develop abscesses or, over a period of years, scar tissue in the hip at the injection site, and absorption of estrogen is consequently poor.

Surgeons often choose to use injections after an oophorectomy (especially in younger women), because women often don't find the doses in the oral tablets or the patch adequate at that time. After about three months, the physician will switch the patient from injections to another form of estrogen.

Peak-and-Valley Experience   One problem some women encounter with tablets and, to a lesser extent, monthly injections, is that they have a peak-and-valley type of effect. Women feel good a short time after taking the pill, but the effect runs out as the hormone levels drop. Their experience is not consistent.

Sometimes hormone levels are more stable when the patch or implant is used.

Wearing the Patch   Because it bypasses the liver, the transdermal patch was hailed for its benefits when it first came out.

It promised better absorption, a more consistent dose of estrogen, and diminished side effects.

A large percentage of women have been pleased with the overall effect of the patch, but some are disappointed for two reasons:

1. It comes off easily, although it can be reattached by gently blowing warm air on the estrogen paste with a blow-dryer.

2. Many women develop a skin allergy, either to the alcohol in the patch or to the patch adhesive, which produces red, hive-like swellings under and around the patch. Some women find that applying the patch to the hip, rather than the abdomen, alleviates this problem. Others find this doesn't help. Another suggestion is to apply a little one-percent hydrocortisone cream on the place where the patch will be applied. Then place the patch where the cream was rubbed in. This will help some women, but there will be some who still can't tolerate the patch. The new Climara patch seems better in this respect.

Estrogen Gel   A new estrogen gel is available in the U.S., a virtually identical product to the one that has been available and widely used in Europe for over a decade. This gel is rubbed on the arm, the inner thighs, or the abdomen daily or twice daily, and apparently provides stable levels of estradiol.[24]

Implanting Estrogen Pellets   The implantation of one or more estradiol pellets, by a minor surgical procedure, into the fatty subcutaneous tissue of the abdomen or hip works very well for women with severe estrogen deficiency. Sometimes testosterone pellets are used with the estrogen. Like the patch, the implant gives continuous and constant estrogen levels and bypasses the liver. According to Dr. Phillip Warner, the blood levels of estrogen available from the pellet are greater and last much longer than those from the patch.

The implant is particularly appropriate for women who have tried every other way of taking estrogen, who respond positively to estrogen, but who cannot maintain stable levels. This includes women who have had their ovaries removed, and some women with hysterectomy (removal of the uterus) only. It may also be appropriate for women without surgery who have estrogen-related depression and need high doses for relief.

The estrogen in this form goes directly to the estrogen receptors in the brain and has a wonderful effect on the emotions. For some women, taking estrogen by implant is far superior to taking it any other way.

The beneficial effects of the implant last three to six months, and, for some women, up to a year. The disadvantage of implants is that once they are in, they are not easy to remove if a woman experiences any side effects.

The pellet was, I believe, FDA-approved at one time, but is not at the present time. However, approval of a pellet in gel form is imminent. The studies necessary for its approval have been submitted, but it will take a few years for approval to come through. A few researchers presently have permission to do estrogen-implant surgery.

How Much Estrogen?   The severity of symptoms strongly influences the amount of estrogen a woman should take, and individual rate absorption and metabolism are also important variables. A physician might, for example, suggest that a woman take a low dose on alternate days if she seems to be getting overdose symptoms such as nausea. Or her dosage might be increased if the lower dose does not alleviate her hot flashes. If a higher dose still does not relieve the symptoms, the doctor might switch to another brand or method of taking estrogen. Height and weight also make a difference. Generally, women who need estrogen before menopause need a higher dose than those who take it after menopause. The standard practice, then, is to give premenopausal women about twice the amount given to postmenopausal women.

The following is a list of the more common forms of estrogen with dosages.

Oral tablets

Estrace (estradiol): This comes in 2 mg (green tablet), 1 mg (violet-blue tablet), and 0.5 mg (white tablet) doses. One milligram of Estrace is roughly equivalent to 0.625 mg of Premarin, though they vary in their potency in different organs.

Premarin (conjugated estrogens): The standard dose is 1.25 mg (a yellow, football-shaped tablet) per day. A smaller dose, given to postmenopausal women, who don't need as much estrogen, is 0.625 mg (a red-brown football-shaped tablet). Other doses are available for women who need more or less estrogen: 2.5 mg (a purple tablet), 0.9 mg (a white tablet), and 0.3 mg (a dark green tablet).

OgEN (estropipate): This is available in 1.25 mg (orange tablet), and 0.625 mg (yellow tablet) doses. A 2.5 mg (blue tablet) is also available.

Injections: More than one brand of injectable estrogen is available. Delestrogen, Depo-Estradiol, and Depo-Testadiol (with a little testosterone) are various brands of long-lasting estrogen injections, usually given about once a month. For instance, 0.5 cc of Delestrogen (40 mg per cc) can be given intramuscularly in the hip. Dosage can be adjusted up or down, depending on the need.

Estraderm and Climara Transdermal Patches: There are two strengths, 0.1 mg and 0.05 mg.

Pellets: Typically, two to five 25-mg estrogen pellets and one 75-mg testosterone pellet are implanted separately (i.e., north, south, west, and east of a specific point), using a trocar in the groin, lateral thigh, or buttocks. If they are inserted too close to the skin's surface, the site may swell and the pellets may be expelled. Also, scar tissue may form when the site is too close to the surface, and absorption will be hindered.

Using several pellets is better than using one large one, as there is more surface area. For example, a woman will get 0.25 mg of estradiol daily from one 100-mg implant, but she will get 0.40 mg of estradiol daily from four 25-mg implants.[25] Depending on a woman's metabolism, the implant's effectiveness lasts for about three months to a year, after which symptoms will abruptly or slowly return. Taking oral estrogen concurrently with the pellet, after the pellets have been inserted for a while, may help lengthen the potency of the implant.

Vaginal Ring: This has been submitted for FDA approval. It will provide a steady dose of estradiol each day to the uterus and vagina, but will not enter the bloodstream. Blood levels of estrogen would remain the same as in normal, untreated postmenopausal women. This would be appropriate for women with severe vaginal dryness who do not wish to have extra circulating estrogen. It might be used, for instance, in a women with a past history of breast cancer who has had treatment that put her into menopause but who did not wish to take estrogen that works systemically.

Different Ways of Taking Oral Tablets   Women on estrogen who have not had a hysterectomy are always given enough progestin to avoid too great a buildup of the uterine lining. While this is common practice, and necessary to prevent uterine cancer, the FDA has not yet officially approved of using Provera for this purpose, and the long-term effects of progestins are still unknown.

The standard way to take hormone replacement therapy has been to use estrogen from day one to twenty-five of the calendar month, and progesterone for ten days, from day sixteen to twenty-five of the calendar month, which corresponds with a woman's menstrual cycle. The woman then stops taking hormones for the rest of the month. This protocol is now considered outdated. Many women experience a "kickback" from going off estrogen for five or six days a month. Because of this, some physicians suggest they only go off of it for two or three days a month, or stay on the estrogen all the time. Taking estrogen all the time is probably best to maintain emotional stability. As long as the woman also takes adequate progesterone, taking estrogen continually is not a problem.

Some women take both estrogen and progesterone daily for five days each week, and stop taking them on the weekend (sometimes resulting in pretty miserable Sundays). This suggestion was made for women with breast problems, to avoid overstimulation with estrogen; simply lowering the daily dose without stopping estrogen also overcomes these problems. So this method, too, is rarely used.

As mentioned before, other women have been put on a daily dose of both estrogen and progesterone. This method works well for women who have completed menopause because, generally, it stops the annoyance of having periods after menopause (a major reason many women dislike estrogen therapy). After the first three or four months, menstrual-type bleeding often stops.

Women Who Still Have Menstrual Periods   There is some difference of opinion here. Some doctors will not prescribe estrogen for women who still have periods; they say that if the women have periods, they still produce enough estrogen. Others believe that women can produce enough estrogen to have periods yet still be functionally low in estrogen.[26]

Some doctors, such as John Arpels, M.D., will put women with estrogen-deficiency symptoms on estrogen alone while their periods continue to be normal and regular. These doctors will watch the patients carefully, and maybe even do occasional endometrial sampling; if these women continue to ovulate, they are presumed to be producing adequate progesterone themselves. These doctors believe that estrogen has more impact on elevating the mood and that progesterone (even sometimes the natural type) tends to lower the mood. When these women begin having bleeding irregularities and irregular periods, these physicians will add progesterone to the protocol.

Other doctors are concerned about putting women on estrogen alone because of the possibility of adverse changes to the endometrial lining, ultimately leading to cancer. The ongoing PEPI study supports these concerns. It abandoned the group of controls with premenopausal women on estrogen alone because of the high number of women who developed adenomatous hyperplasia (abnormal thickening of the uterine lining). Other doctors choose to treat women who still have menstrual periods with daily estrogen and cyclical progesterone to match the woman's own cycle. Taking estrogen and progesterone continually doesn't work as well for them because this tends to cause breakthrough bleeding.

Taking Estrogen—A Summary

- Find a type of estrogen that controls your symptoms and doesn't create new ones. You may need to experiment with different brands.

- Find a method of taking estrogen—oral, injectable, cream, patch, gel, or implant—that suits you and does the job adequately. You may even need to take it by two routes, if your physician agrees.
- Take the lowest dose that will cover your symptoms and still protect your bones and heart.
- Be consistent in taking your medication. Don't stop and start it sporadically.
- If you are taking estrogen for 25 days each cycle and experience a return of symptoms whenever you stop it at the end of each month, try taking it every day without a break. Women commonly experience a "kickback" during the time when they are off estrogen until a few days after taking it again.
- Take adequate progesterone if you still have your uterus (see next section, "The Necessity of Taking Progesterone"). Even if you have had a hysterectomy, you may still wish to take the progesterone to protect your breasts against estrogen stimulation.
- If you find that you are depressed or have other adverse symptoms from taking synthetic progestins, ask your physician if you can try natural progesterone instead of, or with, the synthetic progestin.
- See your physician if you have abnormal bleeding, and return for an annual checkup. Ask him or her to check your hormone levels each year to make sure that you are absorbing what you take.
- If you have been on estrogen a long time and want to go off it, do so over several months, not all at once. This will help you to avoid the recurrence of hot flashes.

The Necessity of Taking Progesterone

Women on estrogen therapy must also take progesterone to avoid hyperplasia (thickening of the uterine lining) or endometrial cancer. An exception is that, when women are still ovulating and having normal bleeding, some doctors will give them estrogen only until the bleeding becomes erratic, monitoring them carefully for hyperplasia. I still think that it's better to take progesterone if you can.

Progesterone therapy is particularly important for post-menopausal women who still have their uterus. But it's a good idea for women who have had a hysterectomy to take progesterone as a protection against estrogen's breast-stimulating properties, even though evidence, to date, does not indicate that estrogen is a direct cause of breast cancer.

How Much Synthetic Progestin Is Needed?   Women who have never had PMS may do perfectly well taking a synthetic progestin along with estrogen. General recommendations in the U.S. are to give women Provera or, less commonly, Norlutate, Aygestin, or Cycrin for 13 days at the end of each cycle. Dr. Lila Nachtigall suggests 5 mg of Provera (a synthetic progestin) for ten days each month, or 10 mg for seven days. Some women who bleed heavily or have hyperplasia need to take 5 to 10 mg for 13 days.

If women wish to take estrogen and a synthetic progestin each day to avoid menstrual bleeding, the usual dose of the progestin is 2.5 mg to 5 mg daily. After three or four months on daily estrogen and progestin, menstrual bleeding usually stops if a woman is well past menopause.

Some Women Can't Tolerate Synthetic Progestins   Some women have problems tolerating the synthetic progestin part of their therapy.[28] Provera and other synthetic progestins may cause mood alterations, particularly in women who have a genetic tendency toward PMS. The combination of Premarin and Provera is the most common regimen of hormone replacement therapy and the most researched, and it is considered "tried and true."

If it works for you, and you don't have side effects on it, you should probably stick with it. If you have completed menopause, you may take Premarin and Provera on a daily basis. When the dose of Provera is halved and taken daily (usually 2.5 mg), it is less likely to produce mental irritability. And after a few months, bleeding will cease, except for occasional breakthrough bleeding. (This doesn't always work, however!)

But if you just can't tolerate Provera, natural progesterone may suit you better. And, personally, I think natural progesterone should be the first choice, not the last.

Doses for Natural Progesterone   Doctors resist giving natural progesterone as a part of hormone replacement therapy, because they feel uncomfortable about the lack of studies done on its ability to make the necessary changes in the uterus. But some studies have been done.[28] Some physicians prescribe 100 mg of natural progesterone twice daily for 13 days. Others say that this is not enough, and give 100 mg in the morning and 200 mg at night for 13 days of the menstrual cycle. The dosage in suppositories suggested by Dr. Don Gambrell is 25 mg, used twice a day for 13 days of the menstrual cycle.

Recent studies have shown that capsules containing both micronized estradiol and natural progesterone, taken daily, prevented hyperplasia in postmenopausal women; after six months, these women had no more menstrual periods.[29] The dosage is 0.5 mg of estradiol and 100 mg of oral micronized progesterone, taken two or three times a day.

Schering Laboratories has begun an FDA trial for natural progesterone. Until it is available, natural progesterone can be obtained from compounding pharmacies. See Appendix 2.

When a Synthetic Progestin May Be Better Than Natural Progesterone   Synthetic progestins can be mass-produced and marketed much less expensively than natural progesterone. Their effectiveness in protecting the lining of the uterus has been widely studied, and doses are well established. Drug companies have a strong financial interest to protect in promoting synthetic progestins, and they are much more widely available.

While some physicians believe that an annual endometrial biopsy should be done as a matter of course for all women on estrogen therapy, even if they are taking Provera, other physicians have had so much experience with Provera and have so much confidence in it that they feel an annual endometrial biopsy is unnecessary.

Because natural progesterone has a poor absorption rate and is rapidly metabolized, it is necessary to take higher, more frequent doses than with a synthetic progestin to effect similar changes. Natural progesterone is also much more expensive than synthetic progestins such as Provera, costing from about 65 cents to a dollar per dose at present.

When Natural Progesterone May Be Better Than a Synthetic Progestin   If a woman has had a long-term battle with PMS, she will probably find that the synthetic progestin component of her estrogen replacement therapy gives her side effects.

Many susceptible women, who react adversely to synthetic progestins, may wish to try natural progesterone, because they tend to be less depressed and irritable on natural progesterone. For those women who find that synthetic progestins, such as Provera, aggravate their emotional symptoms, using natural progesterone may be a necessity.

Changing to natural progesterone doesn't always prevent adverse mood changes. Some women may choose to take progesterone less frequently (for 13 days every two to three months). If they take estrogen long-term, they may find that they develop changes in their uterus. This needs to be watched carefully. Eventually, they might opt, as I did, to have a hysterectomy, so that they no longer needed to take progesterone.

Another advantage of taking natural progesterone is that it does not reverse estrogen's beneficial effect in reducing high-density lipoproteins. Synthetic progestins do reduce HDL levels to some extent, thereby reversing the beneficial effect of estrogen on the heart. Dr. Winnifred Cutler, in her book *Hysterectomy: Before and After,* mentions a study from Sweden showing that the adverse changes in lipids produced by taking 250 mg of Levonorgestrel or 10 mg of Provera per day, did not occur when 100 mg of natural progesterone was taken twice a day instead.[30]

Dr. Kathryn Morris writes:

The 3-year [PEPI] study was the first large study to incorporate natural progesterone in its trials. It involved 875 women, divided into study groups who 1) used estrogen alone, 2) used estrogen with Provera, 3) used estrogen with natural progesterone, and 4) a placebo group. As was expected, all groups on estrogen had significant increases in the

HDL, the good cholesterol, and decreases in the LDL, the bad cholesterol. Also as expected, the addition of Provera had a detrimental effect, lowering the HDL level to less than half of that which had been gained by the estrogen. The surprise was that the natural progesterone had little or no detrimental effect on the cholesterol level and hence didn't appear to promote heart disease as Provera does. Dr. Suzanne Oparil, president of the American Heart Association, estimated that the increases in HDL in either the estrogen alone group or estrogen combined with natural progesterone group would cut the risk of heart disease by almost 25 percent. On the other hand, the women on estrogen and Provera were estimated to have only a 12 percent reduction in their risk of heart disease.[31]

Dr. Phillip Warner says:

Evidence that postmenopausal estrogen replacement therapy reduces cardiovascular risk grew substantially with the announcement of findings from the Postmenopausal Estrogen and Progestin Intervention (PEPI) trial. In that trial, five treatment groups were utilized, including one group using estrogen and micronized (natural) progesterone. The group having the best degree of favorable lipid patterns was the group using estrogen alone. This group developed a high degree of potential uterine cancer. The estrogen and natural progesterone group came closest to the favorable pattern of estrogen alone and still protects against uterine cancer. This study confirms the advantage of using natural estrogen and progesterone to achieve benefits in women on hormonal replacement therapy. The positive lipid benefits confirm the principle of replacing those hormones normally produced by the human ovary.[32]

Progesterone Helps the Bones Progesterone often helps women with fibrocystic breasts, and it is also good for the bones. A study on marathon runners and osteoporosis found that the "normal" women (average age 35) who acted as controls were losing bone density too. Each month, the researchers checked the hormone levels and the bone density of both groups—the controls and the marathoners. They found that when the "normal" women didn't ovulate (that is, did not produce progesterone), they lost up to 2 to 4 percent of their bone mass.[33]

Since it is normal not to ovulate every month from your thirties on, because the egg supply lessens as the years progress, this means that all women begin the process of osteoporosis earlier than has been expected. Another interesting conclusion of the study highlights the importance of progesterone, not just estrogen, to treat osteoporosis.

While estrogen helps reduce calcium loss, studies are showing that natural progesterone actually increases bone mass. Partly because of this positive effect on the bones, I believe that natural progesterone, as an alternative to Provera and Norlutate, will soon be accepted as a superior treatment at menopause.

Having a Period Is Not the Issue   Don't think that if you are having regular periods and the lining of the uterus is being sloughed off, you can't have problems with the cells in your uterine wall. Endometrial cancer can occur where there is no nontypical bleeding.

Some women are severely emotionally affected by having a period, no matter which type of progesterone is used. These women, understandably, are often tempted to lower the dose of progesterone they take and shorten the number of days when they take it.

Women who are ultrasensitive to having periods, yet who need to induce them to ensure protection for their uterus, might talk to their doctors about inducing a period every second or third month, and taking the progesterone for 13 days then. Your doctor may wish to perform an annual endometrial biopsy or an ultrasound to determine the thickness of the lining. The lining should ideally be less than 5 mm and no more than 8 to 10 mm thick, and the X-ray technician has to be well trained to know what to look for.

Do You Need Testosterone?

When a woman's ovaries are removed, she loses the major source of her female hormones and the male hormone, testosterone. Sometimes the addition of a little testosterone to an estrogen shot, or the use of both testosterone and estrogen pellets, makes the estrogen work better and longer. It also helps those women with sore muscles and a flagging libido.

Testosterone levels also decline in women with ovaries, often beginning in their thirties. We find this true of the majority of women patients over 35 who come into Her Place at All Saints Center for Women's Health in Fort Worth, Texas. Levels should ideally be 35 to 50 pg/ml. They are routinely less than 10 to 20.

The physician has to decide whether adding testosterone will be beneficial. If a woman has a stressful job—for instance, as a trial attorney or a business owner—she will not be as successful in situations that cause confrontational stress after having her ovaries removed. Treatment with testosterone makes some women aggressive and sexually excited and may give them violent dreams. Other side effects are the growth of excess facial and body hair, deepening of the voice, and enlargement of the clitoris. These usually do not occur on replacement doses.

Hormone Replacement Therapy— A Typical Protocol

ESTROGEN: If a woman is premenopausal, doctors might prescribe from 0.25 mg to 2 mg of Estrace per day. This could be taken in divided doses twice daily, under the tongue or vaginally (these routes are recommended by John Arpels, M.D., Kit Morris, M.D., and Elizabeth Lee Vliet, M.D.).

On the lowest dose, the patient would cut the 1-mg Estrace tablet into quarters and take 0.25 mg twice a day. On a subsequent month, she might try taking 0.5 mg in the morning and 0.25 mg at night (increasing in one-quarter-tablet increments). The upper average dose would be 1 mg twice a day, but I have known doctors who prescribe more under certain circumstances. Dividing the dose helps avoid the peak-and-valley effect. Use the minimum that works.

Some women who exercise hard find that they metabolize the estrogen they take in the morning, and then have none left in their bloodstream by night. These women should divide their dose and take it morning and night. Women with migraines could divide the dose even further and take it 3 to 4 times a day. If a woman has nausea on even the lowest dose of estrogen, she might take it once at night to see if she can sleep off the symptoms.

If Estrace is not effective, a woman might try Ogen or Premarin in equivalent doses. Another alternative would be to use the estrogen patch, first trying the low dose (0.05 mg), then the higher dose (0.1 mg). Some women may feel better on the low-dose patch along with a low dose of oral estrogen—that is, taking it by two routes.

PROGESTERONE: A woman who still has her uterus will mainly be taking progesterone to make the necessary changes in the uterine lining. But she might also take it if she has a history of PMS or has other symptoms that progesterone alleviates.

While a woman is still menstruating, and if her doctor decides that she should take progesterone along with estrogen, she will probably want to take the progesterone from ovulation until menstruation. That is, she would take the estrogen every day, adding progesterone during the second half of her cycle. To determine when she should start taking the progesterone, she would first determine how long her cycles are (say 28 days), and subtract 13 (the number of days she needs to take progesterone). In a 28-day cycle, then, she would begin taking progesterone on day 15.

She could take 5 to 10 mg of Provera once a day for 13 days, and then stop to allow menstrual bleeding. A woman who experiences side effects from using Provera or Norlutate, or who wishes to use a progesterone that better matches the body's chemistry, may prefer to use natural progesterone. She would take 100 mg of natural progesterone in the morning and 200 mg at night, or use 25-mg vaginal or rectal suppositories twice a day, again for 13 days.

Some women near menopause who take hormones and still have difficulty around the time of menstruation may choose to take both hormones continuously to level their moods. This is not the best plan, since it tends to cause breakthrough bleeding. However these women prefer to feel better and disregard any spotting that may occur.

Postmenopausal Women   If a woman is postmenopausal, she could take the progesterone every day. It can be difficult to determine whether she is postmenopausal if she is already on hormone replacement therapy. She could have an FSH test, but taking hormones will probably result in a false reading.

A postmenopausal woman could take 2.5 mg of Provera each day. Or she could cut the dose of natural progesterone in half and take it each day—that is, 100 to 150 mg per day. The major side effect of natural progesterone is sedation, and usually this can be controlled by lowering the dose or taking it with food. Or she might take progesterone at night since it helps bring on sleep.

Brittle Menopause   Some women have what I call "brittle" PMS or menopause, and they are similar to brittle diabetics whose blood sugar levels are extremely hard to control. These women have severe hormone deficiencies that are extremely difficult to control, caused by poorly understood factors—possibly fluctuating blood sugar levels, altered rate of metabolism, or allergic reaction.

I know this is true because of my own problems. After 15 years of contact with numerous women with severe problems, I consider myself fortunate to have found a hormone protocol that works well for me, though I find fine-tuning my hormones is a process that requires continual adjustment.

QUICK TIPS FOR MENOPAUSE

1. Don't dread menopause. For many women, it's no big deal. Their periods stop overnight, and they have few symptoms. Even if your menopause is uncomfortable, severe problems are often temporary. For some, it may be like going through heavy surf, but eventually you will land on the beach. (However, call for help if you are about to drown.)

2. Read all you can about the subject of menopause so that you can make an educated decision about whether you're likely to need hormone replacement therapy or

can manage your symptoms in other ways. Ask yourself
if the particular author you are reading seems to have
any prejudices. Is their information current?

3. Remember that the body is like a machine. It has necessary parts, and it needs the correct fuel. These are two
different issues. Your particular hormone problem may
respond to giving the body better fuel, because the body
makes some of your hormone supply from nutrients. Lack
of sunshine, too much stress, being overweight, poor nutrition, lack of exercise, too much exercise, the use of
stimulants—all these are factors over which you have
some degree of control. You can sometimes make significant changes in the function of hormones by changing
your habits. Hormone replacement could also be considered a natural fuel.

On the other hand, some body parts just don't work
properly. Some women have parts missing. Others have
parts that break down. The hormone system can break
down for many reasons—heredity, the changes of pregnancy, the use of synthetic hormones (the pill, Provera,
Clomid, Lupron—though for many women these are not
a problem), or surgery (tubal sterilization, hysterectomy,
loss of an ovary or part of one). Problems such as endometriosis, pituitary tumors, polycystic ovaries, ovarian
cysts, and fibroids can also interfere with the mechanism
and predispose women to having problems at menopause.
Also, the immune system can affect the menstrual cycle
via stress, toxins such as pesticides, bacterial infections,
and viruses.

4. Take care of your general health. Those habits will help
your hormones. Eat whole, largely vegetarian foods that
have not been overprocessed. These include lots of vegetables and fruits, whole rather than processed grains, and
lots of legumes and beans. Monitor your intake of sugar,
fat, and caffeine. Try herbs and supplements known to be
helpful for hormone disorders.

5. Live a balanced life—get moderate, regular exercise and
adequate sleep. Go outdoors, allow adequate daylight to
enter your eyes (you don't have to be in bright sunshine,

but glass windows and eyeglasses shut out some beneficial rays). Don't let your life become too stressful. Give up smoking and avoid alcohol and street drugs, all of which deplete adrenal function and prematurely age your glands.

6. Find a support system. For instance, talk with other women going through the same problems that you are having. See if there is a local menopause support group in your area.

7. Find a well-informed, thorough, sympathetic physician who believes in hormone-related symptoms—one who will monitor your physical and emotional progress through the years, and who believes you when you describe your problems and successes. Do not tolerate callous, chauvinistic, uninformed care. Medicine is a business. Ask yourself whose body it is and who is paying the bills. On the other hand, remember that a doctor carries heavy responsibilities and liabilities, and may be unfamiliar or uncomfortable with certain treatments. It is the doctor's right to refuse to dispense certain medications to you.

8. Weigh the information on estrogen and breast cancer. Almost uniformly, the best researchers believe that estrogen does not cause endometrial or breast cancer when balanced with adequate progesterone. In fact, because the hormones strengthen the cells, the present swing is to believe that a combination of estrogen and progesterone generally prevents cancer.

9. Remember that normal blood test results and the absence of symptoms do not guarantee that you are free of hormone imbalance. Not everyone who has hormone deficiency knows about it. You could have heart disease and osteoporosis and yet have no overt menopausal symptoms. This is one reason why women need to contemplate their family and personal history and weigh their health risks. Is osteoporosis common in female family members? Does heart disease commonly occur before the age of 65 in female family members? Have your total cholesterol, HDL, and cholesterol ratio recently become elevated with no other apparent cause than menopause? Are

you losing your physical strength and sex drive? You may need some help with your hormones.

10. If you do need hormones, ask your doctor to prescribe natural hormones that best match your body chemistry. If the first type you try doesn't work or causes side effects, don't be afraid to ask to experiment with other brands and forms of the hormones. Sometimes, just switching to estradiol (Estrace or the Estraderm or Climara patches), with natural progesterone, will bring great improvement. Natural testosterone is often helpful when a woman has low sex drive, muscle weakness, and loss of well-being, especially in women who have lost their ovaries.

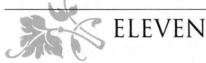

ELEVEN

ESTROGEN AND DEPRESSION

Just as thyroid affects moods because it targets the brain and interacts with brain neurotransmitters, so does estrogen. But this interaction is not as well researched. When I did a Psych-Line (psychology database, similar to Med-Line) search on thyroid and depression for this book, I retrieved 169 abstracts. When I did a search on estrogen and depression, I found only one.

But there are a number of experts who believe that changes in estrogen levels are linked with depression.

Dr. Mark Gold, in his book, *Good News About Depression*, points out that women are more likely to have symptoms of depression during their perimenopausal years, when ovarian hormones are changing, than after menopause, when hormone levels stabilize. And he notes that women who have their ovaries surgically removed are more likely to be depressed.

Dr. Gold sees a link between such types of depression and estrogen's tendency to lower serotonin levels and affect serotonin receptors. Estrogen also plays a role in regulating levels of monoamine oxidase (MAO) enzymes (a brain chemical which affects mood adversely when high).

In Dr. Gold's own words:

> The question naturally arises: If changing estrogen levels affect mood, might estrogen work as a treatment for depression? It's a controversial topic; but preliminary evidence offers some tantalizing clues. Some studies have found that estrogen acts on neurotransmitters and receptors in a way that is similar to antidepressants. In fact, in some patients, estrogen apparently enhances the effects of some antidepressants.[1]

Dr. Gold is not alone in seeing the link between estrogen levels and depression. The following authors and researchers expand on this theme.

Judith Bardwick, Ph.D.

In *The Psychology of Women*,[2] Judith Bardwick wrote that she had ". . . taken the apparently eccentric position that the body makes direct contributions to the psyche of the individual." In studying the physiological basis of behavior and the effects of the sex hormones, she looked at the possible psychological effects of the menstrual cycle, pregnancy, menopause, and the use of oral contraceptives. Bardwick did an amazing job in capturing the reality and the essence of all these problems as women experience them. Considering that it was written 25 years ago, she displayed remarkable insight.

As an example, she describes a study that she, Melville, and Ivey performed in 1968 on a group of 26 normal female students, spanning two menstrual cycles. Twice at ovulation, or mid-cycle, and twice at premenstruation, the women were asked to describe an experience that they had been through. Their replies were tape-recorded and later scored using an anxiety scale. The researchers scored themes related to death, mutilation, separation, guilt, shame, and diffuse anxiety. When the scores were combined, the premenstrual anxiety scores turned out to be significantly higher than those taken at ovulation.

At ovulation, a common theme was self-satisfaction about the ability to cope, high self-esteem, and positive feelings. Before menstruation, the feelings changed to hostility, thoughts of death and separation, anxiety, and depression. The difference in tone in conversations recorded at ovulation and before menstruation in the same woman was remarkable.

Note the following samples taken from the same woman. The contrasts were common throughout the group.

At ovulation:

"Talk about my trip to Europe. It was just the greatest summer of my life. We met all kinds of terrific people everywhere we went and just the most terrific things happened."

Before menstruation:

"Talk about my brother and his wife. I hated her. I just couldn't stand her. I couldn't stand her mother. I used to do terrible things to separate them."

Bardwick concluded that women feel at their best around ovulation when the estrogen level is high and progesterone is absent. They feel at their worst premenstrually when estrogen (and progesterone) levels are low.

Turan Itil, M.D.

Dr. Turan Itil, a clinical professor of psychiatry at New York University Medical Center, wrote a significant article called "The Rebirth of Hormones in Psychiatry" in 1976. Even though this article is 20 years old, it accurately summarizes the situation in medicine today:

> Although male and female hormones have for a long time been recognized as the cause of some of the psychological disturbances in men and women, surprisingly few studies exist to investigate this relationship. It has been advocated that climacteric depression may be the result of diminution of androgen in men, that menopausal depression is due to a decrease of estrogen in women, and that premenstrual depression and irritability seem to be related to the progesterone-estrogen ratio. However, not a single double-blind controlled investigation exists concerning the effects of these hormones in these psychiatric syndromes.[3]

Dr. Itil gives an excellent summary of attitudes toward the hormone/brain issue. I have asked his permission to quote extensively from his article, because it describes the problem so well.

Hormones are organic, biologically active compounds synthesized within the organism. These substances are essential for the control of normal health and growth. A deficiency or excess secretion of hormones causes a variety of physical and behavioral disorders. During alterations of hormonal balance, not only temporary behavioral disorders, affective and emotional problems, but severe depression and exogenous (toxic) psychosis have been reported. This fact, particularly in recent years, has been overlooked in most psychiatric clinics.

The possibility that a patient's psychiatric problems may be the result of a hormonal imbalance has not frequently been considered, unless the typical, well known, physical symptoms are seen and then confirmed by laboratory data. However, it is known to the practicing psychiatrist, to the gynecologist, and to the endocrinologist that behavioral disorders may occur as a result of hormonal deficiency or imbalance, without "typical" somatic symptoms or abnormal laboratory results. In the early stages of their illness, some patients may only have behavioral problems which escape attention, the physical symptoms not appearing until late in the course of the disease. In other patients a chronic deficiency of a hormone may result in the occurrence of psychiatric symptomatology without the development of a "typical" clinical syndrome. In some others the physical signs of hormonal deficiencies may never occur.

A natural (physiological) decrease of the hormonal level, such as a decrease of the male hormone in elderly men (climacteric state) or a decrease of estrogen in elderly women (menopausal state), is frequently associated with behavioral alterations. In most elderly men and women the behavioral problems remain at the "borderline" [subclinical] level and can be compensated for without requiring a psychiatric consultation. A considerably large group of men and women do, however, suffer and seek help. Partly for social and cultural reasons, patients, if they are not specifically asked, report to the doctors only the somatic [of the body] aspects of their problems and hesitate to present their behavioral problems and psychiatric symptoms. The significance of the borderline psychopathology is overlooked most of the time.

Without any justification, it is accepted that the hormonal changes during the physiological aging process are associated with the attenuation of physical and mental ability, resulting in somatic and psychological disturbances. While explanations of the problems are easily made by endocrinological facts and dynamic hypotheses, the suffering of a patient is considered to be the price to be paid in the process of aging, and attempts to correct them are looked upon with considerable suspicion.

Although the discovery of drugs effective in human behavior and the beginning of "classical" psychopharmacology significantly changed the hospital scene, the treatment of psychiatric problems is still rather arbitrary and not individualized. Since the modern psychotropic drugs rather rapidly alleviate psychopathological symptoms, they are being widely, but frequently indiscriminately, used. The classical medical model for seeking the cause of an illness has almost been absent in the drug treatment of psychiatric patients. Frequently patients receive drugs even before a diagnosis is made.

It is well known that none of the psychotropic drugs cure any of the psychiatric illnesses. Despite this, only a limited amount of research is being done to develop better and specifically effective psychotropic drugs. The symptomatic treatment is too easily accepted as a routine procedure because it provides comfort to the family, hospital staff, physician and last, but not least, the patient.

Despite our long-standing knowledge of the occurrence of behavioral problems and psychotic symptoms due to hormonal imbalance, investigations of hormonal levels and applications of hormone treatment in psychiatric patients were reported much more frequently prior to 1954, before the routine use of psychotropic drugs became fashionable. A variety of psychiatric disorders have been related to hyper- or hypo-secretion of hormones and the relief of psychiatric symptoms after the administration of hormones has been reported.[4]

Edward L. Klaiber, M.D.

Drs. Edward Klaiber, Donald Broverman, and William Vogel have written two important articles about estrogen and depression.[5] In the first study they describe, patients were diagnosed as depressive by a clinical psychologist and by the use of written tests. The study comprised 40 women, 25 of whom had made serious suicide attempts prior to inclusion in the study. There were 23 premenopausal and postmenopausal depressive women in the treated group and 17 similar women in the placebo group. The 23 treated women were given high doses of Premarin—5 mg or more daily. If the initial dose did not alleviate symptoms, the dosage was gradually increased to 25 mg daily.

Of the 23 women who received estrogen, five received a maximum dose of 15 mg; six, a maximum of 20 mg; and twelve a maximum of 25 mg daily. The premenopausal women were also given 2.5 mg of Provera from day 21 to 26 of their menstrual cycles.

Compare these study doses to the normal postmenopausal dose of 0.625 mg., and you will see that the highest dose in the study is about 40 times higher than would normally be given after menopause.

The women were repeatedly tested, and the final Hamilton ratings (a test for depression) were significantly reduced in the group taking estrogen, but not in the placebo group. Though there was a statistically significant improvement in the Hamilton ratings after three months, the results were still relatively high, indicating some residual depression. So it was improvement, not cure. Also note that two women became even more depressed when taking estrogen.

Concern about an increase in endometrial hyperplasia and thrombosis (blood clotting) as a result of taking high doses of estrogen is valid, but could not be calculated in such a short time because hyperplasia takes about eight years to develop into cancer. However, these possible threats were considered to be less of a hazard to these women than their suicidal depression.

Drs. Klaiber and Broverman suggest that depression involves an impairment of central chemical functioning in the brain. Estrogen may enhance brain function by increasing norepinephrine synthesis. It may also inhibit chemicals that inactivate norepinephrine, such as MAO. This MAO inhibition increases norepinephrine levels. Estrogen may also stimulate serotonin receptors.[6]

Dr. Klaiber's study on estrogen and depression is the main controlled study that has been done using estrogen, and, if you read the research literature, you will see it quoted frequently. This work needs to be corroborated by longer studies on more women, preferably using other estrogens (such as estradiol) and lower doses.

David Keefe, M.D., and Frederick Naftolin, M.D.

In "Brain Neurochemistry and Mood,"[7] Drs. Keefe and Naftolin look at the biological factors that affect mood, and the way in which steroid hormones affect brain chemistry. They note that symptoms of mood disorder respond to ovarian hormones, and that some patients will have a worsening of their continual symptoms premenstrually. There is a common coincidence of mood disorder and PMS, and the two probably involve related neurobiological mechanisms. They point out:

> Research on the neurobiological basis of mood disorders has uncovered disorders of: (1) neurotransmission, (2) receptor function, (3) intracellular signal transduction, (4) psychophysiology, including sleep architecture, (5) biological rhythms, and (6) brain structure, especially hemispheric dominance. Although clinical study of the effects of ovarian steroids on these parameters has been limited, basic research shows that ovarian steroids can influence practically every one of these systems. In addition, recent studies on the neurobiological basis of steroid action within the central nervous system have uncovered a number of steroid-sensitive brain mechanisms that could underlie sex steroid modulation of mood, and

possibly elucidate the biological basis of premenstrual syndrome and sex differences in the incidence of mood disorders.[8]

Roger Smith, M.D., and John Studd, M.D.

These British research OB/GYNs have collaborated on two articles about estrogens and depression in women.[9] They point out that, while research psychiatrists generally hold the view that there is no increase in the incidence of depression among menopausal women,[10] gynecologists believe that depression is one of the most common presenting symptoms of menopause.[11] Added to depression are other psychological symptoms: difficulty in making decisions, poor concentration, memory impairment, anxiety, loss of confidence, and feelings of unworthiness. They comment on the paucity of well-controlled studies on this subject, but particularly mention work by the following researchers:

- Montgomery and others:[12] This study showed statistically significant reductions in depression and anxiety scores for women on 50-mg estradiol implants or 50-mg estradiol and 50-mg testosterone implants, when compared to a placebo group.
- Ditkoff and others:[13] In this study, using Premarin, the women on estrogen were significantly less depressed than those not on estrogen, even though they were not considered clinically depressed.
- Sherwin and Gelfand:[14] This study showed that intramuscular administration of either estrogen and testosterone, or estrogen alone, after surgical menopause resulted in lower depression scores than a placebo when the hormones reached normal premenopausal levels.

    Smith and Studd note that estrogen functions similarly to antidepressants in the way it acts on neurotransmitters. For instance:

- It increases the availability of norepinephrine (increases its release and inhibits the action of monoamine oxidase);
- It alters adrenergic and serotonergic activity (the activity of the brain neurotransmitters norepinephrine and serotonin) by modulating receptor sensitivity;

- It enhances the dopaminergic system (another brain neurotransmitter).

Smith and Studd conclude that you can use physiologic doses (i.e., those normally found in the human body) of estrogen to treat PMS, postpartum depression, perimenopause and menopausal depression. And you can probably use pharmacological doses (higher than normal) to effectively treat major depression, though this needs more study.

In recent correspondence Dr. John Studd wrote to me:

> We have continued this work with high-dose oestradiol patches 200 mg in a cross-over study, showing that this treatment is more effective than placebo in all of the Moos' clusters [a written form for objective mood testing] for PMS. I have no doubt that percutaneous [via the skin] oestrogens by patch or implant is a very convenient way of raising the oestradiol levels and effectively treating one of the "triad" of hormone responsive mood disorders. That is: 1) Postnatal depression; 2) Premenstrual depression; 3) Climacteric depression.

Elizabeth Lee Vliet, M.D.

Dr. Lee Vliet is a clinical associate professor in the Department of Family and Community Medicine at the University of Arizona College of Medicine, and the founder and director of HER Place, both located in Tucson, Arizona. She and I also work together at HER Place at All Saints Center for Women's Health in Fort Worth, Texas. In 1991, she published an excellent article about the relationship of hormones to affective disorders during perimenopause.[15] In this article, Dr. Vliet describes perimenopause and menopause as normal phases of a woman's reproductive life cycle. She points out that many women find these phases an easy transition. However, 30 to 40 percent of women experience "worsening PMS," irritability, and depressive moods prior to menses, along with migraines, insomnia, mood swings, fatigue, and lowered sex drive. Dr. Vliet points out that there has been little recognition of the role of declining hormone levels in these symptoms. Most medical studies that have tried to address the question of hormonal links have focused on women at menopause, or just after it. Almost no studies have looked at these issues in the premenopausal phase, when such symptoms are actually more common.

Dr. Vliet has continually suggested that the rate of change in estrogen, progesterone, and testosterone levels may be a greater trigger for negative mood changes than is the actual hormone level. Dr. Vliet presented her clinical work on the role of estrogen in mood changes at the 1992 meeting of the North American Menopause Society.[16] In this presentation, she was a pioneer in pulling together research from many different fields. Each of these studies had investigated different aspects of the effects of estrogen on the brain. Dr. Vliet synthesized what was known at the time about the effects of estrogen on various neurotransmitter systems (such as serotonin and norepinephrine) which are involved in regulating mood, memory, and sex drive.

Barbara Sherwin, Ph.D.

Barbara Sherwin is a professor in the Departments of Psychology and Obstetrics & Gynecology at McGill University, in Montreal, Quebec, Canada. She is a well-known authority on the psychological and sexual effects of estrogen and testosterone. She says that sex steroids may exert direct action on parts of the brain that control emotions and sexuality.[17] Dr. Sherwin summarizes some known effects of estrogen:

- Estrogen increases, and progesterone decreases, the excitability of the brain.
- Estrogen induces the synthesis of ribonucleic acid (RNA) and proteins. This leads to changes in genetic products, such as enzymes that synthesize neurotransmitters.
- Estrogen interacts with hormone receptors in important areas of the brain—mainly the pituitary, hypothalamus, limbic forebrain, and cerebral cortex.
- Estrogens can directly alter the electrical activity of neurons in the hypothalamus.
- Certain neurotransmitter systems have been suggested (but not all demonstrated) to be responsive to estrogen. For instance, estrogen increases the rate of degradation of MAO

in rat brains. MAO catabolizes serotonin, so estrogen indirectly increases serotonin levels in the brain.

- L-tryptophan, an amino acid that is a precursor to serotonin, is displaced from its binding to plasma albumin by estrogens; more free tryptophan thus becomes available to the brain, where it is metabolized into serotonin.
- Imipramine binding sites, which appear to modulate serotonin uptake, are fewer in depressed women. Estrogen appears to increase the number of these sites, and consequently improves mood.
- Specific receptors for testosterone have been found mainly in the hypothalamus, and to a lesser degree in the limbic system and cerebral cortex. The brain contains aromatizing enzymes necessary to convert androgens to estrogens.

Sherwin also cites Klaiber's aforementioned article as possible evidence that very large pharmacologic doses of estrogen may significantly alleviate clinical depression. However, she says that her findings support the clinical observation that giving estrogen alone to postmenopausal women helps to alleviate mild psychiatric symptoms, rather than true clinical depression.

However, I think that there are many women like me, who have had significant clinical depression and who did respond well to estrogen therapy.

John Arpels, M.D.

John Arpels is an associate professor of Obstetrics and Gynecology at the University of California at San Francisco. He has written several excellent articles about the effects of estrogen on the female brain.[18] He points out that a survey of menopausal women, taken in 1991 by *McCall's* magazine, showed that women were more disturbed by problems with memory and concentration than by hot flashes and night sweats. Also, problems that were cyclical in women when they were younger become continuing problems during perimenopause. At that time, depression may become constant, and there may be an increase in symptoms such as insomnia, loss of ability to memorize, inability to perform more than one task at a time, and inability to find needed items on a regular basis.

Arpels points out that the centers that control sleep, memory, emotion, cognition, and temperature regulation are all in the brain, and that these centers are rich in estrogen and testosterone receptors. Estrogen increases the number of synaptic connections between these centers of control and other parts of the brain. It also plays a major role in increasing the number of receptors for certain neurotransmitters and the quantity of neurotransmitters themselves—particularly serotonin, the β-endorphins, and dopamine.

Women vary tremendously in their personal need for estrogen in the central nervous system. But when estrogen levels drop below a particular estrogen set point, Arpels says that circuits start to "unplug," and mental and emotional changes can occur.

Testosterone is also important, both in the emotional center of the hypothalamus and in the areas that control libido in the limbic area of the brain. It is needed for a sense of well-being and mental energy, which has been termed "female aggressiveness." In order for testosterone to do its work, a certain amount of brain estrogen is needed, because estrogen creates testosterone receptors.

Arpels lists the stages when a woman's estrogen levels may dip suddenly. The most dramatic instance is with loss of the placenta at childbirth. Estrogen levels can drop one hundredfold, and the rate of decline may be as important as the amount lost. With her estrogen levels suppressed by lactation, and problems compounded by sleep deprivation and the stress of caring for a baby, a woman may begin to experience menopause-like symptoms. Eventually, the ovaries will overcome the initial suppression of estrogen production, and the problem will usually be resolved. Estrogen therapy can help lessen the symptoms greatly.

Arpels describes PMS as the time in each cycle, after ovulation, when women say that they feel their lights have been dimmed. Many patients respond dramatically to low-dose estrogen supplementation begun a couple of days before symptoms begin. He says that estrogen works by increasing the levels of serotonin and all the other neurotransmitters. It also promotes "circuit rewiring," increases blood flow in the central nervous system, and opposes the inhibitory action of micronized natural progesterone on GABA receptors ("GABA" stands for "gamma aminobutyric acid," a brain neurotransmitter).

Ovarian production of estrogen also declines gradually during the perimenopausal years. Dr. Arpels says that progesterone and Tamoxifen are both capable of shutting down estrogen receptors. He also sees some PMS as being caused by high levels of progesterone. Because Provera can shut down estrogen receptors, Dr. Arpels gives women on hormone replacement therapy slightly more supplemental estrogen during PMS, adding a diuretic (low-dose every 2 to 3 days), if necessary, to counteract the mineralocorticoid effect of progesterone.

Dr. Arpels says that replacing estrogen improves cognition, short-term memory, and abstract reasoning in postmenopausal women. Similar positive effects are seen when low-dose estrogen is given to women going through perimenopause; a woman may continue to produce sufficient hormones to have a menstrual cycle, but not enough for optimal brain function. He might give such a woman continual low-dose estrogen, but raise the dose in the luteal phase.

Arpels mentions the positive effects of estrogen in reversing dementia, giving a 40-to-60 percent protective effect against Alzheimer's disease. He also mentions its positive effect in treating cyclic migraine headaches.

James Alexander Hamilton, M.D.

In his book, *Postpartum Psychiatric Illness: A Picture Puzzle*, Dr. Hamilton (in a chapter co-authored with Deborah Sichel) discusses the preventive use of estrogen in treating postpartum depression.

In the late 1950s, Dr. Hamilton met Dr. Emory Page, who investigated the effects of giving estrogen to prevent lactation in women who couldn't or didn't want to breastfeed. Dr. Page observed that, in his experimental group, patients were remarkably free of maternity blues.

Because of this chance observation, Dr. Hamilton tried giving preventive injections of long-acting estrogen at delivery to a patient who had a previous postpartum psychosis. The treatment was successful, and she remained free of psychosis. Dr. Hamilton treated other similar patients with estrogen at delivery. Eventually, he treated a total of 50 such patients with estrogen. None had a recurrence of psychosis.

Dr. Hamilton's treatment consisted of a single injection of long-acting estrogen, given immediately after delivery. This was later extended with oral estrogen, taken for two weeks then gradually reduced.

Dr. Hamilton had no incidences of thrombosis (clotting) among the women he treated with estrogen, but he expresses some concern about this possibility. Women at delivery are more prone to developing blood clots, and the use of estrogen to prevent lactation has resulted in a number of women having fatal embolisms (blood-vessel obstructions) in the past. Dr. Hamilton now suggests using the estrogen patch rather than the injection, because the patch can be removed if there is a problem. Also, the type of estrogen in the patch (estradiol) is considered unlikely to cause blood clotting.

In the 1940s, Dr. Robert Greenblatt also used estrogen shots at delivery to prevent and treat PPD, in combination with natural progesterone. Dr. Hamilton has some concern about using natural progesterone alone for postpartum psychosis, because he has seen cases in which the psychosis returned during treatment.

Summary

As you can see, a number of researchers have looked at the effects of hormones on the brain, and on how they influence mood and sexuality. Estrogen is one of these hormones. If estrogen can alleviate hormonal depression in women, it may be a more natural first choice than an antidepressant.

CHAPTER

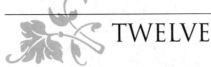 TWELVE

TUBAL STERILIZATION, HYSTERECTOMY, AND OOPHORECTOMIES

 Some women's hormone problems begin after having abdominal surgery that affects either the blood flow to the ovary or the hormone feedback system to the brain.

TUBAL LIGATIONS

Nancy and her husband, Ron, decided that Nancy should have a tubal sterilization after they had their third child. The surgery was performed the day after the baby was born.

Before the surgery, Nancy had never had anything but the mildest mood swings before her menstrual periods. In fact, she had no patience with women who said they had PMS, and felt they were making a mountain out of a molehill.

But after her surgery, there were some gradual but significant changes in her cycle; about six or seven years after the surgery, they became difficult to tolerate. Her periods, which had been accompanied by only minor cramps, became very heavy, and she had significant pain on her right side before and during her period.

When she went to her doctor, he said that these symptoms had nothing to do with the tubal ligation. His nurse practitioner, however, thought otherwise, and sent Nancy to me. I showed Nancy several books containing information on the adverse effects of tubal ligations, and explained that I commonly see women with these side effects after a tubal ligation.

I mentioned a physician friend in southern California who told me, anecdotally, that about 60 to 70 percent of women who have had tubal ligations go through premature menopause six or seven years afterward and have symptoms of declining estrogen and progesterone levels. I told Nancy that I find this to be true in my practice as well; when I speak publicly on hormonal issues, there is always a significant number of women in the audience who only started having symptoms after they had a tubal ligation.

Nancy asked if reversal of the tubal ligation would set her hormones straight. I told her that I didn't know, but I doubted it. I thought that once the blood flow had been damaged, the remaining scar tissue would continue to cause problems.

When the doctor put Nancy on hormone replacement therapy, she soon felt much better.

Tubal Ligations—a Frequent Cause of PMS

About 650,000 American women per year have a tubal ligation. Many of the women I see have had problems after a tubal ligation, and there is no doubt in my mind that this process of sterilization brings on some degree of hormonal dysfunction in a significant number of women. Many women with no history of chronic depression or hormonal problems begin having problems after a tubal ligation, and it can be a very unpleasant awakening for them. I have heard such women say that they used to think PMS was just an excuse that women used for their bad behavior. Now they realize that PMS is real, and they are furious that their physicians told them there would be no side effects.[1]

Some physicians attribute the side effects from a tubal ligation to the fact that the women have just been pregnant or have stopped taking the birth control pill, both of which can cause PMS. However, many women I see waited for a year or so after being pregnant, and were not on the pill before having a tubal ligation. It seems that the surgery itself causes hormonal problems, and research studies and popular books by physicians seem to agree.

Problems with Tubal Ligations Are Nothing New

Many doctors still tell women that there are no side effects, and that they will have no problems following a tubal ligation. But other doctors have been sounding warnings for years.

Ten years ago, Niels Lauersen, M.D., wrote about this in one of his popular gynecological books. He cites case histories of women who developed pain in the area of their fallopian tubes after the surgery, causing severe cramping prior to and during menstruation. He also mentions women whose periods became either much heavier or lighter, and who began to suffer from cyclical PMS or symptoms of premenopause after the surgery.

Lauersen says that up to 15 percent of women who undergo tubal ligations report complications during the first month after the operation. Side effects of post-tubal-ligation syndrome (PTLS) include pelvic pain, irregular menstrual bleeding, severe PMS, and galactorrhea (a milky discharge from the nipples). Sometimes the pain of PTLS is so severe that women undergo further surgery, including hysterectomies.[2]

Lauersen says that tubal ligation should not be considered minor, inconsequential surgery. He concludes that the pain of PTLS is probably caused by nerve damage, and that the PMS is probably due to a hormonal imbalance caused by lessened blood flow to the ovaries, shrinking of the ovaries, abnormal ovulation, irregular periods, and, possibly, formation of ovarian cysts.

Australian Physician Discusses Tubal Ligations

Dr. Sandra Cabot, an Australian physician and a hormone expert, has written some excellent books on hormonal problems.[3] She includes a whole chapter on tubal sterilization, and cites several research articles that discuss the side effects.[4]

Cabot lists the different methods of closing off the fallopian tubes: cutting, tying, burning, or clipping them with metal or plastic rings or clips. She says that the method that causes the fewest problems is using clips. Cutting, tying, and burning produce more side effects and are more likely to damage surrounding blood vessels, which affect blood flow to the ovaries. When the blood flow to the ovaries is diminished, says Cabot, the ovaries become impaired and produce less estrogen. She believes that the problem occurs because of damage to the blood supply to the ovary, since the ovarian blood vessels run beside the fallopian tubes on their way to the ovary and could easily be compressed or cut during surgery to the adjacent tube. This may lead to high blood pressure in the ovary, which could result in damage to the ovarian tissues. She says that if this occurs, the ovary may not function normally and its production of estrogen and progesterone, which need an adequate blood and oxygen supply, may be lowered.[5]

Drs. Guy Abrahams and Joel Hargrove have completed a study on the hormonal effect of tubal ligations, saying that estrogen levels are raised and progesterone levels lowered.[6] I believe that their conclusions fit the presupposition that PMS is caused by high estrogen and low progesterone levels, and I personally think that Dr. Cabot's view is more correct: that the levels of both hormones, particularly estrogen, are lowered.

Symptoms mentioned by Dr. Cabot as a result of tubal ligation are: fatigue, difficulty in losing weight, vaginal dryness, bladder problems, loss of libido, reduced orgasms, poor memory, muscle aches and pains, and more rapid aging of the skin—all mainly due to estrogen deficiency.

Surgeon Resists Doing Tubal Ligations

Dr. Vicki Hufnagel, in her book, *No More Hysterectomies*,[7] says that her patients have to fight her to have a tubal ligation, because she has seen so many side effects from this surgery. Patients who have tubal ligations, she says, complain of heavier, longer menstrual periods, more severe cramps, dysfunctional uterine bleeding, pain with intercourse, and other pain. Examination of the surgery site may show abnormal swelling or enlargement in ovarian veins, resulting in hormonal imbalances, and fistulas[8] associated with endometriosis in the fallopian tubes.

She mentions three main theories as to why tubal ligations are a problem:

1. Tubal ligation destroys the blood supply to the ovaries;
2. Certain types of tubal sterilization procedures are likely to result in endometriosis;
3. An increase in the blood pressure within the ovarian artery can create an estrogen-progesterone imbalance.

Dr. Hufnagel, like Sandra Cabot, prefers clipping the tubes closed, because there are fewer postoperative problems. Both women say that, in the future, more sophisticated methods of microsurgery may prevent these side effects from tubal ligations.

Indeed, Dr. Daniel Fischer, an OB/GYN living in Stockton, California, told me that he has no problems with post-tubal-ligation syndrome among his patients, because he uses microsurgery.

Conclusion

Women who think that their menstrual problems started after having a tubal ligation are probably correct. If their symptoms are cyclical, with physical and emotional problems recurring before each period, they probably need to be treated with natural progesterone. If these symptoms occur during most of the month, and indicate premenopause, they may need estrogen as well.

HYSTERECTOMY AND REMOVAL OF THE OVARIES

Amy was a divorced 44-year-old woman, teaching at a medical university when her doctor told her that she had fibroids. He put her on shots of estrogen with no progesterone— a strange treatment, since taking a lot of estrogen can make fibroids grow.

Amy's fibroids did grow, and she began to bleed continually. When she visited her internist, he told her that the fibroids had enlarged, and that she should have a hysterectomy (removal of the uterus).

Amy didn't want a hysterectomy and, subsequently, went to five different OB/GYNs practicing near the Medical Center. Each of them told her that she needed both her uterus and ovaries removed, even though there was no known problem with her ovaries. The reason given was a common one: if the ovaries are left in, they can become cancerous. The evidence that there is increased risk of this is questionable,[9] and removing the ovaries can have a profound effect on subsequent hormone production.

After hearing the same story from five gynecologists, Amy felt that she had no choice but to have the hysterectomy and oophorectomy. After the surgery, she was given 0.625 mg of Premarin daily, but this did not relieve her symptoms.

I met Amy about 10 months later, when I gave a lecture on menopause at the university's women's center. As she talked to me afterwards, she was crying uncontrollably because she was so terribly depressed. After the surgery, she had developed vaginal pain and was told that she had granuloma (granulated nodules of inflamed tissue) of the vagina. She also had pain in her bladder, burning eyes, and shooting pains in her ears, in addition to crippling depression. She had been to a number of doctors since the surgery because of the physical and emotional problems she was enduring. Incredible as it may seem, no one had linked the symptoms she was having with the hysterectomy, or increased her dosage, or changed the brand or form of estrogen.

During this time, Amy even asked a referral service for the name of a menopause expert, and went to see him at the university hospital. An internist, who did an examination before the doctor arrived, said that he only had to look at her to see that she was estrogen deficient. Nevertheless, the menopause expert disagreed with the internist's opinion, and would not increase Amy's dose of Premarin, though he did give her some additional vaginal cream.

By the time Amy came to see me, she had doubled her estrogen dosage on her own volition; by simply increasing her dose, she had controlled her depression enough to stop her crying jags.

The next woman I saw that day had also had a hysterectomy and an oophorectomy. Her surgeon had given her 2.5 mg of Premarin—four times Amy's dose. This woman seemed to be experiencing symptoms of overdose.

These two case histories illustrate the fact that women are frequently treated according to the whim of the particular physician they are seeing at the time. While many women receive satisfactory treatment and experience success with taking hormones after a hysterectomy, many other women don't. Some doctors give low doses only; some give high. Some are willing to experiment with hormones until satisfaction is reached; some are not. The treatment women may expect after hysterectomy is often not uniform.

Two Basic Concerns About Hysterectomies

One main concern about hysterectomy is that it is often offered as a treatment for severe premenstrual syndrome. While this sometimes works, it doesn't always, and there is the potential for worsening the problems. It's rather like playing Russian roulette.

Another concern is that some women who have hysterectomies never feel the same emotionally and physically again, even if only the uterus was removed. Even when they go to a physician who is an expert in hormone replacement, some hysterectomized women seem unable to balance their hormones. I have talked to many women who blame the breakdown of their health on a hysterectomy. This may represent only a minority response, but it does happen.

Hysterectomy Is Sometimes Necessary

On the other hand, some hysterectomies are absolutely necessary; I am sure that there are many women who have had heavy bleeding or chronic pain for years, who are thrilled to lose their uterus and ovaries. My mother, now 85 years old, says that she never had good health *until* she had her uterus removed (she didn't have hormone replacement). My sister and I have both had hysterectomies (mine recently), and it was a good choice for both of us.

The majority of women who need a hysterectomy will do fine on normal protocols of replacement hormones after the surgery. But I know many others who regret having had a hysterectomy because it marked the onset of their present symptoms of hormonal depletion. Now, several years away from the surgery, their physicians have "forgotten" that these women had a hysterectomy, and believe their present symptoms are all in their heads.

Women Doctors Perform Hysterectomies for PMS Too

It's not only male doctors who do routine hysterectomies. I recently talked with two women doctors who both ran menopause clinics. One was an OB/GYN, the other a reproductive endocrinologist. Both performed hysterectomies and oophorectomies as treatment for severe cases of PMS. One would first give the woman Lupron to put her in chemical menopause for a year or two, to see how she would cope.

While this is a fairly well-accepted treatment, I think it should be a last-ditch effort, not a first choice.

Jeffrey L. Rausch says:

> Although there is evidence that there is already an excess of psychiatric illness among women presenting for hysterectomy, there is data to suggest that the most common symptom following surgical menopause is that of depression.[10]

This is the problem with hysterectomies. You may be depressed, have a hysterectomy, and then not be depressed. Or you may not be depressed, have a hysterectomy, and then become depressed. Both occur in a small percentage of cases. But what guarantee is there that you won't be in this small group?

Perhaps your close relative's response to a hysterectomy might be one indication.

Some Women Need Hysterectomies; Many Do Not

Researchers have frequently stated that, especially in the past, too many women have been given hysterectomies—half to three-quarters of a million women a year in the U.S. alone. Doctors often have the attitude that, when a woman is past her childbearing years, the uterus and ovaries have outlived their usefulness. Though some doctors are conservative about performing hysterectomies, others do it fairly routinely.

This situation has changed and continues to change. If the pathology after the surgery does not reveal a valid reason for the surgery, the physician can come under question about unnecessary surgery. Also, HMOs are becoming more and more reluctant to give permission for hysterectomies without there being a good reason. This is not completely for the benefit of the patient—it's also because they don't want to spend the money!

A Surgeon Defends the Uterus

Dr. Vicki Hufnagel is critical of the number of hysterectomies being performed on women. Dr. Hufnagel's book, *No More Hysterectomies,* is helpful for a woman contemplating hysterectomy. She says that, in 1983, 13,000 hysterectomies were performed to treat PMS. Hysterectomies, she says, are generally performed because of cancer (a valid reason), fibroid tumors, endometriosis, or prolapse (slipped uterus). She feels that there may be alternative treatment for the last three.

Rather than perform hysterectomies on fibroids, Dr. Hufnagel performs early myomectomies, a surgery in which the fibroid is shelled out of the uterus. She feels that these should be performed early on because, once the fibroid grows to a certain size, hysterectomy might be inevitable. She has also developed what she calls "female reconstructive surgery," which tightens up the loose ligaments that caused a uterine prolapse—another attempt to avoid hysterectomy.

It is interesting that, in France, surgeons are trained to perform myomectomies; hysterectomies are rarely performed there for fibroids. By contrast, in the U.S., where performing myomectomies is more of a specialty, fibroids are a major reason for having a hysterectomy.

Reproductive Biologist Researches the Facts

Researcher Dr. Winnifred Cutler's book, *Hysterectomy: Before and After,* is must reading for all women who are advised to have a hysterectomy or who have already had one. Here are some of the points that Cutler makes in her book:

- Fifty percent of women in the U.S. and Canada will have a hysterectomy in their lifetime, compared with 10 percent in Sweden. In the U.S., the average age for premenopausal hysterectomy is 35; in Scandinavia, it is 45. By the age of 44, 21 percent of women in the U.S. will have had a hysterectomy, compared with 4 percent of women in six European countries. Half of the women over 40 who have a hysterectomy will also have their ovaries removed.
- Immediately after surgery, women are often very happy that they had a hysterectomy, but as the years go by, the satisfaction rate drops drastically.
- The effects of a hysterectomy, especially if the woman is not on an optimal hormone therapy, include: alteration of the hormonal environment, earlier aging, high risk of post-operative depression, deterioration of bone health, increase of atherosclerosis and coronary heart disease, reduction in sexual functioning (libido, arousal, lubrication, orgasm),[11] increased urinary incontinence, premature menopause (when only the uterus has been removed), and instant menopause (when the ovaries have been removed).
- Accumulating evidence shows that the role of the uterus and ovaries has been highly underestimated. The uterus plays a large part in keeping the ovaries working (consequently, when they are removed the cycling of the ovaries is affected). Also, the uterus produces hormones that affect brain function and help reduce heart disease. The ovaries are factories for hormones and many other substances.

- Most of the information in Dr. Cutler's book has surfaced since 1983, and is not yet disseminated to medical schools, medical practices, and health centers. She says that when women go to a doctor for help, even the well-informed physician may be limited in giving effective answers, partly because the information is not all collected.

Dr. Cutler suggests that you avoid having a hysterectomy unless you really need it. Dr. Cutler's book includes a helpful chapter called, "Sexual Life After Hysterectomy." I found this chapter interesting because I have counseled a number of women who have experienced significant loss of their drive after having a hysterectomy. Cutler says this is because of the loss of the pudental nerve in the cervix which fires at the height of lovemaking and provides deeply satisfying orgasms. Many women report a lessening of their orgasms after surgery. (On the other hand, this is apparently not universal. Some women who have suffered from pain because of gynecological problems report a dramatic improvement in their sex life after a hysterectomy.)

Difficulty in Treating Hysterectomized Women

In the treatment section for menopause in this book, there is a section that deals with what I call "brittle menopause." Women who have had a hysterectomy and who have a real struggle balancing their hormones should read this section.

Further Information

To contact Winnifred Cutler, Ph.D., and obtain her books, write or call the Athena Institute for Women's Wellness, Inc., located at 1211 Braefield Rd., Chester Springs, PA. This is a research organization delivering state-of-the-art, academically-grounded scientific information to improve women's well-being. Its focus encompasses hormones, nutrition, exercise physiology, and psychoneuroendocrine (the effects of hormones on the brain) aspects of women's health.

The Athena Institute was founded in 1986 by Dr. Cutler, who is a prominent biologist and author on women's health.

She earned her Ph.D. from the University of Pennsylvania and did postdoctoral work at Stanford University.

Dr. Cutler co-discovered human pheromones in 1986, holds several patents, and has published over 30 research papers in medical and scientific journals. Her books include: *Menopause: A Guide for Women and the Men Who Love Them; Hysterectomy: Before and After; Love Cycles: The Science of Intimacy;* and *Searching for Courtship: The Smart Woman's Guide to Finding a Good Husband.*

The Institute provides wellness examinations, workshops, and a "DocFinders" service to help women who need to identify medical specialists in their area. Athena also markets a unique women's cosmetic fragrance additive, Athena Pheromone 1013™ (nicknamed, "The Love Potion"), containing human pheromones designed to promote sexual attractiveness.

CASE HISTORIES

Barbara's Story

Barbara, a cheerful 41-year-old dental hygienist, began noticing problems about six or seven years after she had a tubal ligation, which was performed the same day she delivered her second baby at age 27. Her family history showed good health, with no serious hormonal problems in the women on either the maternal or paternal side.

When Barbara's menstrual periods first began, they were regular, about 28 days apart, but long—generally seven to ten days of flow. She went on the birth control pill at age 19, and took it for a couple of years, even though it caused difficult side effects such as mood swings and bloating. Subsequently, she developed an ovarian cyst, which her doctor thought was related to the pill. At age 21, she used a Dalkon Shield, which caused erosion of her cervix, and, two years later, a wedge resection was done on her ovary because of the cyst.

Her two children were born when she was 25 and 27. Both pregnancies were fine, aside from low blood pressure and frequent fainting spells. Both babies were delivered by C-section and, as mentioned, the tubal ligation was performed after the second delivery. She had no postpartum depression with either baby, but she had problems breastfeeding both children because, despite continual leakage from her breasts, she could not seem to provide enough milk; when she stopped nursing, the milk dried up overnight.

Barbara's problems gradually increased. Always a high-energy person prior to the tubal ligation, she found herself frequently exhausted. She had severe, incapacitating migraines just before her period, for which she often had to be taken home. Her head and skin itched and crawled and was so irritating that she wished she could tear her skin off. She had horrible panic attacks and suffered from allergies.

She also seemed to lose her sex drive, which had never been high. She now had no libido at all, and tried to avoid sex since it was uncomfortable due to vaginal dryness. Despite the dryness, she had a constant, heavy, watery discharge; she had been treated for this with cryosurgery on her cervix, but it did not relieve the discharge problem.

She also had two other unusual problems: what looked like an open sore on her areola (the pigmented area of the nipple), and a recurrently swollen Bartholin gland (a tiny gland near the mouth of the vagina that provides lubrication during foreplay and sexual intercourse), which swelled to the size of a marble. The swelling only lasted for about an hour at a time and then receded, which her physicians thought was unusual because that type of lump usually remains swollen.

Barbara consulted a physician who prescribed a combination of Estratest (esterfied estrogens and methyltestosterone) and natural progesterone. The estrogen relieved her vaginal dryness and fatigue and, with the progesterone, stopped her monthly migraines. The testosterone helped her flagging libido and low sex drive. Barbara had a tremendous response to hormone therapy and felt like a new woman.

Because she had no family history of hormonal problems, and had never really experienced them herself prior to the tubal ligation, she responded wonderfully to treatment.

What's Happening Now After a number of years of taking hormones, Barbara is now off them, and the menstrual problems that began at puberty are now minimal in her forties. She is not having as many migraines (when we first met they were daily, swinging from headache to migraine and back again continually).

Barbara said that I listened to her at a time when the 15 doctors she went to wouldn't. She was at her wits' end and felt terrible about herself.

After I saw Barbara, she went to a doctor who gave her estrogen and natural progesterone, and this combination worked remarkably well for a couple of years. Then she started having a few problems and wasn't feeling as well. She switched her progesterone to one from a local source, and it didn't agree with her.

She decided to go to her previous HMO physician, who was critical of her for taking natural progesterone. He threatened her with an annual endometrial biopsy (she was only about 40). He talked her into trying synthetic progesterone, and she went on Provera. This was a financial decision; the medication cost only $2.00 compared to a much higher figure for natural progesterone. Barbara told me that she felt awful on Provera, like Dr. Jekyll & Mrs. Hyde. She gained weight, and had horrible headaches and mood changes. But she toughed it out it for several months.

She did not like who she was becoming, so she went back on natural progesterone for another four months. Around that time, she had an injury involving her arm and neck, and had to stop working. Her arm kept getting more and more numb. She was having migraines every month, but the timing in her cycle kept changing. Because of the injury, she began going to a female chiropractor who helped not only the injury, but the menstrual problems.

Barbara says that when she has bad days and can't even recognize a door, she goes to the chiropractor, who gently balances her. By the time the office visit is over, Barbara can function again. She is not using hormones at this time, and still has some mild premenstrual changes. But things are much better. She quit her job because of the injury, and this reduced her physical and emotional stress tremendously.

Barbara is now 43 years old. She is still having menstrual periods, and her bleeding is normal (it was heavy and clotting when we first met). In fact, her periods are more normal now than they have ever been. She feels "kind of goofy" around her period, but it is not as intense as it used to be. She is not having swelling of her vulva, and her nipples are not cracking open before her periods as they were years ago.

Now she has no panic attacks. She doesn't wake in the night, ripping off her clothes and bedsheets and wanting to run away without knowing where to go. She notes that she has lost most of her body hair except on her head.

Barbara still has headache days, but they don't compare to those in the past. Typically, she has a headache two days out of every four months, but they are not the emergency-room type.

She told me that the hormones she took were a lifesaver. She doesn't know how she would have survived had she not taken them. When she stopped, she didn't stop slowly, but went off them cold turkey, though she did take them around her period for a while. For the first five months off hormones, she had some hard times. Then she began to feel all right, and she seems to have regulated.

Now Barbara is working twice as many hours for the state government as she was in her former job. She is really doing very well. Her story shows that a woman can have horrible problems beginning at puberty, appear to be going through early menopause, and yet have relief from her symptoms. In fact, after taking hormones for months or years, the menstrual cycle may regulate, and it may not be necessary to continue taking them.

Mona's Story

Mona, 40, had a family history full of hormonal problems. Her mother and sister both had menstrual disorders, thyroid problems, and trouble with their pregnancies, and both, like Mona, ultimately had hysterectomies.

Mona was fairly healthy until puberty, but there her good luck ended. She had horrendous menstrual periods, during which she would bleed for ten days, stop for four, bleed again for ten days, and so on. The flow was extremely heavy, and her cramps were severe. At age 16, a doctor put Mona on birth control pills to regulate her cycle and control the bleeding. She was later diagnosed as having polycystic ovaries and endometriosis, and she was told that her chances of becoming pregnant were very small.

Mona had a miscarriage before the age of 20, which left her with severe postpartum depression. She had difficulty conceiving again, so she took Clomid and became pregnant, but was dreadfully sick the whole nine months and was hospitalized because of vomiting and dehydration. The delivery was very difficult and, afterward, she had milk fever (an infection in the breasts that can occur during lactation; it killed many women in earlier centuries). The penicillin treatment caused her to develop a violent reaction and a fever of 106° that lasted 10 days. She needed surgery on her breasts, which had to be pumped afterward. The bleeding and the pain were unendurable, as was her depression.

The second child was unplanned, and this pregnancy was a similar nightmare. The delivery was, again, very difficult, with severe vaginal tearing and a great deal of hemorrhaging.

Two years later, her uterus was removed because of heavy bleeding, and she was given a low dose of Ogen. After many visits to the emergency room for continually rupturing ovarian cysts, both ovaries were removed two years later. Her estrogen dosage was doubled, but it did not alleviate her symptoms, and the hormonal protocol was never adjusted to meet her needs.

After the hysterectomy, Mona's physical and emotional health deteriorated. She became more and more depressed and was, finally, admitted to a psychiatric ward. Over a period of three years, she was given almost every available antidepressant, including monoamine oxidase inhibitors, tricyclics, and Prozac. She became violent as a result of taking all this medication and, at one point, tried to commit suicide after being on Prozac. She was also treated with electric shock therapy, and when I saw her, she told me that her doctor wanted to give her a course of twelve more shock treatments.

Mona's problem, it seemed to me, was basically hormonal and worsened by the hysterectomy; she needed an endocrinologist, not a psychiatrist. Adequate treatment with the right combination of estrogen and thyroid restored much of Mona's emotional balance and helped her to avoid further shock therapy.

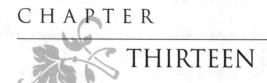

CHAPTER

THIRTEEN

BREAST CANCER

One day, as Sylvia examined her breasts, she came upon a hard, painless lump that she had not felt before. Her doctor sent her to a surgeon, who performed a biopsy on the lump and found that it was malignant, but self-contained; he performed a lumpectomy.

Sylvia was then put on a course of radiation treatment and given Tamoxifen, a drug that acts as an anti-estrogen. The surgeon told Sylvia that there were estrogen receptors in the tumor that he excised. Estrogen, he said, might accelerate the return of the breast cancer, and this was the reason for using Tamoxifen.

Sylvia was 50 at the time when she developed breast cancer. She had her uterus removed at age 36 because of large benign fibroids, which had caused excessive menstrual bleeding. She had been experiencing symptoms of estrogen deficiency prior to the discovery of her cancer, but had not been on any estrogen therapy.

After she had been on Tamoxifen for a while, her menopausal symptoms became more pronounced. Her OB/GYN told her that her vagina was as dry and fragile as that of a woman 20 years older.

But when she questioned her surgeon, he re-emphasized his position that she couldn't take estrogen.

THE CANCER SCARE

Estrogen has received a lot of bad press concerning its possible connection with breast cancer. From time to time, the media put out scare reports about women on estrogen replacement therapy having higher rates of breast cancer. Actually, there have been studies that produced the opposite conclusion; taking estrogen may either increase or reduce the incidence of breast cancer.

Other studies suggest that estrogen does not *cause* cancer but may act as a growth-promoter for pre-existing breast cancers, particularly those containing estrogen receptors.

Putting It in Perspective

To balance this out, it's important to remember that cancer of all types and in both sexes is on the increase. Also, lung cancer (mainly from smoking) kills 53,000 women annually, compared with 46,000 deaths in women from breast cancer, according to present statistics. While breast cancer is the most commonly occurring female cancer, lung cancer is the leading cause of cancer death in women. You may not realize this because the news media exaggerate the threat of breast cancer, and because magazines do not like to offend their cigarette advertisers.

Experts like R. Don Gambrell, Jr., M.D., say that if estrogen does increase the risk of breast cancer, the incidence should drop dramatically after menopause, when estrogen levels drop. This is not the case. The incidence of breast cancer increases dramatically after age 55. By contrast, the incidence of endometrial cancer, which *is* an estrogen-related cancer, does drop after menopause. Fewer than 20 percent of women take hormone replacement therapy, and they only take it for an average of nine months. But the number of cases of breast cancer is much greater in women over 50, and this increase takes place in women worldwide who have not had estrogen replacement.

John Edens, M.D., a prominent Australian endocrinologist and an expert on breast cancer, told me that women like his grandmother, who had 16 children, rarely developed breast cancer in old age. He said that this is because the high levels of hormones in pregnancy, including estrogen and progesterone, protect women from breast cancer. The age when a woman first conceives is a major factor in cancer risk. Women who have had multiple pregnancies early on are better protected against breast cancer. The theory that high levels of hormones in pregnancy protect a woman against breast cancer also opposes the idea that estrogen increases breast cancer risk.

Significant researchers such as Drs. Gambrell and Eden believe that estrogen, with progesterone, is actually protective of the breast, because the hormones support the immune system and help it ward off cancer. Their view suggests that preventing the drop in hormones may help delay the aging process, and that these hormones are anticarcinogenic.

When the estrogen level drops at menopause, it causes other hormone levels to also drop (melatonin, DHEA, and growth hormone). These other hormones are related to the onset of aging, so estrogen loss acts as a catalyst to the aging process. As men and women age, the immune system becomes less efficient, increasing the likelihood of developing cancer. That's why men get more prostate cancer as they get older, and women get more breast cancer as they age.

Environmental chemicals that simulate the function of estrogen in the body may be a bigger factor in causing hormonal cancer than hormone replacement therapy, because there is growing evidence that these xenoestrogens are increasing breast cancer in women and prostate cancer in men, and lowering male sperm count worldwide. (See the next section for more information on environmental estrogens.)

These facts all need to be taken into account when contemplating the risk of breast cancer from taking estrogen. Graham Colditz, M.D., a Harvard physician and a major figure in breast cancer research, does not interpret the data in the same way that Drs. Gambrell and Eden do. Colditz reports that estrogen replacement over five years increases the incidence of breast cancer by at least 30 percent. This is the viewpoint that attracts media attention. But others with equally impeccable credentials disagree and believe that hormone replacement therapy in normal doses does not increase—and may decrease—the risk of breast cancer.

At the last meeting of NAMS, epidemiologist Trudi Bush, M.D., said that it is going to be very difficult to come up with the final answer on how much risk there is for women taking estrogen. This is because the breast cannot easily be biopsied like the uterus, making investigation difficult. But she stated that the increased risk of breast cancer due to taking estrogen would not be more than 30 percent. This seems a dramatic risk, but remember that it is 30 percent of 4 percent of the total causes of death. That increases the figures for breast cancer to 5.6 percent of total deaths of women.

If you are a part of that 5.6 percent, of course, it is not a trivial figure. But doctors compare the 5.6 percent who die from breast cancer to the same number who die from osteoporosis, and to the 53 percent who die from heart disease and strokes. Estrogen helps to prevent osteoporosis and heart disease. That is why some researchers advise weighing these factors in any decision about whether to take estrogen.

Estrogens in the Environment

One factor which has received relatively little attention from researchers is the role of industrial pollutants in over-estrogenizing the population. The *Washington Post* featured an article by Rick Weiss in the Health Section of the January 25, 1994 edition, entitled, "Estrogen in the Environment: Are some pollutants a threat to fertility?" The article stated that there are both good and bad foreign estrogens in the environment, and went on to outline some concerns about the bad estrogens. Here are some of the conclusions:

- Though estrogen is commonly thought of in the singular, there are many kinds of estrogen.
- The three major varieties of estrogen made in the body are 17-beta estradiol, estrone, and estriol (the strongest, weaker, and weakest female estrogens, respectively).

- In the environment, many chemicals and pollutants resemble harsh estrogens in their effects on the body. These include industrial chemicals such as polychlorinated biphenyls, and plastics such as those used in water bottles and baby bottles.
- In the West, men and women have been saturated by these industrial estrogens. The effects may not be known for decades because the research is only preliminary.
- Estrogens make physiological changes in the body by attaching themselves to the body's cells. Scientists are finding that these receptors are not especially picky. The impostor estrogens in pesticides and other chemicals can attach to these receptors. Some can even block a person's own good estrogen and prevent it from doing its job. Others magnify the effects of human estrogen, becoming potent super-estrogens.

The article notes that concern is being voiced about changes now observed in animals and humans. For example:

- In Florida, alligator eggs are failing to hatch, and many male alligators have abnormally small penises.
- In Denmark, endocrinologist Niels E. Skakkebaek, M.D., found that sperm counts in men have fallen 50 percent worldwide during the past five decades, while the number of testicular cancers has doubled and tripled. He and his colleagues proposed that this results from maternal exposure to environmental estrogens during pregnancy.

The article names the following chemicals that are suspect:

- DDE, a major breakdown product of DDT;
- Nonylphenols in spermicides, hair coloring products, and other toiletries;
- Polychlorinated biphenyls (PCBs), a family of chlorine-containing industrial compounds no longer made in this country but still in use;
- Endosulfan, a pesticide;
- Bisphenol A, a breakdown product of polycarbonate plastics (water bottles and baby bottles).

None of this hypothesis is proven, but there are a number of top researchers who are concerned about this trend. The article also points out that some scientists are wondering if estrogen-mimicking pollutants are also contributing to the increase in breast cancer in women. This theory is being investigated at the National Cancer Institutes.

Clarification of the Statistics

In a recent UC Berkeley *Wellness Letter,*[1] the statistic that one woman in nine will get breast cancer was clarified. The article pointed out that only at age 85 is the risk factor one in nine. Actually, at age 50, the risk is 1 in 50; by age 60, the risk is 1 in 23; by age 70, 1 in 13; by age 80, 1 in 10. The article mentioned that the statistic that one in nine women will get breast cancer has terrified many women and made them feel doomed. The American Cancer Society has heavily publicized the "one in nine" figure to convince more women to have mammograms. Sometimes the statistic is reported erroneously as saying that one women in nine already *has* breast cancer. Women need to know this, because these false statistics give women the idea that breast cancer is pandemic, fuel the accusation that estrogen increases breast cancer, and discourage women from taking estrogen.

ESTROGEN AND BREAST CANCER— SOME MAJOR QUESTIONS

The first question is: Will estrogen or estrogen/progestin replacement therapy increase the risk of breast cancer? While studies have produced conflicting conclusions, the majority of current studies support the position that HRT does not increase the risk of breast cancer over the short term (i.e., if you take HRT for less than five years).

The second question is more difficult to answer: If I have a present or past case of breast cancer, can I safely take estrogen? The FDA position is that no estrogen should be given to women with a history of breast cancer. But thought on this question is rapidly shifting. Some doctors are putting women on estrogen and progesterone to counteract their postmenopausal symptoms one to three years after successful treatment of breast cancer. They believe that the benefits of taking estrogen far out-weigh the risk of getting breast cancer again.

The third question is: What about taking Tamoxifen, a treatment that works by inhibiting estrogen in the cell recep-tors of the breast? If Tamoxifen treatment is successful, doesn't that support the idea that estrogen stimulates cancer?

A Researcher's View

Dr. Winnifred Cutler takes the position that hormone re-placement therapy actually reduces the incidence of breast cancer. Those interested in the subject should read her books: *Hysterectomy: Before and After,* pp. 135–37 (with Celso-Ramón Garcia), and *Menopause: A Guide for Women and the Men Who Love Them.*

Here is a summary of Dr. Cutler's conclusions about breast cancer:

- Breast cancer is an older woman's disease, and is most common in the postmenopausal years after age 55, when hormone levels decline.
- While breast cancer is said to be a widespread problem for women, competent statistical studies have not been done to prove this.
- The chance of a 40-year-old woman getting breast cancer some time in the following year is extremely low.
- About 46,000 women a year die of breast cancer, as compared to 500,000 who die per year from strokes or heart disease (often directly related to estrogen loss after menopause).
- According to a study by Dr. Don Gambrell, women who are not taking hormones at menopause have over twice as great a chance of getting breast cancer as those on estrogen-progestin replacement therapy.
- Women on estrogen-progestin replacement therapy have optimal breast health with a reduced risk of breast cancer. Women on estrogen alone have neither an increased nor decreased risk of breast cancer.

Fat and Unbound Estrogen Are the Culprits

Apparently, the incidence of breast cancer increases in women who produce higher levels of estrone. Estrone levels are much higher in postmenopausal women, especially in women who are apple-shaped (overweight around the waist), rather than pear-shaped.

Men tend to get fat around their waist and stomach, yet keep their thin arms and legs. They are very susceptible to heart disease. Women, by contrast, tend to gain weight all over, particularly around the hips and thighs (pear shape). But certain women have the male type of fat pattern and gain weight around the waist (android obesity). These women are most at risk for breast cancer and heart disease.

After menopause, the ovaries and adrenal glands produce higher levels of androgens, the male hormones that break down into estrone in the fat cells. The more body fat women have, the more estrone they are likely to produce. Some think that fat globules carry carcinogens through the bloodstream to the breast, where they stick to the estrogen receptors.

This is why, generally, women over 55 who are overweight around the middle are at highest risk for breast cancer.

REDUCING THE RISK

Some researchers believe that diet during the years prior to puberty determines the hormonal health of the breast. The nearer the diet is to vegetarianism, the less likely it is that breast cancer will develop. Females of all ages should particularly avoid too much fat in their diet.[2] They should eat adequate fiber and avoid salt, fat, and smoked foods. Excessively processed and fatty foods trigger most Western diseases (heart disease, diabetes, breast and bowel cancer, diverticulosis, osteoporosis, etc.). In summary, women should eat more vegetables, fruits, whole grain cereals, and legumes. Smoking should be eliminated, and alcohol used only moderately.

Early diet can affect the age at which a woman's menstrual periods begin and end, because menstruation is not triggered until the body achieves a certain proportion of body fat. Thin, active women tend to begin menstruation later. Women who eat more animal fat tend to start menstruating earlier and to finish later than those who are on a vegetarian diet. The more years a woman menstruates, the more likely it is that breast cancer will occur.

Controllable Risk Factors

- Eat a low-fat (particularly low-animal-fat) high-fiber diet. Fat intake should be less than 25 percent of your calories. Cheeses, for instance, which have most of their calories in fat content, should only be eaten in small quantities and at every third or fourth meal.
- Body fat should be less than 25 percent of total body weight.
- Body mass index (your weight divided by your height) should be less than 25 percent).
- Waist-to-hip proportion should be 75 percent. For example, a 30-inch waist and 40-inch hips. Over 80 percent increases your chances of breast cancer.
- Exercise aerobically (at least three times a week for 30 minutes each time).
- Stop smoking (ten or more cigarettes a day increases your risk).
- Reduce alcohol consumption to fewer than three drinks a week.
- If you need to take hormones, even if you have had your uterus removed, estrogen and progesterone taken together is the best regime.

Other Factors

You should take into account other factors that increase the incidence of breast cancer (most of these you can't control):

- Twenty percent of women who have breast cancer have a family history of cancer.
- Having had a previous case of breast cancer increases your chances of getting it again.

- Being black or white increases your chances—Asian, Hispanic, and American Indian women have a lower incidence of breast cancer—possibly because of lifestyle (unrefined foods, less meat and animal fat, more exercise).
- Women over 5'5" tall are at greater risk of getting breast cancer.
- Having other cancers (ovarian, endometrial, bowel) increases your chances of getting breast cancer.
- Having atypical hyperplasia of the breast (fibrocystic breast disease—the proliferative, not the nonproliferative, type) increases your chance of breast cancer. (Ninety-five percent of women have fibrocystic breast disease, and most of it is benign.)
- Going through menopause later than age 55 increases the chances of getting breast cancer.

Breast Examination and Early Detection

Self-examination of one's breasts, when done according to professional methods, is sometimes helpful in early detection of tumors. However, most of the time early detection of breast cancer does not guarantee greater longevity.[3] Scientific literature suggests that the longer survival time may only reflect the earlier discovery of breast cancer, not an improved rate of cure. Breast cancer is usually slow-growing and may take 20 to 30 years to form.

Mammograms   Some researchers conclude that there is no value in having routine mammograms before the age of 50.[4] Some women doctors who specialize in breast care feel that mammograms before the age of 50 are helpful because they occasionally indicate an early cancer. Even though this is an uncommon occurrence, they feel that the screening is worth it for those individuals. One retrospective review showed that earlier mammograms do not increase the survival rate of women with breast cancer; this study, however, was seriously flawed and has been discredited. Women in their forties who are at high risk because of family history may be an exception. Some doctors who specialize in breast health observe that mammograms before the age of 40 are worthwhile because they do occasionally help in finding an early cancer.

Exposure to radiation does increase the risk of breast cancer. However, today the newer mammogram detectors only use a quarter of a rad of radiation and are considered safer than older machines which emit more radiation.

If you decide to have regular mammograms, it is important to go to a breast-care center that specializes in mammograms and has up-to-date equipment, regularly tested for efficiency by outside inspection, and well-informed, professionally-trained operators.

Instead of having routine mammograms each year, some physicians suggest having a base-line mammogram done (this depends on the individual's risk). This base-line mammogram can be used later as a comparison if a problem arises.

CHOOSE CONSERVATIVE TREATMENT

Currently, most breast cancer is considered systemic. This means that by the time there is a palpable lump, the cancer has usually spread microscopically throughout the lymphatic system and has already metastasized (been transmitted) at distant sites. This is why radical mastectomies—the removal of the entire breast and surrounding lymph nodes—often do not guarantee greater longevity than a local lumpectomy.

This is terrible when you consider how many radical mastectomies were performed in the recent past, even decades after researchers knew that they didn't really improve survival rates for most women. With the removal of the lymph nodes from under the armpit, the lymphatic fluid runs down into the arm tissues and causes frequent swelling and pain. A woman who had had a mastectomy couldn't wear a blood pressure cuff, and the surgery restricted her arm movement.

The original radical mastectomy surgery has been modified and is not now as drastic or as extensive. But the whole idea behind it is based on the premise that breast cancer is a local disease, and that if you can get the lump out, the problem is cured. Mastectomy is sometimes performed on some women with high familial risk for breast cancer who don't actually have the disease yet.

Says P. Skrabanek, "The 'simple' solution of surgery—cut everything out, and you will get rid of the tumour as well as the problem—has been found wanting . . .".[5] Skrabanek finds the evidence that breast cancer cannot be cured with present methods to be overwhelming. He comments that "it is surely complacent to continue our current practice of subjecting . . . women with primary disease to a futile mutilating procedure," and quotes Lowe's assertion that survival is much more closely related to the intrinsic malignancy of the tumour than to early diagnosis and treatment.

Lumpectomy, the Treatment of Choice

Lumpectomy is the treatment of choice in most cases. Many of the 100,000 mastectomies performed each year in this country should not have been done. One *Science* article says:

> For many kinds of cancer it doesn't even make much difference what kind of treatment is used. Most studies seem to reveal no difference among the treatment outcomes.

> These conclusions are well illustrated in the history of breast cancer management. Between 1950 and the late 1970s dozens of studies compared the survival of patients treated with various kinds of surgery from radical mastectomy to mere "lumpectomy," with and without radiation or drugs.

> The results have shown little survival advantage for any treatment. Since the less radical treatments are just as helpful as the most radical, the trend has humanely been toward the less disfiguring procedures.[6]

Nevertheless, doctors remove local cancers in the breast because they may either grow into the chest wall or form an abscess on the surface of the breast. At that point, they become very difficult and unpleasant to manage.

If a woman has radiation therapy in conjuction with a lumpectomy, the lump is now considered less likely to return at that spot (which doesn't mean that a lump won't grow elsewhere).

Having said all this, remember that there are women who had breast cancer in their forties and younger who are still alive in their seventies. Breast cancer can take a long time to develop. And there are a fortunate few who have a lumpectomy and experience no return of symptoms.

Tamoxifen

Tamoxifen is not a form of chemotherapy, but a nonsteroidal compound similar to Clomid; it is said to extend the survival rate of older women with breast cancer considerably. Some consider it so successful that widespread research trials are currently in progress in which even young women with a high rate of breast cancer in their families are given Tamoxifen as a preventive treatment.

Women who are considering Tamoxifen treatment should read the paper called, "Tamoxifen: Special Considerations for Clinicians," by Leon Speroff, M.D.,[7] because taking Tamoxifen has its pros and cons, like every medication. Dr. Speroff concludes that Tamoxifen is particularly helpful for postmenopausal women with breast cancer that contains estrogen receptors. As women move beyond menopause, it also seems increasingly helpful to those whose breast cancer is without estrogen receptors. Dr. Speroff thinks that Tamoxifen is less helpful for women prior to menopause, and may actually exacerbate certain estrogen-related problems. He appears to question the benefits of putting younger, high-risk women on Tamoxifen as a prophylactic because of these side effects.

While Tamoxifen functions as an estrogen antagonist in the breast cells, it also increases the effect of estrogen in other parts of the body.

On the positive side, Tamoxifen theoretically slows down the growth or return of breast cancer. There is a 20-percent increase in survival rate after five years on therapy, and the ten-year survival rate is even more significant. Tamoxifen, like estrogen replacement therapy, stabilizes bone density and increases the beneficial HDL cholesterol levels.

Negative Effects of Tamoxifen On the negative side, however, taking Tamoxifen may increase estrogen stimulation of the vaginal and endometrial tissues, leading to an increase in endometrial cancer and endometriosis. The FDA has issued a warning about increased risk of uterine cancer with Tamoxifen use (2 to 3 times higher). Since uterine cancer is a relatively minor killer of women, the FDA still approves the use of Tamoxifen for patients, but suggests that women have regular vaginal exams and watch for bleeding irregularities.

Uterine cancer caused by Tamoxifen is more likely to occur in premenopausal women, because many women who go on Tamoxifen end up experiencing an increase in their estrogen levels, and many stop ovulating. Also, the type of endometrial cancer that occurs in patients using this drug is not the benign type seen with hormone replacement therapy, but is often fatal.

Also, while doctors stress the estrogen-like benefits of Tamoxifen on the bones and heart, there are significant numbers of women who do experience severe estrogen-deficiency symptoms such as hot flashes, nausea, vomiting, vaginal irritation, arthritis, muscle cramps, and pains—all classic menopausal symptoms.

Keep in mind that it is mainly postmenopausal women over the age of 50 who benefit from treatment with Tamoxifen. As with many other issues in hormonal health, women need to read significant articles, ask questions of their doctors, and, in the end, weigh the pros and cons before deciding on a treatment.

Testosterone and Breast Cancer in Women

Pentii Siiteri, M.D., a Professor Emeritus of the National Cancer Institutes in Rockville, Maryland states:

> Eighty percent of breast cancer is modifiable by . . . factors related to diet.

> Increase in breast cancer after menopause is not secondary to estrogen as this is decreased relative to a few years earlier. But there is a far more significant decrease in androgens in the menopause, which are protective and the probable cause of the increase in postmenopausal breast cancer is more related to the lost androgen protection.

[There is also a] . . . significant drop in DHEA [dehydro-epiandrosterone] parallel with aging. DHEAS [dehydro-epiandrosterone sulfate] is not usually transformed into estrogen, but it is a major precursor of testosterone and DHT (dihydrotestosterone) in the normal female.

Androgens are very protective of breast cancer. DHT has 1,000 times the protective effect on breast cancer in comparison to progesterone.

Many studies have shown that androgens are potent antagonists of estrogen-stimulated cell proliferation. Similar effects by low levels of androgens in women may be important in determining ultimate breast size and cancer risk.[8]

Breast Cancer Rare with Estrogen/Testosterone Pellets

C. W. Lovell, M.D., has a menopause clinic in Baton Rouge, Louisiana, and has treated approximately 4,000 patients, almost exclusively with subdermal estradiol and testosterone pellets or with injections of estradiol and testosterone cyprionate. He found a marked statistical difference (a lower incidence than the national average) in the rates of breast cancer in his patients on testosterone. (Dr. Phillip Warner of Los Gatos, California, also a 25-year pioneer in giving estrogen and testosterone pellets, has also had very little if any breast cancer among his patients receiving pellets long-term.)

In Dr. Lovell's study (of approximately 50,000 woman-years' experience), conducted from 1985 to 1994, the incidence of breast cancer among women receiving estradiol and testosterone (mainly in pellet form) was roughly half the national rate. In general, doctors tend to see one malignancy for every 100 mammograms. In Dr. Lovell's practice, they find only one malignancy in every 1,000 mammograms. He has had one patient contract endometrial cancer in the past 10 years. He feels that testosterone has a preventive effect against breast and endometrial cancer.[9]

Dr. Rick Wilkinson compares Tamoxifen, with its negative effect on mood and libido, with testosterone. He comments that some are considering the use of testosterone instead of Tamoxifen, as it produces similar benefits without the negative side effects.

Apparently, in Canada, Europe, and Australia, large doses of Provera (about 1,000 mg per day!) are being used in place of Tamoxifen with at least as much success. Dr. John Eden, head of the department of endocrinology at the Royal Hospital for Women, in Paddington, N.S.W, Australia, told me that natural progesterone could be used instead.

Treatments Come and Go

The treatment of the moment is always a miracle cure, but only time will tell what the side effects will be, and, in the meantime, what will happen to you? Always remember that what was used for treatment 10 years ago is now obsolete; in retrospect, it may have been the wrong treatment, even though it may still be in use. It's wise to be more than a little skeptical, remembering that often HMOs and insurance companies may have more say in the treatment recommended than does the clinician, and their information may be out of date. And, incredible as it seems, a doctor may be legally liable for not following a standard course of treatment, even if he knows that the patient is not going to be any better off with the treatment and that her condition may actually be worsened.

Breast Cancer and Menopause

Some of the treatments for breast cancer, including Tamoxifen, can throw women into the symptoms of menopause: vaginal dryness, night sweats, sleep disorders, and typical emotional changes. The FDA position remains the same: that women who have had breast cancer should never take estrogen. This is a problem. Women exchange the symptoms of having breast cancer for the symptoms of going through menopause. This seems fine on paper, if you believe that menopause is a minor event. But as we have mentioned before, some women have a rough time with menopause, and only estrogen will help. What does a woman do if she has had both breasts removed because of cancer, and her uterus and ovaries have been removed as well? Apparently a lot of women in this position choose to take estrogen. The way they feel overpowers their fear of estrogen.

Current Opinion on Estrogen Use Is Rapidly Changing

Despite the FDA position, the tide of opinion is rapidly turning in regard to the use of estrogen for women who have had breast cancer in the past. Now some doctors—including Dr. Don Gambrell, of the Georgia School of Medicine in Augusta, Georgia[10]—are treating women who have menopausal symptoms with estrogen and progesterone within a year or two of successfully treating their breast cancer.

This opinion has been repeatedly voiced at the annual meetings of the North American Menopause Society. A number of experts in the area of hormone replacement therapy and breast cancer stated that giving estrogen did not increase the likelihood of the cancer returning,[11] and significantly improved the woman's quality of life. But this is still a highly debated issue. Because adequate research studies have not been done, the answers are not yet known.

Whether a woman would consider taking hormones might depend on how severe her menopausal symptoms were. Apparently 50 percent of women who have had breast cancer, and who also have menopausal symptoms, choose to take hormone replacement therapy even if they are not sure of the risk. They are too miserable without it.

A Difficult Decision   When a woman has an obviously hormone-related cancer such as breast cancer, doctors treat it by reducing estrogen levels in the body. This is because estrogen is known to cause breast cells to proliferate. Also, certain types of cancer can proliferate quickly during pregnancy under the influence of high levels of hormones. This suggests a strong relationship between breast cancer and hormones (although, conversely, women who have had multiple pregnancies tend to get less breast cancer).

It is not easy to test whether or not a breast cancer has estrogen receptors in it. Even if a breast cancer test indicates no estrogen or progesterone receptors, specialists may be skeptical. They believe that even a breast cancer without estrogen receptors may later produce a tumor that does have estrogen receptors in it. Also, when biopsies are done by electrocautery methods, the heat process can destroy estrogen and progesterone receptors that were originally there.

Actually, the survival rate is better among women who do have estrogen receptors, probably because estrogen receptors are more common in the earlier stages of breast cancer.[12] The women who have breast cancer without estrogen or progesterone receptors may have a poorer prognosis because the cancer is often more aggressive.[13]

For these reasons, some cancer specialists put all women with breast cancer, with or without estrogen receptors, on Tamoxifen. They hesitate to put any woman with a current case of breast cancer on estrogen replacement therapy, and think twice about putting anyone with a past case of breast cancer on it either. However, as mentioned earlier, the tide of opinion is changing on this. Some physicians believe that small postmenopausal doses of estrogen can make a tremendous difference to a woman's general health and will not shorten her life expectancy as regards the cancer.

John Arpels, M.D.   Dr. John Arpels summarizes this point of view well by stating that fully 80 percent of postmenopausal breast cancer develops in women not on hormone replacement therapy. Most of the studies show no increase in risk. Some even show a slightly decreased incidence of breast cancer. A few studies show that, at worst, one percent of the patients may have a 30-to-60-percent increase in risk after 10 to 15 years of using the higher-dose estrogen. Although this sounds like a significant risk increase, it must be put into proper perspective as in the following example:

Risk factor at age 60 to 70: 4 percent
60 percent increase: 6.4 percent

This risk is distributed over a 10-year period, and for each year spent without developing breast cancer, the risk for that year is dropped and the remaining risk is lowered.

Compare the percentage increase of cancer due to specific risks:

Cause	Cancer	Risk
Tobacco	Lung	30 percent
Diet	Colon	28 percent
Hormones	Breast/Uterus	1 percent

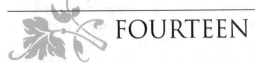

C H A P T E R

FOURTEEN

CHRONIC FATIGUE SYNDROME AND MULTIPLE CHEMICAL SENSITIVITY

Sheila, 28, was a well-paid executive in a large computer company. She worked long hours, and her job was intense and demanding. Even at home, her time was highly self-regulated; she stuck rigidly to her exercise schedule, and jogged three miles twice each day.

One day, Sheila developed what seemed like a persistent case of the flu. She had a sore throat and a mild fever, and she ached all over. The lymph nodes in her neck were swollen. She took a few days off, but the illness continued. She struggled to return to work, but found herself more and more exhausted. Finally, she stayed home and spent most of her time lying around, unable even to raise her head off the pillow.

She stopped jogging when she became sick, and found that she no longer had any energy for exercise. At night she had intense sweats, nightmares, and insomnia. During the day, her mind became more and more cloudy. She started forgetting things, and found it impossible to concentrate.

When she went to her doctor, he asked her if she had ever had mononucleosis (also called the Epstein-Barr virus or EBV). Sheila said that she'd had it when she was 15, at which time she had needed two months' bed rest. Her doctor measured the EBV titer in her blood and found it very high. He said she had chronic fatigue syndrome (CFS), for which there was no known cure. He told her to do all she could to support her immune system, including plenty of rest, and offered her an antidepressant.

When Sheila came to see me, she had improved somewhat from her original condition; she had enough energy to work four to six hours a day. During the two years when she had been most sick with CFS, her boyfriend had supported her financially, but now she wanted to be independent again. Sheila told me that her mind was working well, but that her low energy levels hampered her. She was looking for a part-time job because she felt that she couldn't cope with an eight-hour workday. But her former employers weren't interested in letting her work part time. When she interviewed for other jobs, she learned to keep quiet about her CFS. Nobody wanted to employ somebody whose sickness might interfere with her work.

Sheila's symptoms were much worse before her menstrual period, so it seemed reasonable to investigate the possibility of a hormonal link. Her physician responded to the suggestion that a combination of cyclical natural progesterone with low-dose thyroid might help (her thyroid level was borderline low). He gave her both medications to try.

Within three months, Sheila called me from her new job. Still struggling with mild symptoms, she nevertheless felt much better. She had found the hormones to be very helpful in diminishing her symptoms, enabling her to go back to work.

HORMONAL PROBLEMS AND IMMUNE SYSTEM DYSFUNCTION OCCUR TOGETHER

Elizabeth Lee Vliet, M.D., points out in her book, *Screaming to Be Heard: Hormonal Connections Women Suspect, but Doctors Ignore,* that there are a number of diagnoses that share common symptoms. These illnesses include hypothyroidism, premenstrual syndrome (PMS), hormonal problems at mid-life, systemic candida (yeast) infections, allergies, multiple chemical sensitivities (MCS), and chronic fatigue syndrome (CFS). All of these illnesses are more common in women than in men. For example, CFS is 70 percent more common in women than in men.

In each of these diseases, both the hormone and immune systems are out of balance, but the ratio of how much each is involved varies with the type of problem and the individual reaction. Sometimes the main problem is hormonal imbalance, and the person has impaired immune-system function causing fatigue, allergies, and recurrent yeast problems. Other times, the basic problem is centered on the immune system, and this can cause damage to the ovaries and thus affect hormonal status. This is true with CFS (virally caused), and MCS (caused by environmental toxins)—the immune system is compromised, and the hormones are also frequently out of kilter.

Normally, the main hormones (estrogen, progesterone, testosterone, thyroid, cortisone, DHEA) all strengthen immunity. Generally, taking the appropriate hormone can help a lot, but sometimes taking hormones can aggravating allergies in vulnerable people.

Chronic Fatigue Syndrome

Chronic Fatigue Syndrome (CFS, also called CFIDS), was originally thought to be a recurrence of mononucleosis (also called Epstein-Barr virus, EBV, or glandular fever). But other viruses, such as herpes simplex (related to EBV) and cytomegalovirus (CMV) are now known to be involved. CFS occurs when the body's immune system breaks down as a result of viral assault, usually in people who overexert, overstress, and overtire themselves.

The Centers for Disease Control presently define CFS as "new onset of persistent or relapsing, debilitating fatigue lasting at least six months in a person with no previous history of similar symptoms."

The body's immune system, called upon to attack the virus, overreacts and begins to produce too many killer cells (a specific kind of cell that fights cancer). Somehow, the mechanism that starts the killer cell action gets stuck in overproduction mode. The exhaustion, lack of concentration, depression, and muscle and joint pain that characterize CFS are considered to be side effects of killer cell action.

Usually, doctors say that there is no known treatment for CFS. Rest is particularly important, with adherence to a simple, healthy lifestyle with minimal (but some) exercise. This gives the body a chance to heal itself. People with CFS need to continue resting even when their condition is improving. Unfortunately, the "type-A" personality most prone to contracting CFS finds it almost impossible to slow down. As such individuals improve, they often overdo things again, and tend to keep having relapses. Counseling on behavior modification may be an important part of their treatment.

Testing for CFS Doctors suspecting CFS usually check a patient's blood to find out if he or she has ever had mononucleosis; sometimes they check for other viruses. These tests are not conclusive, and CFS is a disease that is partly diagnosed by the presence of clinical symptoms and by ruling out other diseases. This makes its diagnosis vague.

The EBV titer is often high in people with CFS, but the test does not tell the doctor if the mononucleosis is current or past. Sometimes the patient recalls having had mononucleosis. But often they weren't aware they had it; in a mild case, it appears just like a case of influenza.

Multiple Chemical Sensitivities

MCS also involves a breakdown of the endocrine and immune systems, but in this case the trigger is toxic chemicals (called xenobiotics) that overpower the system, rather than a virus. The liver and kidneys become unable to cope with eliminating these chemicals, which then keep circulating in the blood and creating havoc. People with MCS become intolerant of many substances, and often have extreme reactions when exposed to perfumes, paint, formaldehyde, gas fumes, and other chemicals. The symptoms include exhaustion, depression, joint pain, headaches, allergy reactions, and behavior changes.

Sudden Toxic Assault   MCS is more likely to develop in people who already have depressed immune systems, but sometimes toxic assault can be so sudden and overwhelming that it happens to quite healthy people. For instance, when police raided a building where illegal drugs were being manufactured, the fleeing criminals threw PCP dust directly in the faces of the police, causing MCS. As another example, Gulf War veterans experience many side effects from exposure to pesticides and anti-nerve-gas chemicals. You may recall Norman Cousins, the famous author of *Anatomy of An Illness,* who became sick after being caught in a blast of jet exhaust.

There are special centers, called "detox clinics," set up in many major cities in this country to help people recover from serious toxic chemical exposure.

Past Approaches to MCS   Theron Randoph, M.D., first coined the term "chemical sensitivity" in 1967. His approach to treating MCS was to isolate patients from the chemicals to which they were hypersensitive. That sometimes meant that they had to live in isolated locations, or in houses with walls sealed off by aluminum foil and other protection against exposure to toxic substances. This isolation technique has been effective for some people with MCS, but it does not directly address the source of the problem.

Another attempt to deal with MCS was to do skin testing for the patient's allergies, and to give antigens under the tongue as treatment. This has been a controversial approach, but some have found it helpful.

Total Body Load   The phrase "total body load" is used to describe how multiple factors affect a person's reaction to toxic chemicals. These factors include stress on the job, sensitivity to molds, food allergies, allergies to trees and grasses, genetic factors, relationship problems, frequent travel (exposure to radiation, interruption of circadian rhythms from jet lag), lack of sleep, and eating junk food. A person's body can cope with a variety of stressors, but when too many accumulate, that person may be pushed over the edge into MCS.

Other factors making MCS more likely are poor diet, intestinal parasites, the repeated use of anti-inflammatory medication or antibiotics, and the use of narcotic drugs. These can all disrupt the friendly bacteria in the bowel and cause chronic inflammation or even perforation of the bowel. The resulting problem is called "leaky gut."

As a result of leaky gut, items that should pass through the bowel cannot, and items that should not get through the bowel get through. A lot of food remains undigested and leaves long chains of amino acids—harsh, undigested proteins that can cause severe allergic reactions. These proteins cause high levels of toxins in the bloodstream, which in turn overwhelm the liver.

Liver Toxicity, a Key Factor   During the past four to five years, doctors have recognized the importance of detoxifying the liver. Currently, the most common test for detecting liver enzymes only shows up gross abnormalities of liver function, such as hepatitis or cirrhosis of the liver. It doesn't show how well the liver is working at detoxification.

Within the past few years, a more helpful liver test has been developed, but it is only available at a research level and is not yet commercially available. The test measures two different ways in which the liver detoxifies and is performed by giving the patient a specific dose of caffeine and a specific dose of sodium benzoate. The output of these two substances is measured, and the results show how well the liver is eliminating toxins.

Conjugation Dependent on Molybdenum   One of the newer approaches to treating MCS is the use of the element molybdenum. The liver marks toxins for destruction by a process called conjugation. In conjugation, a marker molecule made by the immune system attaches to the toxin and accompanies it through the bloodstream, where it is eliminated in the waste. The marker molecule cannot attach without a particular enzyme, and this enzyme is dependent on the element molybdenum to work.

Therefore, when molybdenum is deficient or missing in the human body, the conjugation process is defective. Toxic chemicals continue to circulate in the bloodstream and are not passed out of the body. Molybdenum can be replaced by using a supplement, and this can often enable a person to eliminate toxic chemicals more efficiently.

Antioxidants (for instance, vitamins A, C, and E, and herbs such as Ginkgo Biloba) are helpful. I recommend Carolyn Reuben's excellent book, *Antioxidants: Your Complete Guide* (see Recommended Reading). Also helpful are zinc, glutathion, and special sulfur-containing supplements.

MCS Requires Professional Help   Much of the information in this chapter was provided by Richard S. Wilkinson, M.D., who, with his brother, runs an allergy clinic in Yakima, Washington. Dr. Wilkinson stresses the fact that self-help treatment is not appropriate for MCS, because the condition is too complex. This is why no specific doses of the suggested supplements are given. There are multiple approaches to treatment, and different patients respond to different methods. People with severe cases of MCS need specialist supervision.

The Hormonal Link

Dr. Wilkinson has seen a crucial hormonal connection in both CFS and MCS and uses a variety of hormones to help his patients. He investigates the levels of the main sex hormones (estrogen, progesterone, and testosterone), but he also checks thyroid and adrenal function. He does not depend solely on routine blood tests for thyroid and cortisol; he finds that while they are useful they have limited value. He prefers using the ACTH-stimulating test and the Broda Barnes Foundation urine analysis.

ACTH stands for adrenocorticotropin, the pituitary precursor of cortisol. In this test, urine is collected for 24 hours. Then the patient is given a shot of ACTH to stimulate the adrenal glands. The urine is collected for another 24 hours. The report will show the levels of cortisol and various other adrenal hormones, including DHEA. The levels measured in the first 24 hours represent a resting level. The second 24-hour test reflects a stressed level. It is also possible to tell from this test whether the problem is an adrenal problem or a hypothalamus/pituitary problem.

The Broda Barnes Foundation analysis is a 24-hour comprehensive urine collection.[1] This test analyzes urinary output of thyroid, cortisol, aldosterone, and androgen levels. A report is prepared by Jacques Hertoghe, M.D., a prominent Belgian endocrinologist. The Hertoghe family (four generations of endocrinologists) took over the work of Broda Barnes, M.D., after his death.

Different People Need Different Hormones   Dr. Wilkinson says that using low physiologic or replacement doses instead of suppressive doses of natural cortisone and thyroid can produce miraculous results in some people. He also uses the main sex hormones—a mixture of estrogens (estradiol, estrone, estriol), natural progesterone, and sometimes a little testosterone in women. He uses testosterone replacement for some of his male patients, and occasionally uses DHEA for both sexes.

In some cases, Dr. Wilkinson finds that just replacing the main sex hormone will correct the chemical sensitivity. Some women respond better to estrogen, and others to natural progesterone.

Dr. Wilkinson recommends finding an expert who will:

- Take a good, comprehensive history;
- Check out the function of the gut and liver;
- Check whether you are nutritionally sufficient;
- Suggest ways to identify and remove the stressors;
- Check out the hormones.

CASE HISTORIES

Ken's Story

Ken, a cross-country trucker in his late fifties, had always had good health, but he continually worked long hours on the road and was often tired. His father had died the previous year, and he had been feeling rather depressed ever since. One day a pest control operator came and sprayed Ken's house. When he drove home that day, he immediately re-acted to the spray; his chest and eyes hurt, and he had diffi-culty breathing. He was so uncomfortable that he left the house after about 20 minutes and slept in his truck. But after this experience, Ken began having classic symptoms of MCS.

Ken's wife, Julie, often went with him cross-country. She noted that when he drove through certain areas, he would be-come suddenly angry and upset. It was noticeable because he was usually calm and easy-going. They talked about it and re-alized that it occurred only in places where there had been commercial spraying. Ken was reacting to the pesticides.

Ken visited an allergist who tested him for chemical sensi-tivity. But, to the doctor's surprise, the tests didn't show much. Because the doctor knew that hormones might be a factor, and because Ken complained that his sex drive was diminishing, the doctor checked Ken's testosterone levels and found them very low. When he began treating Ken with testosterone, it made a dramatic difference in how Ken felt.

Often cases are multifactorial, and Ken's was one of these. The lack of sleep, the stress from the death of his father, and the exposure to pesticides were all factors, but the main key was hormonal.

Rosemarie's Story

Rosemarie was 43 years old when her doctor advised a hys-terectomy. She had large fibroids and had been bleeding con-tinously for two months. The doctor had tried to stop the bleeding, but had been unsuccessful. Rosemarie was looking forward to the surgery, because several friends had told her how much better they felt after their hysterectomies, and she was tired of having cramps and bleeding.

Rosemarie's ovaries were cystic, so the surgeon removed them, too. Recovery was uneventful, and Rosemarie initially felt fine. She was given 0.625 mg of Premarin daily after her surgery. After several months, she became symptomatic of es-trogen deficiency because the dose was not adequate. Her physician did not suggest any alterations to her medication. In Rosemarie's case, her main symptom was a compromised immune system. She became highly sensitive to many substances, and began having reactions to substances in her house, such as carpet and paint. Her life became a miserable round of hay fever, constant post-nasal drip, headaches, joint pain, lassitude, and depression. She developed food allergies and became unable to eat many foods without a worsening of her symptoms.

She tried many forms of treatment, even going to live in Arizona for a couple of years, but the allergies affected her even there. She came back to live in San Francisco in an environmentally-safe house, covered with aluminum. She became a recluse, unable to venture out into society because of her reactions.

When Rosemarie read about the role of hormones in treating MCS, she found a physician in San Francisco who specialized in hormone balancing. When she was given natural estradiol, building up the dose gradually to prevent sensitivity, she began to feel some resolution of her symptoms.

Immunity is a new area of study. The immune system is as complex as the brain. It's like a large, unexplored country that researchers are entering only at the borders. This is why much of the treatment of MCS and other immune system problems focuses on supporting the ability of the body to heal itself. That involves, rest, diet, mild exercise, supplementation, sunshine, pure water, adequate sleep, possibly an antidepressant, and hormones.

FIND AN EXPERT

For thyroid and adrenal testing, contact the Broda Barnes Foundation at 203-261-2101, or write to them at P.O. Box 98, Trumble, CT 06611.

To find a specialist in MCS, call the American Association of Environmental Medicine (AAEM), in Kansas City, Kansas. The phone number is 913-642-6062.

Another helpful source of physicians who practice alternative medicine is The American College for Advancement in Medicine (ACAM), located in Laguna Hills, California. Their phone numbers are 714-583-7666 within California, and 1-800-532-3688 elsewhere in the U.S.

CHAPTER

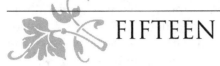

FIFTEEN

ANDROGENS IN MEN AND WOMEN

 Ron was age 20 and serving in the military. Once, while on leave, he stayed with his brother whose son had chicken pox, and Ron caught chicken pox from him. When Ron returned to the army base, he was placed in the infirmary; he was the only person with chicken pox, so he was put in a private room. But it was only two doors away from a large ward where a number of soldiers were sick with the mumps. After having chicken pox, Ron also developed the mumps and felt sick for several months. After recovery, he was told by the army doctor that he might never have children, because mumps can make men sterile. Despite the dire prediction, he later married and had five children! But Ron now believes that having had the mumps caused damage to his testes, which prematurely diminished his testosterone production.

Ron's health began to deteriorate at about age 49. He became extremely allergic to certain foods—pickles, chocolate, coffee, milk, and wheat. At age 54, the fourth lumbar disc in his back became weak; it ruptured, pressing on the sciatic nerve in his left leg. He said it was like having 1,000 needles stuck into his leg at once. Any movement was excruciating. Ron had an operation on his back that cost $25,000. In retrospect, he believes that he had early-onset osteoporosis. The back surgeon told him that he would need back surgery again within five years, and that the problem was genetic and due to aging. Eventually, the surgeon said, Ron would need surgery to fuse his spine.

At age 55, Ron began having severe cardiac arrhythmia. He was put into the hospital twice for monitoring of the variation in his heartbeat, so that the correct medication could be prescribed. He often carried a heartbeat recorder for later analysis. Sometimes his heart would stop. Fear of imminent death would make cold sweat appear on his forehead.

Ron's allergies were worsening. His nose ran constantly, his eyes burned, his headaches didn't stop. Eating became a miserable process, and he would often fast for three to four days to avoid having to go through the symptoms that accompanied eating.

At age 55, looking 70, Ron attended his youngest son's wedding. The photographs show him as a shell of his former self. He had lost two clothing sizes, his face was pallid, and his hair was prematurely white. He had many symptoms, his libido was very low, his body temperature was 96.4 degrees, and he was so cold that he needed to wear sweaters all the time. Worst of all, his ability to think logically in his work as a scientist was disappearing, and he was finding it impossible to focus on details.

He went to a famous national clinic to see if they could help him find the problem. This was a three-day, in-depth hospital examination that should have uncovered any major problems. They did extensive blood tests, took thorough medical histories including genetic data on his close family members, checked for diabetes, and ran many other tests. But they did not check his testosterone level. They told him that he was just aging faster than normal!

A physicist by training, Ron decided to find some answers to his health problems. First, he investigated nutrition and supplements and addressed his allergy problems. Food avoidance was difficult, as he had such a small range of options at that time. If he ate any food on the prohibited list or drank a cup of coffee, his problems came back immediately.

He kept studying, and by age 57 he had the data, the facts, and the theory about what was happening. In the process, Ron became an expert on the function of the human cell. He came to the conclusion that he mainly needed testosterone, but had a lot of trouble finding anyone who would prescribe it for him. Eventually he found a physician who treated him with hormones, and from then on his health began to improve.

Ron now takes testosterone, thyroid, DHEA, and melatonin. He says that his temperature is now normal, his skin is healthy and ruddy, his allergies have disappeared, and he has put on the weight that he formerly lost. His heart is strong and healthy, and his blood pressure is normal. His cholesterol level dropped from 190 down to 150. Also, his long-lost libido returned. He has not needed the surgery on his back. In the past three years, Ron has added three new patents to his list of discoveries—his thinking ability is back to normal!

In summary, Ron says that the answers can be found in the medical literature, but you have to search hard for them—and ignore some of the myths about the negative side effects of hormones. He says the central problem is that hormonal deficiency throws out the nitrogen balance—the process that controls the rate of the production and destruction of proteins or amino acids. When testosterone levels drop in men, nitrogen balance and protein production are adversely affected, and this can lead to many health problems.

MALE HORMONES ARE IMPORTANT

Just as estrogen is important for female development, so is testosterone important for male development. Men and women both have estrogen and testosterone, but in opposite proportions: women need a little testosterone, and men need a little estrogen. According to researchers, the presence of many xenoestrogens (chemicals containing phenols that act like harsh estrogens) in the environment has increased men's estrogen levels dramatically and may have caused the drastic drop in the amount of sperm produced in men living in Western countries.

The action of testosterone in males at puberty is spectacular, transforming the child into a youth, then a man. It is present in a number of organs, and it regulates protein production.

Testosterone receptors are present in the muscles, skeleton, reproductive organs, brain, nervous system, and sebaceous sweat glands. Testosterone is the best bone-builder of all the sex hormones. Red-blood-cell levels increase under the influence of testosterone, but white blood cells contain receptors for testosterone. So testosterone levels influence the white blood cell count, and higher levels increase immunity. Testosterone stabilizes blood sugar levels, increases HDL cholesterol levels, and lowers triglyceride levels. It gives a feeling of well-being, and it fuels the sex drive.

Sexual Physiology in Men

Semen is made up of sperm plus secretions from the seminal vesicles, the prostate, and other glands. Sperm are produced by primitive germ cells called Sertoli cells (the male equivalent of eggs) in the testes. These germ cells do not become depleted, as women's do at menopause. They keep producing sperm, but production does decline with age. Sperm production is at its highest between age 25 and 30, and diminishes from then on.

Testosterone, which is the main male hormone, is produced by the Leydig cells (or interstitial cells), which are also found in the testes. The testosterone produced goes into the bloodstream, but most of it is bound by sex-hormone-binding globulin. So a small part of the testosterone is free and available, but most of it is bound and unavailable for use until broken down.

The quantity of sperm and seminal secretion is directly related to the level of male hormones. Without hormonal stimulation, the glands will atrophy and sperm production will cease.

The prostate gland, which you hear about so much in older men, is a fibromuscular organ the shape of a doughnut and the size of a chestnut (about an inch and a half wide and deep). Its major function is the secretion of semen, which makes up 95 percent of the ejaculate (the remaining 5 percent is sperm). The prostate gland encircles the urethra (the tube from the bladder to the end of the penis). As men age, the prostate gland tends to progressively enlarge, which can obstruct the flow of urine. Most men in the Western world end up having some type of prostate trouble as they get older. This is probably due, at least in part, to diet and chemical pollution; it is less of a problem among vegetarians.

Sexual Activity

Ejaculation—the release of semen out of the penis—takes place when sperm fill the genital passages and the resulting swelling stimulates nerves centers to orgasm. This happens two to three times a week in men under the age of 30. If there is no sexual activity, ejaculation will occur naturally, often at night, resulting in nocturnal emissions called "wet dreams."

Testosterone is responsible for heightened libido and aggressiveness, and testosterone levels are at their highest during a young man's late teens. This explains the recklessness of some pubertal men and the fact that they may have a fairly constant erection during those years. A young man can develop a full erection in a few seconds, while it can sometimes take several minutes to half an hour for older men. It is unusual for a young man to lose an erection unless startled, but in later years, an older man is more easily distracted and may occasionally have erection failure during sexual intercourse.

According to Dr. Aubrey Hill, men's sexuality begins to wane slightly from age 30 until age 40. Then it decreases rapidly for the next twenty years. A man's sexuality is waning as his wife's is increasing in her forties to fifties. Pentii Siiteri, M.D., an expert endocrinologist, says that most men's sexuality begins to taper off in their mid-fifties to sixties, and sooner or later most men go through male "menopause." These changes, added to the man's fear of sexual failure, can cause marital rifts if not understood.

At age 80, a man's testosterone levels are at about one-fifth of the peak level of his youth.[1]

Changes with Aging

As men age from 40 to 50 and onward, the function of the testes slows down. Their primitive germ cells continue to produce sperm, but at a slower rate. The Leydig cells in the testes produce less testosterone. The blood levels of testosterone remain much the same because testosterone clearance from the body also slows down, but the binding globulin level increases, and so less testosterone is free and available. Men begin to lose testosterone receptors in their heart, brain, gastrointestinal tract, and penis (but apparently not in their prostate gland). On the other hand, stress control, exercise, and having regular sex can increase testosterone levels. For many men, andropause will only become a problem after age 65 to 70, but it can occur earlier than the norm, as shown by Ron's experience.

This aging process can be accentuated by stress causing adrenal burnout, or by trauma, injury, undescended testicles, or damage from viruses and autoimmune processes. Other factors that affect testosterone production are: illness, some medications (cortisone, some cholesterol-lowering drugs), psychological state, obesity, lack of exercise or overexercise, malnutrition, and alcohol or drug abuse. Additional factors that cause osteoporosis in men include: reduced level of exercise, poor nutrition, medications such as cortisone, diabetes mellitus, reduced growth hormone levels, and accidental falls.

The reasons for changes in sexuality and a man's lessening ability to have erections are more complex than just having lower testosterone levels.[2] Erection failure is more connected to vascularity—having enough blood, fluid, and oxygen in the penis. Stress, hypertension, vascular problems from arteriosclerosis,[3] cigarette smoking[4] (which constricts the blood vessels in the penis), consumption of alcohol, obesity, and, possibly, vasectomy[5] can contribute to loss of male potency. When erectile failure begins to happen, it is so connected to a man's self-esteem that fear may bring repeated failure.

Symptoms Are Similar to Menopause in Women

Men do not have the abrupt ceasing of reproductive capacity that women do. They do not run out of eggs the way women do. Nevertheless, there are changes that have been variously termed "andropause" and "viropause." The symptoms of andropause are remarkably similar to those experienced by women with declining estrogen levels.

This lessening of testosterone and other androgen levels can lead to fatigue, irritability, mental depression, mood swings, loss of visual and cognitive ability, forgetfulness, loss of well-being and vigor, sleep disorders, dry skin, progressive aging of the face, a decrease in muscle mass causing muscle weakness, and increased body fat. Osteoporosis can also occur, though later than in women, with varicose veins, hemorrhoids, arteriosclerosis, hypertension followed by hardening of the arteries, increasing fragility of bone causing rheumatism in the shoulder and arthritis of the spinal column, and declining sexual performance (both lower libido and fewer and poorly sustained erections). Since the heart is a muscle, the loss of muscle strength, combined with the tendency to put on weight, spells bad news about heart disease.

According to Georges Debled, M.D., a Belgian endocrinologist, there are familial and individual variations in the capacity of the sex glands to produce hormones, and this phenomenon is linked to life expectancy.

Other Hormonal Factors in Aging

Aging is also associated with decreases in the levels of other hormones—melatonin, DHEA, and growth hormone—in both men and women. It is not so much the actual levels of growth hormone that are problematic, for these do not alter much; rather, the pulsatory waves and peaks in growth hormone production change with age.

Melatonin is a hormone secreted nocturnally by the pineal gland. It helps regulate the body's clock. Production drops off gradually, beginning around age 20 to 30. Melatonin may well play a prominent role in the aging processes. Treatment with melatonin seems to stop insomnia in some older people, and helps restore body rhythms. It has also been used for preventing jet lag, and is available as a supplement in many health food stores.[6]

DHEA (dehydroepiandrosterone) is a weak androgen produced by the adrenal glands in men and women. It breaks
down into testosterone and estrogens. Production begins to
decline at about age 30. In animals, it reduces obesity, boosts
the immune system, prevents cancer, increases life span, possibly lowers the risk of heart disease, and increases a feeling of
energy and well-being.[7]

There have been some studies done on growth hormone
showing that it may stimulate the immune system, improve
feelings of well-being, improve sexual potency, improve the
quality of sleep, and reduce the toll of cardiovascular disease
by reducing both body fat and total cholesterol levels and
strengthening the heart muscles.[8] However, the long-term
risks associated with overdosing on growth hormone have not
been well studied; they include possible disabling carpal tunnel syndrome, enlarged and tender breasts in men, changing
blood sugar levels, osteoarthritis, and cancer. There has been
some incidence of unconventional viral infections leading to
death as a result of treatment with growth hormone from a
contaminated bovine source,[9] but usually growth hormone is
made in the laboratory.

It is likely that the changes in these other hormones—
melatonin, DHEA, and growth hormone—is initiated by a prior
drop in the main sex hormones, but this also has not been studied in depth.[10] If this is so, it shows how the drop in sex hormones acts as a catalyst to the aging process and illustrates the
importance of sex hormone replacement in some men and
women. These hormones are all being studied at present; they
may eventually become acceptable additions to hormone replacement therapy and the prevention of frailty in the elderly.

Prostate Problems

Because of its position, the prostate gland has poor circulation. It is called the crossbar, because it cuts across the urethra. As men age, the prostate gland is prone to swell and
become inflamed. This swelling or enlargement of the tissue
is called "benign prostatic hypertrophy," or BPH. When the

prostate gland is enlarged, it narrows the urethra, which leads to obstruction and inability to urinate; this causes urinary urgency, hesitancy, decreased pressure behind the urine stream, and frequent urination, particularly at night. This is a common problem in men over 55. Its effect is to cut the stream of urine and make it more difficult to have an erection.

By the age of 70, 80 percent of men will have BPH, often leading to obstruction and urinary problems that require surgery. By about the same age, 50 percent of men will have microscopic prostate precancerous changes—but this progresses into clinical cancer in only a small percentage of men. The incidence of prostate cancer varies among ethnic groups, and this means that other factors than hormones are at work (for example, environment, genes, and lifestyle).

Testing for Prostate Cancer   Men over age 50 have been urged in the past to have an annual rectal exam to check for prostate cancer. However, this recommendation has been questioned recently in both the U.S. and Europe.

Dr. Philip Warner says:

> At present the PSA (prostate specific antigen) test is really the gold standard of prostate cancer tests. It is much more accurate than a rectal exam. If the PSA test is positive, we then do a prostate ultrasound.

Dr. Rick Wilkinson says that the PSA is also of value if a man is contemplating testosterone therapy, since testosterone can[11] purportedly act as a catalyst for already existing cancer. If a man has a PSA of 8 to 10, he would need to be monitored closely. But note that Jens Møller, M.D., an expert Danish cardiologist, said that he never found a case of prostate cancer in twenty years of treating his male patients with testosterone.

Often, early cases of prostate cancer are being left untreated because the condition is usually slow-growing. Early treatment has been shown to cause more problems than benefits. Men typically die of something else. Many urologists are recommending that if you find an early cancer, you do nothing but monitor it.

Sexual Changes in Men

As men age, they will experience a decline in sexual interest and function, lower libido, more difficulty sustaining erections, less explosive orgasms, and a longer time between erections. They will need more time to achieve an erection, and they will need more help from their partners to stay firm. They will experience a decrease in both the pressure and volume of ejaculate, and will feel less demand to ejaculate. The refractory period (the time between erections) will lengthen from hours to days. However, between the ages of 66 and 77, 80 percent of men are still interested in having sex.[12] Note that between the ages of 66 and 77, 50 percent of women are still interested in having sex.[13]

While many men over 65 are sterile, others can father a child well into old age. According to Georges Debled, here are the percentages of impotent men at different ages:

Age 40:	1.9 percent
Age 50:	6.7 percent
Age 60:	18.4 percent
Age 65:	25.0 percent
Age 70:	27.0 percent
Age 80:	75.0 percent[14]

Sexual attitudes and behavior tend to continue into old age. That means that if you liked having sex frequently when you were young, most times you still will when you are older.

Unisex Plumbing Problems

Both men and women, as they age, can experience lessening kidney function, with narrowing and contraction of the ureter (the tube which carries urine from the kidney out of the body). They can both experience urethritis, repeated bladder infections, inflammation of the ureter, painful or difficult urination, and the triad of urinary problems—urgency, frequency, and incontinence.

This is more of a problem at a younger age in women than in men—possibly due in part to childbirth and the pressure of the uterus on the bladder. Also, the urethra outlet in women tends to change direction because of weakening muscles, and shifts from voiding at an angle to a "straight shot downward."

Incontinence is connected with having less bladder capacity. The bladder feels that it needs emptying without being properly full. The individual is less able to postpone voiding. This is something of a professional hazard of teachers and public speakers, who form the habit of going to the bathroom to urinate before giving a class or speech when the bladder is only half empty. Gradually, the bladder begins to signal the need to go to the bathroom when it is only half full, and this leads to needing to urinate too often.

Other problems involved in incontinence include less urethral closure pressure, less urinary flow rate, more residual volume (the bladder does not fully empty), and more bladder contractions.

Types of Incontinence

URGE INCONTINENCE. Seventy percent of aging women feel a need to go to the bathroom but have some leakage on the way. They may also have bedwetting problems at night. This is a problem of lessened residual volume; their bladder can no longer contain the amount of urine that it formerly could.

STRESS INCONTINENCE. This involves losing urine when coughing or straining (it is often connected with uterine prolapse in women). These people don't have wetting problems at night, but do have a small residual volume.

OVERFLOW INCONTINENCE. This occurs mainly in men, and is usually due to swelling of the prostate gland, which obstructs the passage of urine, as well as to incomplete emptying. These men will have a slow flow, a need to strain, frequent leakage, and a large residual volume. They begin having a sense of fullness or a "need to go," but find that they have trouble actually urinating.

Help for Incontinence   One of the most animated and humorous women's support groups I attended occurred when someone brought up the subject of incontinence. It became quickly apparent that "having to go quickly and not quite making it" was a common problem in women around menopause. Yet bladder dysfunction and decreasing sexuality are problems that women generally keep to themselves.

This is unfortunate, because these urinary problems (in both sexes) can be helped by a good urologist. Also, Kegel exercises[15] can restore muscle tone in both men and women.

Other Ways Testosterone Can Help Women

Androgens also help in treatment of breast tenderness in women as a result of other hormone replacement, hot flashes where estrogen alone does not help, and osteoporosis.[16] Concerns about hirsutism (excessive hair growth) from taking androgens are overstated. The effect is reversible and usually disappears when the dose is lowered. Another concern— adverse cardiovascular effects—does not seem to be scientifically validated, according to Ronald Young, M.D.[17]

Testosterone has been found to be helpful in the prevention and treatment of breast cancer in women. See details in Chapter 13 on breast cancer.

Treating Women with Low Testosterone Levels   Elizabeth Lee Vliet, M.D., and Denise Mark, M.D., both do repeated hormone level tests on their female patients. They have both found that testosterone levels can decline early in women in their mid-thirties and early forties. In fact, it is well known that androgen levels decrease as much as 50 percent following menopause.[18] This may lead to low sex drive, muscle weakness, and loss of a feeling of well-being. When these symptoms occur, if the testosterone levels are lower than 10–20 pg/ml, they may add natural testosterone to the hormone replacement program.[19] Dr. Mark might also use DHEA because it tends to break down to testosterone in women.

Testosterone and Chronic Disease in Men

In the past, the use of testosterone has been thought to increase the risk of heart disease. But a Danish cardiologist, Jens Møller,

M.D., believed otherwise. Before his death in the 1980s, he was president of the European Organization for the Control of Circulatory disease—EOCCD. He used testosterone extensively in his practice to treat a number of chronic diseases in men, such as cardiovascular disease, diabetes mellitus, and resulting gangrene.[20] In a practice spanning over 30 years, he found very few side effects and no cases of prostate cancer. He also observed a 25-percent reduction in cholesterol levels in his patients on testosterone, and a decreased frequency of angina and stroke (testosterone makes the blood less likely to clot).

A recent study performed at Columbia University,[21] cited by Dr. Richard Wilkinson,[22] supports Dr. Møller's observations; it showed that testosterone, instead of being a causative factor for myocardial infarction, might actually protect men against coronary artery disease.[23] The findings show that low testosterone levels may not only be a risk factor for myocardial infarction, but may also lead to the development of coronary artery disease and thrombosis. This study showed a positive correlation between testosterone and HDL cholesterol levels.

A study by Maurice Lesser[24] in 1946 showed that testosterone propionate, properly used, not only reduces the frequency of attacks of angina pectoris, but decreases their severity when they do occur.

Testosterone may help a considerable number of people with clotting problems. According to Michael Hanson, M.D., who continues the work of Dr. Møller, testosterone treatment can also be helpful in preventing strokes in susceptible men.[25]

Dr. Wilkinson notes that testosterone has also been successfully used, since the late 1930s, for treating mental depression and other psychological problems.[26]

Summary of Good Effects of Testosterone (When Needed)

- Improves libido and sexual performance;
- Increases muscle strength;
- Improves vigor, energy, and zest for life;
- Improves angina;
- Useful in the body's healing process;

- Supports the immune system;
- Improves aerobic metabolism;
- Improves glucose metabolism;
- Stabilizes and improves diabetes mellitus;
- Increases oxygen uptake by tissues;
- Increases protein metabolism;
- Leads to a positive nitrogen balance;
- Increases fibrinolysis and so helps in thrombosis;
- Decreases risk of stroke in those with transient ischemic attacks (TIAs or ministrokes);
- Increases bone density and strength (it is the best bone builder);
- Prevents breast cancer;
- Relieves allergies.

Why Then Is Testosterone Not Used?

If testosterone is so great, why is it not used more frequently? Among men, there are a number of reasons, including: 1) fear of developing prostate cancer, paralleling the fear of breast cancer among women taking estrogen; 2) fear of heart disease; and 3) the fact that testosterone is an anabolic hormone, meaning that it increases muscle mass. Testosterone has been abused by athletes, particularly in its more potent, synthetic forms, and is, therefore, a controlled drug. Women fear using it because of the possibility of androgenic side effects, such as hair growth. As we have shown, these side effects are usually reversible.

The evidence is that these fears are largely ungrounded.

TREATMENT WITH ANDROGENS

The issue of testosterone replacement and prostate cancer in men is similar to the issue of estrogen replacement and uterine cancer in women. Researchers have always been cautious about both because estrogen stimulates the proliferation of uterine (and breast) tissue, and testosterone stimulates the proliferation of prostate tissue. They have thought that decreasing testosterone levels in men who have swelling of the prostate decreases the size of the prostate and improves the flow of the urine. This would imply that giving testosterone would increase prostate problems, but in fact there is no evidence that replacing testosterone in younger or older men will either cause hyperplasia or aggravate a present condition.[27] Dr. Joel Hargrove of Vanderbilt University has been using progesterone successfully to treat benign prostatic hypertrophy (BPH). Progesterone reduces the number of receptor sites in the prostate just like it does in the uterus.

Dr. Norman Beals, Jr., says that inflammation of the prostate or benign prostatic hyperplasia (not equivalent terms), is mainly caused by lowered testosterone levels. But, unlike the rest of the body which tends to lose testosterone receptor sites as men age, the prostate tends to develop more. So large doses of testosterone may irritate this condition, even though the person needs the therapy. He suggests initially beginning with low doses of testosterone and gradually building the level up to allow the swelling to subside. Also, like Joel Hargrove, M.D., he recommends using natural progesterone (100 mg at bedtime) to counter the effects of testosterone on the prostate gland because progesterone reduces the number of testosterone receptors by competing for its sites.

Treatment for Prostate Swelling and Urinary Difficulties

Treatments have centered on inhibiting 5-alpha reductase, the enzyme responsible for the conversion of testosterone to dihydrotestosterone (the byproduct of testosterone that is considered to cause inflammation of the prostate).

There are drugs available to inhibit this enzyme: Finasteride and Terazosin (a blood-pressure-lowering drug). Both of these are only marginally effective and do not slow the progression of the disease. Surgery (called transurethral resection of the prostate, or TURP) is another option, but not without side effects, including perforation of the bladder, hemorrhage, infection, and incontinence. It is not always effective either.

Alan Gaby, M.D., suggests some other better-known alternative remedies for relieving BPH.[28] These include the use of saw palmetto berries (Latin name: serenoa), found in Florida and North Carolina and sold in Europe as Formixin. Saw palmetto berries have been used for nearly a century in treating urinary problems; they relieve BPH by blocking the 5-alpha reductase. According to Gaby, saw palmetto berries are more effective than drugs and produce no known side effects. The bark of the Pydgeum tree acts similarly to saw palmetto berry; it is anti-inflammatory, helps metabolize testosterone, and counters estrogen.

Dr. Gaby also recommends the essential fatty acids found in pumpkin seed oil, zinc, a small amount of copper, and extra vitamin E.

Men's Need for Testosterone

Dr. Beals says that men have three strikes against them as they get older:

1. They have less free (usable) and more bound (unusable) testosterone;
2. They have more sex-hormone binding globulin, which makes testosterone less available;
3. They have fewer receptor sites, except in the prostate gland (which, as we mentioned, creates problems).

He notes that, like estrogen therapy in women, testosterone may act as a catalyst and inflame existing hormonal cancer, but it doesn't cause it. This area of hormone replacement in men has now come into its own, and testosterone has been widely used for cardiovascular disease prevention (Dr. Jens Møller) and for birth control (the Japanese Menopausal Society).

Side Effects in Men

There are few or no side effects in mature men from physiologic or replacement doses of natural testosterone. Unfortunately, men are mainly treated with methyl testosterone, a synthetic. Methyl testosterone is known to have adverse effects on the liver.[29]

Methyl testosterone is also associated with mild weight gain, breast swelling (this is rare, mild, and needs no treatment), excessive oiliness of the skin, and acne. Other side effects can be the aggravation of already existing prostate disease including cancer, changes in lipid and carbohydrate metabolism (a good side effect), sleep apnea, increased red-blood-cell production (can be good or bad), and fibrinolysis (this has to do with clotting factors, and is a good side effect). However, all of these side effects have been questioned. HDL cholesterol levels may be slightly lowered in men on testosterone. It is not yet known whether the increase in red-blood-cell production that accompanies testosterone treatment will increase the risk of thrombosis or not. But testosterone treatment also increases the level of antithrombin III, a natural anticoagulant. This may counter the adverse effect on HDL level and the increased red blood cell problem by decreasing clotting ability.

Androgens do not cause malignancy, but they may promote the growth and intensify the pain of existing prostate and breast cancers in men.

Some doctors are concerned that giving testosterone may cause the testes to atrophy and sperm production to cease.[30] Dr. Beals says that this atrophy is not complete, and that it is reversible. It only occurs in proportion to the amount of hormone that is replaced. A similar effect occurs in women on the birth control pill or on hormone replacement therapy; their ovaries become temporarily smaller, but do not completely shut down. This also occurs with thyroid treatment; it shrinks the thyroid gland—in fact, that is one of the factors that originated the use of thyroid hormones for the treatment of goiter.

Testosterone Treatment in Men

Testosterone treatment has been used in men in the following ways:

- To initiate puberty in young boys with delay of development;

- To treat declining libido (loss of sex drive);
- To treat wasting conditions (such as in victims of Nazi concentration camps) and trauma, such as from battle injuries, burns, surgery, or radiation therapy;
- Formerly, as a treatment for anemia because testosterone increases red-blood-cell count;
- To treat depression and psychosis (from the 1930s to mid-1980s);
- To treat andropause, the male equivalent of menopause;
- As an adjunct to treatment with growth hormone in children who are growth-hormone-deficient;
- More recently, as a treatment for the weakness and muscle-wasting produced by HIV infection and full-blown AIDs;
- As a possible male contraceptive.

Testosterone Treatment in Women

Testosterone may be used in treating women who have low free testosterone levels for the following grouping of symptoms:

- Loss of libido (or lack of sexual enjoyment or orgasm);
- Headaches or migraines that do not respond to estrogen and progesterone by themselves;
- Muscle weakness, loss of strength, and loss of feeling of well-being;
- Low energy, irritability, forgetfulness, crying spells, and hot flashes that do not respond to estrogen alone;
- Loss of female aggressiveness in those who need it (business owners, lawyers);
- Osteoporosis.

   Side effects of testosterone treatment in women include acne and virilization (enlargement of the clitoris, deepening of the voice) or hirsutism (development of male body-hair pattern) in about 5 to 20 percent of patients.[31] This is apparently reversible, and may disappear by lowering the dose. Liver effects are unlikely at low doses, even with methyltestosterone. The adverse effect on lipids is, according to Ronald Young, M.D., insignificant.[32]

Different Protocols for Using Testosterone

Hormone experts recommend not using the higher doses of methyltestosterone for men. Doses for women are lower and may not be as damaging. But natural testosterone is available in tablets, gels, and creams from several compounding pharmacies and is probably a better choice for both sexes. Dr. Philip Warner says that the non-oral forms of natural testosterone are preferred—gels, sublingual tablets, pellets, or injections. These have greater absorption, produce more stable blood levels, and bypass the liver.

Some Protocols for Using Testosterone

Dr. Norman Beals suggests prescribing 0.25 to 1.0 cc injections of testosterone cyprionate (200 mg/cc) every two weeks. He suggests supplementing this with Yohimbe (an herbal sexual stimulant, also called Yocin) and ginseng. Yohimbe has some side effects in sensitive patients, for example palpitations and nervousness. It should be avoided by a person who has high blood pressure or heart arrhythmia. It is recommended for short-term use only. Yohimbe can also be used by women, with the same cautions, but it should not be used during pregnancy.

Dr. Beals recommends the use of natural progesterone to help block testosterone receptors in the prostate gland, help reduce inflammation, and clear the urinary passage. He says that some urologists prescribe Hytrin, a hypertensive drug that reduces internal swelling.

For women, Dr. Beals suggests using testosterone injections of 0.0625 to 0.25 cc (100 mg/cc) every two to four weeks. He says that oral testosterone is usually appropriate for women (0.625 mg to 2.5 mg of natural testosterone once or twice a day), because they don't need as much. Injections may only be necessary for women who have trouble with maintaining steady levels.

Dr. Jens Møller suggested using 200 to 300 mg of testosterone cyprionate or propionate every two to four weeks for men. Alternatively, he suggests applying one gram of testosterone gel twice a day (25 to 50 mg/g).

For women, he suggests applying one gram of testosterone gel twice a day (6 mg/g). He recommends monitoring the blood levels of testosterone because skin absorption varies. The dosage for oral tablets can be 1.25 mg twice a day or more; and it is wise to call specific compounding pharmacies for suitable doses for both sexes (see Appendix 2).

To counteract gangrene, Dr. Jens Møller suggests injections of 250 mg of testosterone three times a week. This would be a rare and unusual treatment, and needs to be monitored by an expert.

Dr. Denise Mark on Testosterone Therapy for Women   Dr. Denise Mark, having done repeated serum level tests over the years on her female patients, says that the first hormones to drop are commonly testosterone and progesterone. She believes that early screening and replacement of both hormones, when necessary, is critically important in a preventive approach to women's wellness.

Dr. Mark uses very small amounts of a soy-based natural testosterone to replenish a woman's levels—anywhere from 0.625 mg to 10 mg daily (Dr. Mark prefers low doses to start). She says that women taking testosterone notice increased libido, less fatigue, improved muscle strength, an overall sense of mental and physical well-being, an increase in mental clarity, and a more purposeful approach to getting things done.

Used locally on the urethra, testosterone can help prevent urinary incontinence in some women and significantly raises systemic testosterone levels. Testosterone may help increase bone density and improve bone mineralization when taken with calcium. It also helps the blood circulate, and builds muscle strength and endurance.

In relation to PMS, testosterone may relieve migraines, mood swings, and joint pain, and balance the effect of estrogen dominance.

Side effects Dr. Mark notes are: acne, body and facial hair growth, scalp hair thinning, and clitoral enlargement. Hypersexuality and aggressiveness are a possibility, but only at higher doses. At the physiologic doses Dr. Mark commonly uses, testosterone is a safe hormone, and she rarely sees any of these side effects.

Reasonable Hormone Blood Levels in Men

Normal testicles produce 7 to 10 mg of testosterone daily.

TOTAL TESTOSTERONE: an average level is 225 to 1,000 ng/dl. Ideal is about 700 to 1,000 ng/ml.

FREE TESTOSTERONE levels should be between 50 and 300 pg/ml. The ideal would be 140 to 300 pg/ml.

DIHYDROTESTOSTERONE levels should be 90 ng/100 ml; 25 ng/100 ml indicates weak activity.

ESTRADIOL reaches 20 pg/ml. ESTRONE levels vary between 40 and 60 pg/ml; a level of 80 pg/ml brings total lack of sexual interest.

Reasonable Testosterone Levels in Women

TOTAL TESTOSTERONE: a normal level should be 25 to 90 ng/ml. Ideal is 35 to 50 pg/ml.

Follow-Up Is Important

Patients need to be monitored carefully. In men, this includes regularly checking the size and condition of the prostate gland by rectal exam, studying urinary flow, and doing blood work to check markers of prostate disease. In women, increase in the size of the clitoris, deepening of the voice, and hirsutism need to be guarded against.

Testosterone treatment in men will often improve sexual function and prevent bone loss. Better studies are needed to confirm the beneficial effects of testosterone on bone and muscle mass, physical well-being, and psychosexual function.

The Use of DHEA

Dr. Denise Mark uses DHEA as part of a balanced replacement therapy at menopause and viropause (male menopause). She says that DHEA is an andrenal androgen reserve hormone, and it is one of the four major hormones that the ovary produces premenopausally. Prior to menopause, the ovary may produce 20 percent of the body's DHEA, and the adrenal gland 50 percent; the other 25 percent is produced by conversion in fat tissues.[33] After menopause, the adrenal gland takes over the bulk of the body's production.

Dr. Mark says that DHEA is a biomarker for aging. Low levels correlate with an increased risk of degenerative diseases, such as cardiovascular disease, arthritis, Alzheimer's, and possibly even cancer. In both sexes, as they age, DHEA levels may become suboptimal. When Dr. Mark gives DHEA replacement to her patients, she is trying to reproduce the levels found in a 20- to 30-year-old. She does blood tests and looks for diagnostic symptoms, such as fatigue, lack of mental clarity, loss of memory, mood swings, depression, recurrent infections, immune dysregulation, and arthritis. She also finds that DHEA increases muscle tone and skin tightness in women.

In using physiologic replacement levels, Dr. Mark finds few side effects, and these side effects are primarily androgenic, rather than estrogenic. She mentions mild acne and hair thinning, with some mild hirsutism that is reversible. These effects can occur even at normal serum levels, so patients need to be followed clinically.

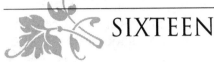

CHAPTER

SIXTEEN

NATURAL PROGESTERONE AND THE WORK OF DR. JOHN LEE

In recent years, John Lee, M.D., of Sebastopol, California, has contributed to our knowledge about hormones by bringing the issue of the use of natural progesterone before the medical world. He has emphasized the role of natural progesterone in reversing the effects of osteoporosis,[1] and he is not alone in seeing this connection.[2]

A side benefit of his emphasis has been that more and more people are thinking of natural progesterone as preferable to synthetic progestins such as Provera, Aygestin, Cycrin, and Norlutate for treating postmenopausal women on estrogen. Natural progesterone generally has a less depressing effect on the mind, and provides other health benefits as well. These emphases are a great step forward for women's health.

Interest Tickled by Mistletoe

Dr. Lee first became interested in progesterone 25 years ago, after reading two articles. One of them was about the Christmas custom of hanging mistletoe; the other was by a doctor who recalled a local gypsy lady who used European mistletoe berries as a morning-after pill to prevent pregnancy. The latter article pointed out that mistletoe berries contain high amounts of progesterone.

In 1978, Dr. Lee heard Ray Peat, Ph.D., lecture on the subject of natural progesterone derived from diosgenin, a hormone-like substance that is plentiful in wild yam root. Dr. Lee had observed in his medical practice that estrogen, calcium, and vitamin D therapy were not the complete answer for treating osteoporosis, and he became intrigued by the idea of using natural progesterone for this purpose.

Using Transdermal Progesterone Cream

Dr. Lee began trying transdermal (absorbed through the skin) cream containing natural progesterone on his female patients who were unable to take estrogen. He performed repeated bone density tests on each individual and found that these women not only did not lose bone, they actually gained it. When he tried his patients who were already taking estrogen on the cream, he found the same improvements with them.

Not only did their bones improve, but the progesterone treatment had other benefits. These women felt better, they had less breast swelling and tenderness, their low thyroid problems improved, their high blood pressure went down, and they had a return of normal libido. Younger women with PMS who used the cream also found relief. Best of all, there appeared to be no side effects.[3]

The details of Dr. Lee's work can be found in his book *Natural Progesterone: the multiple roles of a remarkable hormone.* Dr. Lee is also currently working on a book with Virginia Hopkins about natural progesterone, to be published in spring of 1996 by Time-Life-Warner. It is called *Hormone Balance and Natural Progesterone: What your doctor may not tell you about menopause.*

Not All Agree

Dr. Lee is a retired family physician who has based his ideas not only on his extensive reading but on the women he has treated in his practice. His published studies would be called "case studies," or "anecdotal," in the scholarly world. This means that he has gathered past and present data from his patients and compared the results, but the studies were not controlled.

While this is one way of doing a study, research scientists prefer double-blind controlled studies, wherein they take two groups—the study group and a control group—from the same type of population. The scientists gives one group the medication, and the control group a placebo, for a period of time. They make measurements and draw conclusions, then switch the groups and put them on the opposite treatment. This double-blind, controlled type of study is considered to be more objective than the other type, which can be influenced more easily by both physician and patient bias.

Research scientists would not be satisfied with the conclusions of Dr. Lee's anecdotal studies and will await the confirmation of more scientific studies yet to be done.

Down on Estrogen?

According to his books and lectures, Dr. Lee endorses the use of progesterone much more than the use of estrogen.[4] He feels that estrogen exacerbates PMS symptoms, increases cancer risk, worsens autoimmune disease, and so on. I disagree strongly with this position. This automatically makes estrogen undesirable as a treatment. As a result, many women who hear Dr. Lee lecture or read his books avoid using estrogen.

As I have mentioned before, there are other expert physicians who are more favorable toward the use of estrogen than progesterone (Elizabeth Lee Vliet, M.D., John Arpels, M.D., and John Studd, M.D., are examples). They believe that estrogen is more helpful than progesterone in treating PMS, osteoporosis, and mental depression, and they say that progesterone, whether natural or not, is more depressive. You will find their opinions covered in Chapter 11 on estrogen and depression.

Difference in Emphasis

If you talk to members of both groups, they each acknowledge a use for the other hormone. Dr. Lee would use estrogen for women with vaginal dryness and hot flashes, but he would probably only use it temporarily; he says that many postmenopausal women need only progesterone.

Drs. Elizabeth Lee Vliet and John Arpels both use natural progesterone in their practices. They understand well the differences between natural progesterone and synthetic progestin. But they have both seen that even natural progesterone makes some women depressed.

This difference in emphasis can be confusing for women who are looking for an absolute answer. Because of Dr. Lee's emphasis on progesterone, many women have stopped taking estrogen. This may not be a wise decision. Estrogen and progesterone are not the same hormone, and progesterone will not replace estrogen when it is needed. Dr. Lee acknowledges this in personal conversations, but unfortunately he does not make this clear in his writings and presentations.

Estrogen and Progesterone Types

As I have mentioned elsewhere, I find in practice that there are "estrogen" and "progesterone" types who may respond better to one or the other hormone (or a combination of both) for similar problems. The way a women reacts initially to a particular hormone (presuming that it's the best natural form she can take) is probably the way she will always respond to it. A trial will tell you what's best for you.

I learned this 20 years ago through my own experience. I read Dr. Katherina Dalton's books back then and tried natural progesterone in many forms and doses, but it never worked for me (though I have taken it for 20 years to protect my uterus). I had PMS, but estrogen always worked best for me. However, I have met many women who have had remarkable results from taking natural progesterone for PMS, and some women who actually feel better on progesterone than on estrogen after hysterectomy or menopause.

Because of this, I appreciate both hormones equally. I like the statement of Don Gambrell, M.D.: God made both hormones, and he knew what he was doing. Also, David Zava, Ph.D., a biochemist who is an expert on hormone receptors, says that estrogen and progesterone are like day and night. One is more excitatory, the other more calming. But both are needed, and neither one will replace the other.

When you read research in any area, the more you dig, the more deeply you find experts disagree. They even sometimes use the same facts to prove opposing positions. Breast cancer research is a great example of this; you may find some consensus, but you also find absolutely opposite conclusions.

As I have mentioned elsewhere, don't let the disagreements between scholars upset you. People want simple answers. They want a universal panacea. But people are individual, the body is complex, and the issues are not always simple. It's often not an issue of either/or, but an issue of both/and. If you need estrogen, no amount of progesterone will replace it, in my opinion.

You won't be disappointed if you accept these differences and try to find the solution that works for you.

Love Him or Hate Him

Because Dr. Lee takes a strong stand for natural progesterone, he has both worshippers and detractors. I particularly appreciate him for playing a major role in bringing the issue of natural progesterone to the national attention of menopause experts. This needed to be done, and Dr. Lee has certainly gotten their attention. I also appreciate Dr. Lee's concern about women's health care. However, I do have reservations because many women hearing him have concluded they do not need estrogen, and this has created real problems for some when they stop taking it.

Some of the issues that others question Dr. Lee about, apart from his making progesterone the primary hormone, are: seeing estrogen dominance as a causative factor in cancer, autoimmune disease, PMS, and other problems; giving the impression that women can almost always do without estrogen after menopause; and making statements to the effect that estrogen has no direct effect on the brain, and that thyroid problems are rare and that progesterone will cure most thyroid problems. Some feel that he is overreacting against the past emphasis on estrogen within the medical community and say that he is going too far.

Sources of Transdermal Cream

A number of pharmacists (see list in Appendix 2) will provide compounding of standardized transdermal natural progesterone creams and gels, which are available by prescription only. I encourage you to discuss with your physician whether you might benefit from progesterone and talk with the staff at these compounding pharmacies.

A nonprescription product, Pro-Gest® cream, is also available (again, see Appendix 2). This cream contains progesterone that has been converted from diosgenin, which is derived from wild yams. Another source used in progesterone creams is stigmasterol from soy beans. Progesterone must first be chemically synthesized in the laboratory from these plant products and then put in the cream. This is because the body doesn't convert the yam or soy bean precursors into progesterone on its own.

Pro-Gest® Matches Your Own Progesterone

According to Dr. John Lee, Pro-Gest® contains an exact match of the progesterone manufactured in your ovaries. If you use about 1/4 tsp for 21 days a month, Dr. Lee believes that you will achieve blood levels of progesterone consistent with low luteal phase levels (about 2 to 10 ng/ml).

As with most forms of progesterone treatment (whether oral or topical), absorption will vary tremendously with the individual. Dr. Lee says that Pro-Gest®, as he suggests using it, is sufficient to make the necessary changes in the lining of the uterus, maintain bone density, and help prevent menopausal symptoms, in the presence of adequate estrogen. However, this has not been studied under a controlled situation. More research must be done on transdermal progesterone cream and its effect on the uterine lining before we can say this for sure. At present, Dr. Elizabeth Lee Vliet and I are participating in a double-blind controlled study using Pro-Gest® cream to see whether Dr. Lee's assertion can be verified.

Most scientific studies assessing the amount of natural progesterone needed to make changes in the endometrium have used the oral micronized form administered at 100 mg, two to three times a day. This dose is about ten times higher than that provided by transdermal application. When micronized progesterone is taken in other ways (swallowed, or used vaginally or anally), a majority of it is destroyed in the gastrointestinal tract and during the first pass to the liver.

As with other hormones, natural progesterone is more effectively absorbed transdermally; this route has the same advantages as hormones given by injection or pellet, sublingually or vaginally. These methods allow the hormone to go straight into the bloodstream, without the alteration, interference, or changes that occur when hormones are taken orally.[5]

Creams Are Not All the Same

It is important to note that not all progesterone creams on the market claiming to have natural progesterone in them really do. David Zava, Ph.D., of Aeron/Lifecycles, Inc., has been monitoring the progesterone content of a number of wild yam creams claiming to contain progesterone or the progesterone precursor diosgenin. He finds a remarkable variation in the amount of progesterone actually contained in these commercially available creams; sometimes there is none.

The creams can be categorized in three groups: 1) those that contain high levels of progesterone (about 450 mg/oz); 2) those that contain only trace levels of progesterone (at least 100 times less than the first group); and 3) those that contain no progesterone at all, but very high levels of the yam-derived progesterone precursor, diosgenin. If a cream in category three has any hormonal effect in the body, it would probably be estrogenic, according to Dr. Zava.

Many of the so-called "progesterone" creams on the market have no direct progestational effect in the body. The body is very inefficient in converting diosgenin to progesterone, because diosgenin does not bind to progesterone receptors in the body. The progesterone has to be converted first in the laboratory, and then put in the cream or it won't work. Women who buy wild yam creams without converted progesterone in them will be short-changed.

According to Dr. Zava, this is also true of some DHEA creams made from diosgenin. The fact that these creams contain yam extract does not mean that the body will convert it to DHEA.

Home Hormone Test Kit Available

Aeron/Lifecycles, Inc., has developed a saliva test that you can perform at home to check your progesterone levels. Saliva progesterone levels are lower than in blood serum, but more accurately reflect the biologically active levels of free progesterone (not bound by protein, and therefore usable) available to target cells in the body.

One advantage of this test is that it is noninvasive. The saliva can be collected in your home and sent directly to the laboratory for testing. Another advantage is that you are not dependent on a physician to obtain this information.

Aeron/Lifecycles has also developed other tests to detect saliva levels of testosterone, DHEA, cortisol, and estradiol, as well as plant and synthetic estrogens and progestins.

Who Might Benefit   This test will be useful for:
- Anyone, on or off hormones, wanting to know her hormonal status;
- Women taking herbs, who wish to know if they are getting increased levels of phytoestrogens or phytoprogesterones ("phyto" means coming from a plant source) in their body;
- Women using the transdermal creams or prescription hormones, wanting to know whether they are absorbing them;
- Women with luteal-phase defects, wanting to know if they have ovulated;
- Women taking the birth control pill or Provera, wanting to find out their progestin and progesterone levels (since tak-

ing synthetic progestin tends to suppress the body's own progesterone production);

• Checking a woman's testosterone levels if her sex drive is low (testosterone deficiency is a reality for many women as early as their thirties).

To purchase the Aeron/Lifecycles Saliva Test Kit, contact Transitions for Health at 1-800-888-6814. For more information about other saliva-testing products, contact Aeron/ Lifecycles, at 1-510-729-0375.

Progesterone Is Not a Panacea

My own experience, as I have mentioned elsewhere, is that natural progesterone is not a panacea for everyone. I am one of the women who didn't do well on any type of progesterone in the twenty years before my hysterectomy. I did try using Pro-Gest®, and I could tolerate it better than the oral form of natural progesterone, but I still had side effects. Dr. Elizabeth Lee Vliet says that she has about twenty patients in her practice who have become depressed from using progesterone transdermal creams.

The Uterine Lining

Because the effects of transdermal progesterone cream on the uterus are not yet adequately studied, you may choose to take higher prescription doses of micronized progesterone, as suggested in Dr. Don Gambrell's study or the PEPI study,[6] until thorough research supports Dr. Lee's viewpoint. The former study suggests taking 300 mg per day of oral micronized progesterone, taken in a divided dose of 100 mg in the morning and 200 mg in the evening for 13 days per cycle. The PEPI study used 100 mg twice a day.

An occasional vaginal ultrasound examination to check the thickness of the uterine lining would be a sensible safeguard. And many physicians would want you to have endometrial biopsies, repeated every one or two years, to make sure that the desired changes in the lining are being made.

CHAPTER

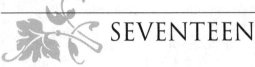

SEVENTEEN

THE OPTIMUM DIET FOR HORMONAL PROBLEMS

 Diet is very important for women with hormonal problems, because the cells in the body are dependent on nutrition for good health and function. Poor diet may be largely responsible for an existing hormonal problem and certainly makes symptoms worse. Changes in diet make a considerable contribution to treatment for some women, particularly those with mild problems who have been on a poor diet for years.

On the other hand, severe hormonal problems probably won't respond to diet alone. The problems we describe in this book are endocrine disorders—chronic medical problems that require that a patient cross the line between natural and hormonal treatment. A good comparison is the treatment for diabetes. At certain stages, and with different types of diabetes, dietary change may be all that is needed to handle the disease. But at some point, with severe diabetes, the patient will need insulin in order to survive.

Women with hormonal problems may not actually die from their symptoms (though they might want to), but the analogy is good. There comes a point at which diet and supplements are still important for general health, but not adequate as treatment.

Excellent Nutritional Guides for PMS and Menopause

Dr. Susan Lark has written two outstanding books, *The PMS Self-Help Book* and *The Menopause Self-Help Book*. Dr. Lark is not only a physician, but she loves to cook. Her books are very practical and informative and contain many recipes with step-by-step instructions for good nutrition, plus information on supplements, herbs, and relaxation exercises that will eliminate or improve many women's symptoms.

Supplements and Diet Not Always Effective

In her practice in the Bay Area, Dr. Lark treats PMS with natural remedies, and rarely uses hormones. I am sympathetic with this approach and feel that it is effective for some women. But if a woman meets with no success after trying natural remedies, she should not feel that she has failed. The next step may be hormone replacement therapy; if she needs hormones, she should not be afraid to take them.

I have seen many women who are on a good diet, who take the right herbs and supplements, and who are on a good exercise program. Yet these measures have made little improvement in their hormonal problems. At my worst with PMS, I was eating an unprocessed vegan diet, taking herbs, and running five miles a day over a period of years, all of which did nothing to relieve my PMS. Admittedly, the women I see are extreme cases, but changes in lifestyle are not enough for them.

Diet Is Important for General Health

The incidence of all chronic diseases, such as heart disease, hypertension, diabetes, and cancer, is much higher in Western countries. Many studies have shown that, when people in other countries with a simpler, more natural diet emigrate to the U.S., within a couple of generations they begin to develop the diseases of the West. Breast and other cancers, heart disease, stroke, and osteoporosis have been strongly linked to a high-fat, high-protein diet, eaten in early childhood and the teen years. Diet in the adult years is also important, but the growing years are more important, and, unfortunately, what we ate in childhood was largely beyond our control.

The Best Type of Diet

What is the best diet for hormonal health? It's the best diet for your general health.

The consensus of 16 world committees on nutrition is that we should be largely vegetarian, using natural, unprocessed foods: whole grains; peas, beans, and lentils, all of which are naturally high in vitamins B and E; and fruits and vegetables, which are rich in vitamins C and A. Though some vegetables need cooking because their starch is indigestible, raw food should comprise a large part of the diet. Foods high in animal protein, animal fat, other fats, salt, or sugar should be seen as concentrates and used sparingly.

Asian women who consume traditional, high-soy diets and drink green tea (which is known to be anticarcinogenic), have lower rates of osteoporosis and breast cancer and fewer menopausal symptoms than women in Western countries. It is believed that genestein, a phytoestrogen (plant estrogen) is responsible for this.[1]

Recent Chinese Study

The China Diet Study began gathering information on the lifestyles of 65,000 Chinese adults, living in 65 countries, in 1983. This ten-year study is now completed. It is the most comprehensive study ever done on the diet of Chinese people.

Highlights of this 920-page study[2] show that:

1. Obesity has more to do with which kind of food one eats than with how many calories one consumes. Chinese natives consume 20 percent more calories than Americans

do, but Americans are 25 percent heavier. This is because the Chinese eat three times the amount of starch and only a third the amount of fat that Americans eat. This is a more important factor than exercise.

2. Cholesterol levels in China are much lower than in America. The Chinese average is 127 mg percent, compared to 212 mg percent in the U.S.

3. For every heart attack in China there are 16 in the U.S.

4. Protein intake in China is one-third less than in America (64 grams per person per day, compared to 100 grams).

5. Female cancers relate to diet. A childhood diet high in protein, fat, calcium, and calories promotes rapid growth and early onset of menstruation. This increases a woman's risk for developing cancer of the reproductive organs and the breast. Chinese women rarely get these cancers, and they begin to menstruate three to six years later than American women.

6. Osteoporosis is rarely found in China, though Chinese women eat only half the calcium that American women eat. Most Chinese eat no dairy products at all and obtain their calcium from plant foods.

7. The Chinese diet is three times richer in fiber than the American diet, resulting in relatively low rates of colon cancer in China.

8. Iron-deficiency anemia is rare in China, though their diet is mainly plant food, and they rarely eat meat.

Dr. T. Colin Campbell says that these findings will challenge our traditional beliefs about protein, calcium, weight control, ideal cholesterol levels, dietary fiber, and vitamin requirements.

Beware of Fads

There have always been fad diets, just as there are fads in medical treatment. For instance, Adelle Davis wrote interesting and influential books on diet in the 1960s. Some of the theoretical material was excellent, and many people still swear by it. Her books make many good points, and they recommend eating lots of fruits, vegetables, and unrefined grains. But the diet Davis recommended was extremely high in animal protein and fat. These are the very food items that lead to Western diseases—heart disease, cancer, osteoporosis, diabetes, diverticulosis, and hemorrhoids.

The Error of the Four Food Groups To show the power of a fad, consider how nutritionists swore by the "four food groups" as a standard of good nutrition for many years. Two out of four food groups were animal products—meat and milk—giving the impression that a person's diet should be 50 percent animal products.

Nutritionists have changed the "four food groups" theory because they now know that eating a lot of animal products leads to heart disease and other Western diseases. Now they use the illustration of a pyramid.

Meat	Milk and Eggs
Grains	Fruits and Vegetables

The base of the pyramid is carbohydrates, because, worldwide, more nations eat more grains than fruits and vegetables. Meat and dairy products have been put at the top of the pyramid. This illustration shows more clearly that animal products are concentrated and should be a relatively small portion of the diet.

I like to reverse the triangle and put fruits and vegetables above carbohydrates. The graphic then shows that people should eat lots of fruits and vegetables, then carbohydrates, then legumes, then concentrates such as meat and animal products, other high-protein and fat foods, sugars, and salt, in descending amounts.

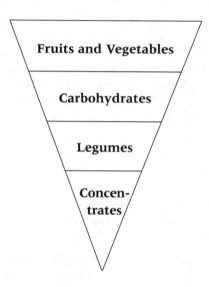

High Protein Diets are Another Fad   Emphasizing the need for protein has led many people to consume far too much of it, and because most high-protein foods are also high-fat foods, they eat too much fat. A lot of protein, especially from animal sources, is extremely difficult for the body to digest. The process of excreting proteins puts a heavy load on the kidneys, because so much more water is needed to excrete protein than other nutrients. Along with the loss of fluid, there is a loss of bone minerals, which are leached out into the urine. This process then brings on early calcium loss and eventually paves the way for osteoporosis.

Meat, milk, and cheese are often recommended as good sources of calcium. Though they have much higher levels of calcium than nuts and vegetables, the high protein and fat in these products inhibits the absorption of calcium. Therefore, it is better to get calcium and other minerals, such as magnesium and potassium, directly from fresh fruits and vegetables.

Vegetarian Fads   Vegetarians who avoid all the problems of meat can run into other problems with fads. For instance, it is easy to eat even more fat if you eat a lot of eggs, milk, cream, nuts, and avocados, and use refined or cold-pressed cooking oils.

When I first became a vegetarian in Australia, I attended cooking schools that taught people to cook appealing meat substitutes, such as "gluten steaks" (made from the gluten in wheat flour). These gluten products, such as gluten mince or gluten steak, could be made to taste delicious.

In reality, gluten is a very poor protein made from white flour. It contains fewer vitamins and minerals than white flour. Since it has no fiber, if people eat it day after day as a meat substitute, they are asking for trouble. Those who eat gluten regularly have been shown to have a higher incidence of bowel cancer.

Read the Package Labels   Other canned meat substitutes were made from soybeans and widely recommended as a nutritional breakthrough. You could buy chicken-like, beef-like, and turkey-like products. Since Australians eat a lot of meat, some people just substituted these gluten and soy products and ate them three times a day.

If you read the nutritional information on many of these products, you would be surprised at the chemical additives used to make them palatable. People who regularly eat these products have a higher incidence of pancreatic cancer.

Many vegetarians, thinking they are being smart in avoiding meat, would be better off eating a little meat, rather than these synthetic meat substitutes with their chemical additives.

Common Sense Can Help You Avoid Fads   The few illustrations given show how diet fads, which are popular for decades, can be dead wrong. Rather than promote good health, they do the opposite and leave a trail of disease. How can you test each theory or fad and know quickly whether a dietary suggestion is good?

1. **Eat simple, wholesome food**—natural foods prepared in as natural a way as possible.

2. **Avoid processed foods as much as possible**—fats, grains, and processed sugars. Simple sugars, such as cane sugar, raise the levels of the blood fats (triglycerides) and increase cholesterol levels.

3. **Be particularly careful of fat intake,** whether processed or not. Fat is fat, whether it's saturated or unsaturated.

4. **Use high-fat, high-sugar, and high-protein foods** as concentrates only, sparingly, in the diet. Consider meat as a condiment—a flavoring agent.

5. **Avoid or restrict anything else detrimental to health,** such as alcohol, caffeine, and tobacco. All of these substances increase glycogen levels in the liver and tend to cause blood sugar fluctuations. Caffeine also increases the level of free fatty acids, which accelerates the development of heart disease and diabetes.

6. **Find out which foods suit your digestion.** Avoid foods that you are allergic to when possible.

7. **Drink about eight glasses of water a day.** People who eat a lot of fruit may not need as much water. Note that the intake of huge quantities of water can be dangerous.

8. **Try to eat high-quality food from good sources** calmly, joyfully, and gratefully.

A Handy Diet Summary

As far as the type of food is concerned, eat:

Fruits and vegetables
ABUNDANTLY

Whole grains and cereals
MODERATELY

Beans, peas, and lentils
OFTEN

Fats and concentrates
SPARINGLY

As far as quantity is concerned:

Eat like a KING for breakfast

Eat like a PRINCE at lunch time

Eat like a PAUPER at supper

Much of the food eaten after 5:00 P.M. is likely to be stored as fat. For women with functional low blood sugar, it may be better to eat smaller meals, including some carbohydrate, every three or four hours.

What Are Concentrates?

Concentrates are foods that are high in either protein, fat, or sugar. Concentrates include meat, butter, milk, cheese, salt, cream, cooking oil, margarine, nuts, sugar, candy, jams, honey, and yeast powder.

Nuts, avocados, and olives contain high fat levels. While this type of fat is not as saturated as that in animal products, it is still a concentrate and should be eaten sparingly. Avoid nuts that have been cooked in oil. It is best to eat small quantities of freshly shelled nuts.

PUBLIC ENEMY #1: REFINED AND SATURATED FATS

Because of the affluence of the Western world and the invention of refrigeration, fat intake has increased dramatically this century. Only a very little fat in the diet is actually necessary for life. The body produces most of the fat it needs by metabolizing carbohydrates and sugars.

When thyroid or estrogen levels are low, cholesterol levels tend to increase. This is a major reason why women with hormonal problems need to be concerned about their intake of fats.

The Essential Fat

The only essential fatty acid that the body cannot make without a dietary source is linoleic acid (and arachidonic acid, but this is synthesized from linoleic acid in the body). The requirement for this fatty acid is small, and it is easily obtained from a starch-centered diet (for instance, there is enough linoleic acid in three tablespoons of oatmeal to meet a day's need). There is very little of this essential fatty acid in animal products.

Therefore, most of the fat we consume is nutritionally unnecessary. We eat fat because it makes things taste good and satisfies hunger for a longer period of time. The main problem with fat is that it clogs the arteries.

Different Types of Fat in Your Diet

Generally, dietary fat can be divided into two groups: naturally occurring fats found in food, and refined or processed fats that have been altered by humans. Both can create problems, but the refined fats are particularly problematic.

Naturally occurring animal and vegetable fats all contain saturated, polyunsaturated, and monounsaturated fats in varying proportions.

Saturated fats are typically solid at room temperature. Sources of saturated fats are animal products, such as beef, pork, and dairy products. Chocolate, coconut, and palm oil are the only common plant sources that are rich in saturated fats. Saturated fats increase cholesterol levels.

Polyunsaturated fats tend to be fluid at room temperature, and are found in high concentrations in vegetables, fish, and poultry. Polyunsaturates do not increase cholesterol levels directly in the body. They do, however, raise the LDLs. While all fats become rancid, polyunsaturated fats go rancid faster. In the body, they break down into free radicals, which are cells that tend to go berserk, metaphorically throwing a monkey wrench in the works.

Monounsaturated fats are in a liquid form. These are found in olives, peanuts, olive oil, and canola oil (the best oils to use if unprocessed).

It's the Proportion That Varies   Both animal and plant foods contain saturated, polyunsaturated, and monounsaturated fats, but the proportions are different.

Meat and animal products contain mostly saturated fats, some polyunsaturated fats, and very few monounsaturated fats. They also contain cholesterol, a waxy, fatty alcohol always found in association with other fat cells in the human body.

Plants contain mostly polyunsaturated fats, fewer saturated fats, and some monounsaturated fats. Palm oil, coconut (both the fleshy part and the oil), and chocolate contain plant fats with a high proportion of saturated fat. Olive, canola, and peanut oil are especially high in monounsaturated fats. Plant foods contain no cholesterol.

Fish contains mostly polyunsaturated fats; otherwise, fish would solidify in cold water. But fish contains as much or more cholesterol as meat.

Refined Fats, Also Called Hydrogenated Fats   These are made by chemically adding hydrogen to vegetable oils—for instance, in making margarine. The hydrogenation process converts the oils into more saturated fats, which are solid at room temperature.

Margarine has been touted for years as being better than butter in the prevention of heart disease because of its "polyunsaturated" fats, but the process of hydrogenization makes the advisability of using these fats very questionable. Such refined fats do not contain cholesterol, but they increase heart disease by raising the LDLs and triglycerides and decreasing the HDLs. To understand this, we need to understand how the body handles the digestion of fats.

Cholesterol and Triglycerides

To determine the amount of fat in your body, a physician will test the amount of cholesterol, triglycerides, and high, low, and very low density lipids (HDLs, LDLs, VLDLs) in your blood.

Cholesterol is a waxy, fatty, alcohol found in conjunction with fatty acids in the body. It is necessary for life and is produced in various places throughout the body, particularly the liver. Therefore, it is not necessary to eat any added cholesterol. Eating large quantities of animal products causes the cholesterol level to rise. The higher the levels of cholesterol, the more likely a person will be to have fatty plaques on the inside of their arteries and the more likely they are to have a heart attack from blockage of the heart vessels, or a stroke from narrowing of the blood vessels in the brain.

A normal cholesterol level for women is 200 mg percent or less, though closer to 150 mg percent is better. Levels below 130 mg percent aren't necessarily good either, but this depends on the diet; 130 is about the average level for native Chinese. Very low levels of cholesterol can interfere with the liver's ability to regulate and convert hormones.

Triglycerides are fatty acids (saturated, polyunsaturated, and monounsaturated fats) that are formed in the body by the breakdown of simple sugars and complex carbohydrates. Simple carbohydrates and sugars raise the level of triglycerides higher than complex carbohydrates do.

Triglyceride levels are part of the overall profile of fats in your body and are frequently elevated in people with heart disease and diabetes.

HDLs, LDLs, and **VLDLs** are different types of cholesterol found in different types of fat cells in the body. "HDLs" stands for "high-density lipids," the "good" cholesterol (called alpha globules); "LDLs" stands for "low-density lipids," the "bad" cholesterol (small beta globules); and "VLDLs" stands for "very low-density lipids," the "worst" cholesterol (large beta globules).

The more high-density lipids or alpha globules of fat you have the better, because they act like a broom in the bloodstream and sweep out excess cholesterol, keeping the blood vessels from becoming clogged. By contrast, the beta globules—LDLs and, particularly, VLDLs—inhibit the effects of HDLs and so encourage the clogging effect of cholesterol. When you have your cholesterol level checked, it's better to have a high HDL level than a low LDL level.

In most cases, except in certain people with genetically high cholesterol levels, the type of fat you eat in your diet has a lot to do with your cholesterol levels. But this is a general rule. Hormone status is also linked with cholesterol levels. When estrogen production drops at mid-life, levels of HDLs also tend to drop and LDL levels rise. Changing cholesterol levels in the thirties and forties, without dietary changes, may indicate a drop in estrogen production. Hypothyroidism is similarly associated with high cholesterol levels.

Summary on Fats

Some fats are definitely worse for us than others, but it is best to concentrate on decreasing overall fat intake. All fats, including cold-pressed vegetable oils, promote the growth of cancers in animals, and there is a definite link between breast cancer and intake of fat.

Meat eaters should cut down on their fat intake. But vegetarians should not think that because they don't eat meat, they can eat large quantities of hard cheese, cream, butter, milk, eggs, salad dressings, margarine, and cooking oils.

On the other hand, don't be too extreme. Some women who go on an extremely low-fat diet start to age rapidly. Because estrogen is produced in the fat cells, a non-fat diet can cause estrogen deficiency, which shows up as wrinkled skin, dull hair, and premature aging. Eat some freshly shelled nuts and avocados.

Refrigeration and Milling
Have Made the Difference

Keep in mind that today we are plagued with diseases hardly known before this century. Massive coronary heart disease, diabetes, and other Western diseases were not the plagues of earlier generations. They have come only with the processing of foods, particularly grains, and the ability to refrigerate fats. Toward the end of the nineteenth century, white flour became a universal product because of the invention of the millstone. With refrigeration, it became possible to store animal fats for long periods of time, and so they became a much bigger part of the average person's diet.

PUBLIC ENEMY #2:
REFINED OR PROCESSED FOODS

As whole grains are processed, the outer bran on the seed is discarded. With it goes most of the nutrients necessary for digestion. Most of the fiber is also removed, and fiber is necessary for rapid transit of food through the digestive tract. For both these reasons, refined foods put a heavy burden on the digestive system and, eventually, cause a breakdown in health.

In countries such as Africa, where people eat a native diet of unprocessed plant foods, diseases caused by lack of fiber in the diet (bowel cancer, diverticulitis, hemorrhoids, and varicose veins) are virtually unknown.

People who eat unrefined, whole grains can handle fat in the diet better, too, because the fiber in whole grains helps sweep the fat out of the system.

It is best to buy the grain yourself and grind it as you need it. Like milk, grains will become rancid soon after grinding and should be refrigerated and used quickly. Bread without preservatives, flour, porridge, wheat germ, and bran will quickly go rancid on store shelves. That's why preservatives are often used.

Refined grains include white flour, white rice, white sugar, tapioca, corn flour, gluten flour, pearl barley, white spaghetti, and all forms of white flour pasta. They all lack fiber and nutrients.

Grains Are Good for Premenstrual Blood Sugar Problems

By contrast, a variety of whole grains is very helpful for women with hormonal problems. Eating some starchy food every three to four hours in the premenstrual week helps maintain a steady level of blood sugar. Since women have functionally low blood sugar premenstrually, eating frequent small meals with some carbohydrate or starchy food can make a tremendous improvement. This practice can prevent violent emotional outbursts, low blood sugar headaches, and the unexpected crying jags that come when a woman has not eaten for several hours. It doesn't require a huge meal; you can divide your meals and eat more frequently. All it takes is eating a couple of crackers, or half a slice of bread, or some potato, or oat biscuits, and so on.

Dr. Katherina Dalton has been an expert witness in several murder trials involving women with severe PMS. She says that, in all cases, these women had not eaten for several hours prior to losing control. She finds that, if women whose blood sugar levels are erratic do not eat regularly during the week before their period, their blood sugar level can drop precipitously and it may take a week to be able to maintain it again.

Grains Contain Magnesium

The element magnesium is especially important in the production of hormones and helps regulate the menstrual cycle. Animal products are especially high in calcium in proportion to magnesium, and this high calcium-to-magnesium ratio tends to interfere with the absorption of magnesium.

Dr. Guy Abraham's research showed that women who live in countries where calcium levels are high in proportion to magnesium (i.e., they eat a lot of animal products) are more likely to have PMS. For instance, Ethiopian women who consume large amounts of animal products have a greater incidence of PMS. Japanese women, by contrast, have a low incidence.

Grains are a great source of magnesium and their magnesium-to-calcium ratio is superior to that in animal products. Millet, for instance, has eight parts of magnesium to one part of calcium. Other grains have at least two parts of magnesium to one part of calcium.

PUBLIC ENEMY #3: REFINED SUGARS

Many symptoms of PMS and other hormonal problems are caused or aggravated by functionally low blood sugar levels. Women with PMS typically have strong food cravings for sugar, starches, chocolate, candy, caffeine, and alcohol, all of which raise the blood sugar level. One might suppose that a high sugar intake would help the problem. Instead, these substances cause the blood sugar levels to drop rapidly soon after eating, and this actually worsens the problem.

There are many types of sugar in nature that are good for you under normal conditions. For instance, fruit is full of a sugar called fructose. But sucrose (refined white sugar) is a concentrate that, if overused, can deplete your mineral supply, depress your immune system, and create havoc with your blood sugar levels. By easily satisfying the appetite but giving you only empty calories, sugar displaces more nutritious foods. Because sugar is bereft of nutrients to help in its digestion, your body has to call on the store of minerals in your bones and teeth. Thus, it contributes to tooth decay and osteoporosis. Because of its high content of calories, eating too much sugar contributes to a weight problem. Refined sugar is converted into triglycerides (fatty acids), and these levels may become elevated.

When you eat sugar, your blood sugar is swiftly elevated, which may make you feel temporarily more energetic. However, the effect is brief, and soon the blood sugar level slumps again. Complex carbohydrates (grains and starches) maintain the blood sugar level better than simple carbohydrates (sucrose). Grains also contain fiber and nutrients that contribute to their digestion, whereas simple sugars don't.

Honey and raw sugar may not be much better than white sugar, as they have only trace nutrients in them. All concentrated sugars should be used sparingly.

PUBLIC ENEMY #4: SALT

Many other symptoms of PMS—seizures, closed-angle glaucoma, varicose veins and hemorrhoid flare-up caused by premenstrual constipation, and emotional changes caused by swelling of the brain—are caused by water retention, rather than by low blood sugar levels. Overuse of salt contributes to hormonal disorders by worsening bloating. Salt also raises blood pressure.

The adrenal hormone aldosterone regulates water retention and controls the sodium/potassium ratio. Premenstrually, this regulator often goes awry. Sodium is absorbed into the cell walls and attracts fluid, causing water retention.

Most vegetables and grains contain sodium, so adding salt to the diet is not generally necessary for nutrition. A little added salt may make food more palatable, and may also be necessary for people who are physically active in hot weather. But you should beware of cooking with too much salt and adding it at the table.

Hidden Sugar, Fat, and Salt

Packaged and processed foods often contain high levels of hidden sugar, fat, and salt to make them tastier. It is a good habit to read food labels. Many packaged foods list white or enriched flour (white flour plus a few vitamins) or sugar as the first ingredient. Many others have high levels of added salt (sodium) or oils.

SUMMARY

Make fruits, vegetables, whole grains, and legumes the staples of your diet. Use fats, sweets, or salty foods as concentrates only—treats to be eaten occasionally. With daily, vigorous exercise, your health should flourish. In most cases, you will lose weight, your blood pressure will drop, and you will feel better.

But remember, if you have severe hormonal problems because of a genetic inheritance or as a result of hormonal interference or surgery, you may find that changing your diet is not enough to relieve your symptoms.

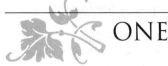

ONE

TREATING PHYSICIANS

**Dr. Denise Mark, M.D.,
Internal Medicine**
San Francisco Preventive Medical
Group
345 West Portal Avenue
San Francisco, CA 94127
415-566-1000

Denise Mark, M.D., is an internal
medicine specialist, trained in the
practice of complementary or natural medicine. Her approach focuses on using nutritional
medicine and provides preventive
care. As part of her practice, she
specializes in natural hormone balancing for women and men, PMS,
perimenopause, menopause, and
andropause. She utilizes the full
range of natural hormones, including estrogens, tri-estrogens, phytoestrogens (plant estrogens),
micronized natural progesterone,
testosterone, DHEA, and natural
thyroid.

**Kathryn Morris, M.D., Family
Practice**
Hormone Balancing for Women
5905 Soquel Drive #300
Soquel, CA 95073
408-464-7777

Kathryn Morris, M.D., is a graduate of Stanford University Medical
School and board-certified in family practice. She is the medical director of Hormone Balancing for
Women, located in Soquel, California. She and her practitioners
are dedicated to the fine-tuning of
hormone programs for women.
They favor the use of natural hormones and emphasize the importance of individualizing the doses
for each woman. Telephone appointments are available for
women who live out of the area.

Ramon Scruggs, M.D.
New Hope Health Partners
1831 Orange Avenue #A
Costa Mesa, CA 92627
714-646-1252.

Dr. Scruggs practices alternative
medicine in Costa Mesa, California, and uses hormone therapy.

Elizabeth Lee Vliet, M.D.
HER Place
1990 Miraval Cuarto
P. O. Box 64507
Tucson, AZ 85718
520-797-9131

413

Also: HER Place at All Saints
1400 8th Avenue
Fort Worth, TX 76132
817-922-7470

Elizabeth Lee Vliet, M.D., is a
Clinical Associate Professor in the
Department of Family and
Community Medicine at the
University of Arizona College of
Medicine in Tucson, Arizona. She
founded and directs HER Place:
the Women's Center for Health
Enhancement and Renewal. This
is a multidisciplinary, wellness/pre-
ventive medicine program located
in Tucson, Arizona and HER Place
at All Saints Health System, Fort
Worth, Texas. Dr. Lee Vliet checks
for the overlooked hormonal connections in many facets of
women's health. These include
PMS, perimenopause and
menopause, menstrual migraines,
depression, anxiety, fibromyalgia,
and chronic fatigue. Since her
background is in both internal
medicine and psychiatry/behav-
ioral medicine, she has long studied the ways in which changing
ovarian hormone levels trigger
changes in physical, emotional,
psychological, and pain-related
symptoms. She approaches these
problems by checking women's
ovarian hormone levels and thyroid function. Then she seeks to
identify the underlying medical
causes of women's symptoms before turning to treatment options
with antidepressant and anti-anxiety medications. Telephone appointments are available out of the
Tucson office.

**Phillip O. Warner, M.D.,
OB/GYN**
The Menopause Institute of
Northern California
700 West Parr Ave., Suite D.
Los Gatos, CA 95030
408-370-1833

Dr. Warner is an OB/GYN with
many years of experience. He
trained under Robert Greenblatt,
M.D., to do pellet implants (estrogen and testosterone), particularly, but not solely, for women
after hysterectomy and oophorectomy (uterus and ovaries removed). Dr. Warner uses natural
estrogens and progesterone.

Philip Weaver, M.D., OB/GYN
Center for Women's Health
840 Hay #321-95
North Lenoir City, TN 37772
615-988 6358

I worked for twelve years with
Dr. Weaver, and he is experienced
in all types of female hormone replacement. Dr. Weaver does not
do telephone consultation.

**Richard Wilkinson, M.D.,
Family Practice**
302 S. 12th Ave.
Yakima, WA 98902

Dr. Wilkinson has an allergy clinic
in Yakima, and he and his brother,
Randall Wilkinson, M.D., also
help people with chronic fatigue
syndrome (CFIDs) and multiple
chemical sensitivities (MCS). Dr.
Wilkinson is also familiar with
hormone replacement therapy.
Dr. Wilkinson does not do telephone consultation.

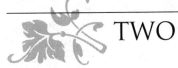

TWO

SOURCES FOR NATURAL HORMONES AND SALIVA TESTING

To purchase the Aeron/ Lifecycles Saliva Test Kit, contact Transitions for Health at 1-800-888-6814. For more information about other saliva-testing products, contact Aeron/Lifecycles at 510-729-0375.

By Prescription Only
Bajamar Women's HealthCare
9609 Dielman Rock Island
St. Louis, MO 63132
1-800-255-8025
(In Missouri: 314-997-3414)

Bajamar Women's HealthCare is devoted exclusively to compounding natural hormone products. These include progesterone, DHEA, estradiol, estrone, estriol, tri-estrogens, pregnenolone, and testosterone. The hormones can be compounded singly or in combination in various forms: sublingual tablets, capsules, oral tablets, suppositories, gels, creams, ointments, or suspensions, at the lowest price in the nation.

Belmar Pharmacy
12860 West Cedar Dr., #210
Lakewood, CO 80228
1-800-525-9473
(in Colorado: 303-763-5533)

Belmar Pharmacy is a quality compounding pharmacy that makes natural hormonal formulations. These include estradiol, natural progesterone, and others. Belmar also compounds a long-acting T3 supplement (T3 is so active that it usually has to be taken in low doses two to three times a day). Belmar specializes in tablets that are swallowed but, like other compounding pharmacies, they can make up any formulation the doctor requires.

College Pharmacy
833 N. Tejon Street
Colorado Springs, CO 80903
1-800-888-9358
(in Colorado: 719-634-4861)

College Pharmacy of Colorado Springs, Colorado is an excellent source for natural hormonal therapies. Their staff is extremely knowledgeable about hormone replacement therapy and are more than willing to answer questions you or your doctor may have. College Pharmacy is unique in that it can prepare virtually any dosage form your doctor may prescribe, including hard-to-find pellet implants. For more information, they can be reached Monday to Friday, 7:30 A.M. to 6:00 P.M. (mountain time).

Health Pharmacies
319 West Beltline Hwy. #112
Fitchburg, WI 53713
1-800-373-6704

HomeLink Pharmacy
2650 Elm Ave., Suite 104
Long Beach, CA 90806
1-800-272-4767
(in Long Beach: 310-988-0260)

Madison Pharmacy Associates
429 Gammon Place
P. O. Box 9641
Madison, WI 53715
Pharmacy: 1-800-558-7046;
PMS Information Access:
1-800-222-4PMS

Marla Ahlgrimm, R.Ph., is a pioneer in compounding natural progesterone options for women. Madison Pharmacy Associates has over 15 years' experience in compounding natural progesterone and other hormones, including DHEA, estriol, and testosterone. In addition to the Women's Health Access newsletter, Madison Pharmacy provides a Women's Health America Infolog of reputable resources nationwide and has an excellent catalog, available upon inquiry. They are also a good resource for vitamins tailored to the needs of women with PMS and menopause.

Professional Village Pharmacy
1701 Professional Drive
Sacramento, CA 95825
916-483-3455

Rite-Price Pharmacy
23653 El Toro Road
El Toro, CA 92630
714-586-7780

Women's International Pharmacy
5708 Monona Drive
Madison, WI 53716-3152
1-800-279-5708
(in Wisconsin: 608-221-7800)

Women's International Pharmacy is the largest compounding pharmacy in the country that specializes in natural hormone prescriptions. They make a variety of hormones in many different bases.

Nonprescription Sources
Pro-Gest® Body Cream
Professional and Technical Services, Inc.
5200 SW Macadam Ave., Suite 420
Portland, OR 97201

Call Professional and Technical Services/Transitions for Health, at 1-800-888-6814 to order Pro-Gest® or to receive a free catalog of natural healthcare products for women. This company also carries the Aeron/Lifecycles Home-Kit for testing salivary hormone levels.

Ray Peat, Ph.D.
P. O. Box 5764
Eugene, OR 97405
503-345-9855

Dr. Peat, a pioneer in the use of natural progesterone, has written a number of books about health, including *Nutrition for Women, Generative Tissue,* and *Mind and Tissue* (these three are $10.00 each), and *Progesterone in Orthomolecular Medicine* ($5.00).

Dr. Peat also compounds a progesterone oil and cream. He invites you to call for consultations or products.

APPENDIX

THREE

AUTOIMMUNE LINKS WITH THE ENDOCRINE SYSTEM

Hashimoto's Thyroiditis— a Central Hub

Hashimoto's thyroiditis is often linked to other coexisting auto-immune diseases.[1] Dr. Boris Catz of Beverly Hills, California, has listed these associations and separates them into two different groups: endocrine and nonendocrine autoimmune dysfunctions.[2]

The first group involves those disease in which autoantibodies attack the endocrine glands (thyroid, parathyroid, adrenals, pancreas, ovaries, pituitary, etc.).

The second group affect other nonendocrine organs or systems (including collagen diseases like lupus).

Sometimes the division is not completely clear, and there may be a mixture of both. But autoimmune thyroid problems are a common denominator of both groups. The extensive footnotes in this section are included to show that these links are a reality.

Local Versus Systemic

Autoimmune disorders can also be divided into those that are local (specific to a particular organ or tissue) and those that are systemic and nonspecific (the autoimmune process is not confined to any single organ).[3]

Schmidt syndrome is an example of a systemic autoimmune syndrome in which antibodies attack and destroy several endocrine glands at the same time. In Schmidt syndrome, you have simultaneous infiltration of the thyroid and adrenal glands, and sometimes other glands too.

Endocrine-Related Autoimmune Diseases

The following is a list of autoimmune diseases that affect particular endocrine glands. Some of them can occur singly (local) or in multiples (systemic). The footnotes after each problem listed cite research articles making a common link with thyroid dysfunction.

- Polyglandular Syndromes (in which more than one endocrine gland is affected by a systemic autoimmune disease; for more information, see the PAS section in Chapter 3);[4]
- Insulin-dependent diabetes (Type 1);[5]
- Addison's disease and Schmidt syndrome;[6]
- Addison's anemia;[7]
- Autoimmune ovarian failure;[8]
- Hypophysitis (swollen pituitary);[9]
- Hypoparathyroidism (the four parathyroid glands are located within the thyroid);[10]
- Graves' disease (autoimmune hyperthyroidism);[11]
- Progressive ophthalmopathy (bug-eyes).[12]

Non-endocrine-related Autoimmune Diseases

The following autoimmune diseases are linked with non-endocrine tissues:

- Lupus erythematosus;[13]
- Multiple sclerosis;[14]
- Myasthenia gravis;[15]
- Rheumatoid arthritis;[16]
- Sjøgren's syndrome, also called sicca syndrome (disease of the salivary glands and dry eyes);[17]
- Pernicious anemia;[18]
- Atrophic gastritis;[19]
- Chronic active hepatitis;[20]
- Primary biliary cirrhosis;[21]

- Malabsorption syndrome (coeliac disease);[22]
- Vitiligo (white patches on the skin);[23]
- Alopecia areata, alopecia universalis (bald patches);[24]
- Chronic mucocutaneous moniliasis or candidiasis (yeast);[25]
- Others (scleroderma, Wegener's disease, thrombocytopenic purpura, Feltys syndrome, etc.).[26]

Watching for Simultaneous Effects of Autoimmune Disease

Since some individuals have systemic problems wherein more than one endocrine gland may fail, it is important to recognize these syndromes in clinical practice. A physician needs to be alert to the possibility of a second major endocrine organ failure after one has been diagnosed. Hall and others caution physicians to watch for the development of other further autoimmune problems in these patients. They especially mention insulin-dependent diabetes mellitus, and suggest that thyroid and adrenal antibodies should be checked in all patients with this type of diabetes.

The Link Between Autoimmune Disease and Early Menopause

Autoimmune diseases have been linked with premature ovarian

failure.[27] Dr. Richard Bronson said that a third of women going through menopause before the age of 40 have autoimmune disease, including Hashimoto's and Graves' diseases.[28] This not only means early infertility for those who may still wish to have a child, but early perimenopause and menopause symptoms.[29]

A study by Mignot and Schoemaker and others discusses this phenomenon:

> In a study of 24 women with signs of early menopause (high LH and FSH), all the women were checked for the presence of autoantibodies. These women had significant levels of autoantibodies (92 percent had signs of autosensitization) for various diseases, but, at that time, premature ovarian failure was the only sign of the problem. Sixty-seven percent of the women studied were positive for non-organ-specific autoantibodies, and 50 percent were positive for organ-specific auto antibodies.[30]

Note that a woman does not have to have autoantibodies to the ovary itself. If an autoimmune dysfunction is going on elsewhere in the body, the ovaries can be affected even before the autoimmune disease is apparent.

While not many women, comparatively speaking, actually go through menopause before age 40 because of the autoimmune problems described above, I have wondered whether many women have partial ovarian failure because of autoimmune activity. This may be one reason why some women's ovaries begin to decline in their mid-thirties to forties, causing perimenopausal symptoms long before menstruation actually stops.

GLOSSARY

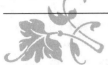

ACTH: abbreviation for adreno-corticotropic hormone, a hormone secreted by the anterior lobe of the pituitary gland which stimulates the growth and function of the adrenal cortex.

Addison's disease: chronic underfunctioning of the adrenal cortex, characterized by weakness, loss of body hair, and increased skin pigmentation.

Adrenal glands: two small ductless glands, situated one above each kidney. They produce a variety of hormones involved in immunity, sodium-potassium balance, sexuality, and the control of stress.

Adrenaline/epinephrine: adrenal hormone which acts to stimulate the heart, dilate the blood vessels, and relax bronchial smooth muscles.

Adrenergic: relating to nerve cells or fibers of the autonomic nervous system that use norepinephrine.

Adrenocorticotropic hormone: See ACTH.

Affect, Affective: the external expression of emotion attached to ideas or mental representations of objects. The influence of emotions.

Aldosterone: the main mineralocorticoid hormone produced in the adrenal cortex, regulating electrolyte and water balance by promoting the retention of sodium and the excretion of potassium.

Allergy: heightened sensitivity to any substance that is harmless to others in similar amounts.

Alopecia: absence of hair from skin areas where normally present.

Amenorrhea: absence of menstrual periods.

Anabolism: the process by which nutrients are built up into the living organism. Opposite of catabolism.

Androgens: hormones that produce male or masculine characteristics. Present in both men and women, but in greater quantity in men.

Anorexia: loss of appetite.

Anorexia nervosa: an eating disorder that leads to excessive loss of weight, bone loss, absence of menses, etc. Also described as a personality disorder manifested by extreme aversion to food, usually occurring in young women, resulting in life-threatening weight loss. Often considered a hysterical illness, through which medium the patient is seeking control of some aspect of her life. At times can resemble or precede a psychosis. Some brain neurotransmitter abnormalities have been noted. Absence of menstruation often occurs before the weight loss.

Antidepressant: drug that alters brain neurotransmitters and stimulates physiological activity, thereby tending to alleviate depression.

Antithyroglobulin and antimicrosomal antibody test: test for thyroiditis which measures the level of these antibodies against the level of thyroid.

APICH syndrome: a polyendocrine immune system dysfunction affecting more than one endocrine gland. Allergies, candida, and respiratory symptoms may accompany it.

Armour Thyroid: an animal thyroid preparation designed by Dr. Broda Barnes and preferred by many alternative physicians since it contains all the components produced by the human thyroid gland.

Atrophic gastritis: autoimmune condition causing inflammation of the stomach.

Autoantibodies: antibodies formed in response to a threatening factor in one's own tissues.

Autoimmunity: the condition in which one's own tissues are subject to adverse effects of the immune system.

Autism: a tendency to total self-absorption at the expense of the regulation of outward reality.

Biliary cirrhosis: autoimmune liver disease linked with nausea.

Bromocriptine (brand name Parlodel): treatment to reduce pituitary tumors and swelling.

Bulimia: grossly increased appetite, marked by gorging, and often associated with purging with laxatives or self-inducement to vomit. Often alternates with periods of anorexia.

Catabolism: the breaking down in the body of complex chemical compounds into simpler ones, often accompanied by the liberation of energy. The opposite of anabolism.

Candida, candidiasis: yeast-like fungi that are part of the normal flora of the mouth, skin, intestinal tract, and vagina, but which can cause a variety of infections if they grow out of control.

Catecholamines: components of the hormonal system which arouse rather than calm (opposite of endorphins).

Celiac disease: autoimmune malabsorption syndrome; gluten intolerance.

Cholesterol: a fat-like steroid alcohol found in animal fats. A large part of most gallstones, it occurs in plaques in the arteries, in various cysts, and in cancerous tissue.

Clomiphene (brand name Clomid): a nonsteroidal estrogen analog used as the citrate salt to stimulate ovulation. A treatment for infertility.

Corpus luteum: yellow patch which is the remnant of the egg that passes from the ovary into the fallopian tubes at ovulation. Manufactures progesterone and some estrogen in the luteal phase (second half of the cycle).

Corticosteroids: any of the steroids made in the adrenal cortex (or synthetic equivalents) divided, according to their biologic activity, into two major groups, glucocorticoids which are chiefly involved in carbohydrate, fat, and protein metabolism, and mineralocorticoids, involved in the regulation of electrolyte and water balance. They are used clinically for hormone replacement therapy, as anti-inflammatory agents, and to suppress the immune response.

Cortisol: the major natural glucocorticoid made by the adrenal cortex. (Hydrocortisone is the form used in treatment).

Cortisone: a steroid isolated from the adrenal cortex, but not in significant amounts. Largely active in humans until converted to hydrocortisone (cortisol).

CRF: abbreviation for corticotropin-releasing factor, the hypothalamic releasing hormone that goes to the pituitary to produce ACTH.

C-section: Cesarean section. Surgical delivery of a baby by cutting through the abdominal wall into the uterus.

Cytomel: brand name for triiodothyronine, T3, an active thyroid medication. Used in psychiatry to potentiate (see potentiate) antidepressants in people who don't respond to the antidepressant on its own.

Danazol (brand name for danocrine): an anterior pituitary suppressant used for treating endometriosis.

D & C (dilettation et curettage): surgery to dilate the cervix and remove the outer endometrial lining of the uterus.

Depo-Provera: intramuscular injection of medroxyprogesterone. Used as a form of long-term (3 months) birth control. Also used, at times, for bleeding problems.

DHEA or DHA, Dehydroepiandrosterone: an adrenal androgen occurring in normal human urine and synthesized from cholesterol.

Diosgenin: a steroid derived from plants such as the wild yam to yield progesterone and DHEA.

Diuretics: substances stimulating the discharge of urine.

Dopamine: a monoamine formed in the body by the decarboxylation of dopa. It is an intermediate product in the synthesis of norepinephrine and acts as a neurotransmitter in the central nervous system.

Encephalopathy: any degenerative brain disease.

Endocrine system: a system composed of ductless glands that release hormones directly into the blood or lymph and that exert powerful influences on growth, sexual development, metabolism, etc.

Endogenous: produced within or caused by factors within the organism.

Endorphins: a group of endogenous polypeptide brain substances that bind to opiate receptors in various areas of the brain and thereby raise the pain threshold.

Endometriosis: the abnormal occurrence of tissue, which more or less perfectly resembles the endometrium (lining of the uterus), in various locations in the pelvic cavity and elsewhere.

Estrace (brand name for micronized estradiol): Estradiol is the main human estrogen. This product is derived from soya beans and yams. See micronized.

Estrogen: female hormone produced by the ovaries during the reproductive years, responsible for female sexual characteristics.

Estrovis: a synthetic estrogen, quinestrol, broken down by the body into ethinyl estradiol.

Estropipate: estrone, a form of estrogen, manufactured under the name of Ogen. Estrone is a weaker estrogen than estradiol, but they convert back and forth into each other as they travel through the body.

Euthyroid: this describes normal thyroid function.

Fallopian tubes: the tubes opening near the ovary and extending down to the uterus as a conduit for sperm to the egg.

FDA (Food and Drug Administration): government agency that regulates foods and medication.

Fibroids: masses of tissue that grow independent of surrounding tissue and have no positive physiological function. Usually benign, but can turn malignant under certain conditions. A common cause for heavy bleeding in women.

Fibromyalgia: muscle pain.

Fiornal: medication for severe headaches. Contains butalbital, aspirin, and caffeine.

FSH (follicle-stimulating hormone): a pituitary-stimulating hormone that travels to the ovary, calls eggs to the surface of the ovary, stimulates them to produce estrogen, "chooses," and matures the egg destined to be evicted from the ovary at ovulation.

FSH-LHRH (follicle-stimulating and luteinizing-hormone releasing hormone): the hypothalamic releasing hormone that travels to the pituitary and causes the production of FSH and LH.

Galactorrhea: excessive, spontaneous, inappropriate milk flow from the breast.

Gamma globulin: component of blood serum that contains various antibodies used to treat some infectious diseases.

Glucagon: a polypeptide hormone secreted by the alpha cells of the islets of Langerhans (see islets of Langerhans) in response to hypoglycemia.

Glucocorticoid: any of the group of corticosteroids predominantly involved in carbohydrate, fat, and protein metabolism (they also have many other functions). The most important glucocorticoids in humans are cortisol (hydrocortisone) and cortisone.

Goiter: enlargement of the thyroid gland.

Gonads: female or male sex glands; ovaries or testicles.

Gonadotrop(h)ic hormone, gonadotropin: substances that stimulate the gonads (sex organs) and are secreted by the anterior pituitary gland. (FSH, LH)

Graafian follicles: any of the follicles in the ovary that contain a maturing ovum or egg.

Granulomatosis: formation of multiple nodules occuring with ulcerated infections.

Graves' Disease: autoimmune hyperthyroidism; a condition in which the body produces autoantibodies against the pituitary hormone, TSH, which in turn overstimulates the thyroid gland.

Gynecologist: physician specializing in the care and treatment of women and their diseases, especially of the reproductive system.

HMO: Health Management Organization; these provide managed health care for groups.

Hashimoto's thyroiditis: inflammation of the thyroid gland, called lymphocytic thyroiditis. Named after the Japanese surgeon who discovered it.

Hirsutism: excess body hair.

Hormone: a chemical messenger substance produced in the body, and having a specific regulatory effect on the activity of certain cells or organs.

HRT: hormone replacement therapy, for men or women needing hormones.

Hyperadenosis: enlargement of glands.

Hyperplasia: excessive production of cells resulting in enlargement of tissue or of an organ.

Hyperprolactinemia: excessive production of prolactin.

Hypertension: high blood pressure.

Hypoglycemia: low blood sugar. Abnormally small amount of glucose in the blood, which can lead to insulin shock.

Hypophysitis: swollen pituitary gland. Common when other circulating hormone levels are low (e.g., thyroid and sex hormones).

Hypotension: low blood pressure.

Hypothalamus: region of the brain below the thalamus, which, with the pituitary, regulates internal organs.

Hysterectomy: surgical removal of the uterus.

Idiopathic: self-originated. Occurring without known cause.

Imipramine hydrochloride: an antidepressant. Estrogen is sometimes used to potentiate Imipramine in women with depression.

Incontinence: inability to control excretory functions.

Insulin: protein hormone made by the islets of Langerhans in the pancreas. It checks the accumulation of glucose in the blood and promotes the utilization of sugar in the treatment of diabetes.

Islets or Islands of Langerhans: irregular masses of small cells located in the intestinal tissue of the pancreas that secrete insulin.

Lability: emotional instability, mood swings.

Laminectomy: surgery on the spine involving the excision of the posterior arch of a vertebra.

Laparoscopy: a surgery wherein a small lighted scope is inserted through the navel to explore the abdominal cavity.

Levothyroxine (brand name Synthroid): thyroid replacement medication (T4).

Limbic: relating to the edge or fringe of a part. The limbic brain refers to the part of the brain that controls emotion, mood, and pain management.

Lithium: a salt used in the treatment of manic-depression psychosis.

Locus ceruleus: melanin-pigmented neuronal cell bodies with norepinephrine-containing axons located under the floor of the brain ventricle.

L-tryptophan: an essential dietary amino acid (precursor of protein), which is converted in the brain into serotonin.

Lumpectomy: removal of a lump, either benign or malignant, from the breast. This procedure is usually preferable to having a mastectomy, which is the removal of the breast itself.

Lupus erythematosus: see systemic lupus erythematosus.

Lupron: a synthetic analog of naturally occurring gonadotropin-releasing hormone (GnRH or

LHRH). Used in injectable form to chemically induce menopause in women with endometriosis or in women with PMS, to see if hysterectomy is likely to help the problem.

Luteinizing hormone (LH): a hormone secreted by the anterior lobe of the pituitary gland, which stimulates a Graafian follicle to release an ovum or egg during each menstrual cycle (ovulation), and converts the follicle into the corpus luteum.

Mammogram: X-ray of the breast to screen for cancer.

Mania: an emotional disorder characterized by great psychomotor activity (excitement and exaltation) but also unstable attention. Characterized by insomnia, pacing the floor, garrulousness (overtalkativeness), supercreativity, violence, etc.

Mastectomy: removal of the breast, usually unnecessary as a primary cancer treatment.

Melancholia: mental sluggishness and depression.

Melatonin: formed by the pineal gland during the hours of darkness, while sleeping. Involved in the aging process. Low levels affect the mechanism of ovulation, causing it to occur days earlier in women with PMS. Its affects are not all understood yet. Taking melatonin may help restore sleep patterns and relieve jet lag.

Menarche: occurrence of the first menstrual period.

Menopause: cessation of menstruation usually considered due to depletion of a woman's supply of eggs. However, there appears to be a separate brain-related trigger for menopause which marks the end of a woman's ability to reproduce.

Menstrual cycle: a woman's monthly reproductive cycle, with stimulation of ovarian follicular growth and ovulation, corresponding hormone production and resultant thickening of the uterine lining, with shedding of this lining as a menstrual period if pregnancy does not occur.

Micronized: to reduce substances to particles that are only a few microns in diameter.

Mineralocorticoids: a class of adrenal hormones involved in the regulation of electrolyte and water balance (aldosterone).

Mitral valve: the membrane between the left atrium and left ventricle of the heart that prevents the backflow of blood into the atrium.

Mononucleosis: infectious disease caused by an excess of mononuclear leukocytes in the blood. Also called glandular fever.

Mucocutaneous candidiasis: candida present with mucous membrane and skin, especially the line of junction of the two at the vaginal and anal orifice.

Multiple sclerosis: an autoimmune degenerative disease of the nervous system.

Myasthenia gravis: an autoimmune disorder of neuromuscular function, causing involuntary weakening of the muscles.

Myomectomy: a surgery in which the fibroid is shelled out or removed from the uterus. A possible alternative to hysterectomy.

Nardil: a monoamine oxidase inhibitor, a class of antidepressant that carries food restrictions (cheese, alcohol, anything that contains tyrosine).

Neoplasia: the process resulting in the formation and growth of a neoplasm (abnormal tumor growth).

Neuron: a nerve cell that conducts nervous impulses from one part of the brain to another.

Neurotransmitter: a chemical that transmits messages between nerve cells in the brain, and between brain and tissues and organs in the body.

Norepinephrine: a catecholamine and a principal neurotransmitter, released from the adrenal medulla in response to hypotension (low blood pressure).

Norlutate: an androgenic progestin (synthetic progesterone-like substance), used sometimes in place of Provera.

OB/GYN: physician specialty. OB = obstetrician, dealing with the care of the pregnant woman and her delivery. GYN = gynecologist, dealing with the treatment of diseases of the female sexual parts.

Ogen: brand name for a natural estrogen, Estropipate.

Osteoporosis: reduction in bone mass and increase in interior space, porosity, and fragility of bone.

Ovaries: female reproductive glands that produce eggs and female sex hormones.

Pancreas: a large gland, situated behind the stomach, that contains the islets of Langerhans which produce insulin and glucagon. It secretes pancreatic juice via small ducts to the duodenum (the first part of the intestine).

Paranoia: a personality disorder in which the individual is extraordinarily sensitive to praise or criticism and subject to suspicions and feelings of persecution.

Parathyroid glands: four small endocrine glands near or embedded within the thyroid gland, usually two per side, that regulate blood calcium and phosphorus levels.

Perimenopause: the period of time before and during menopause.

Periodontal disease: gum disease.

Pernicious anemia: blood disease caused by lack of vitamin B_{12}.

Pituitary gland: small endocrine gland situated at the base of the brain. Secretes vital hormones governing vital body functions such as growth and metabolism.

Placebo: an inactive substance of no medical value, given to humor a patient or as a test in controlled experiments on the effects of drugs.

Polycystic ovaries: characterized by numerous cysts (closed cavity—normal or abnormal—usually containing liquid or semisolid material).

Polyendocrinopathy: a condition in which more than one endocrine gland is involved.

Postpartum depression: mood depression which may follow giving birth.

Potentiate: substances used to enhance or increase the potency of other drugs (in this book, antidepressants).

Premenstrual syndrome (PMS): physical and psychological/ emotional symptoms associated with the post-ovulatory (luteal) phase of the menstrual cycle. Usually followed by a time entirely free of symptoms.

Premarin: conjugated equine estrogens, collected from pregnant mares' urine.

Pro-Gest®: cream containing natural progesterone. Use has been made prominent by John Lee, M.D., who uses it for treating PMS and osteoporosis.

Progesterone: a hormone produced by the ovary after ovulation takes place. Progesterone prepares the endometrial lining for implantation and pregnancy. It fills the lining with starch and protein to feed the early embryo. Progesterone is the pregnancy hormone, and largely maintains pregnancy in the first 7–12 weeks. At term, it reaches levels 300 times those present during the normal luteal phase.

Progestin: synthetic hormone with progesterone-like effects. Used for a variety of problems, including birth control, bleeding disorders, amenorrhea (lack of periods), and as a part of hormone replacement therapy, along with estrogen. Not the same as natural progesterone, and tends to depress the mood.

Prolactin: pituitary hormone that stimulates milk production and also suppresses ovarian function in the early postpartum days. Also has hormone-regulating functions during the menstrual cycle.

Prostaglandin: any of a group of naturally-occurring hydroxy fatty acids that stimulate contractility of the uterus and other smooth muscles. They have the ability to lower blood pressure, regulate acid secretion of the stomach, regulate temperature and platelet aggregation, and control inflammation and vascular permeability. They also affect the action of certain hormones.

Provera: a synthetic progestin, medroxyprogesterone, used to treat a variety of disorders (see progestin), and commonly used as part of hormone replacement therapy along with Premarin.

Prozac: the brand name of fluoxetine, an antidepressant belonging to the serotonin re-uptake inhibitor class (SSRI). Works by making more serotonin available.

Pruritis: intense itching (often used about itching in the vaginal/anal tissues).

Pseudoprolactinoma: swelling of tissue in the pituitary gland, creating a false impression of the presence of a prolactin-producing tumor. Also see hypophysitis.

Psychopharmacology: use of drugs to treat abnormal mental states.

Psychophysiology: study of the interaction between mental and physical factors.

Psychotropic: affecting the mind. Used to describe mind-altering drugs.

Puberty: the time period during which a person reaches sexual maturity and becomes functionally capable of reproduction.

Puerperal psychosis: a morbid condition sometimes associated with childbirth.

Ribonucleic acid (RNA): a nucleic acid, a constituent of all living cells.

Rheumatoid arthritis: autoimmune arthritis marked by inflammation, degeneration, or metabolic derangement of the connecting tissue structures.

Sarcoidosis: a systemic autoimmune disease of unknown cause, especially involving the lungs with fibrosis, but also involving lymph nodes, skin, liver, spleen, eyes, phalangeal bones, and parotid glands with granulomas.

Schmidt syndrome: autoimmune polyglandular disease combining Addison's disease (low adrenal function) with thyroiditis. May lead to other associated autoimmune dysfunction, such as early ovarian failure.

Serotonin: a brain neurotransmitter with calming effects.

Serotonin syndrome: a condition in which a person's system has too much serotonin, leading to anxiety and other severe symptoms. Sometimes caused by use of Prozac and similar drugs.

Sjøgren's syndrome: a disease of the salivary glands and eyes. Also called sicca (dry) syndrome.

Spironolactone (brand name Aldactone): a progesterone-like diuretic that balances aldosterone. Helpful for treating the bloating and water-retention of PMS. Also used in higher doses to treat acne and hirsutism (hairiness)

Steroid: any of a group of organic compounds occurring naturally (can also be produced synthetically). These include the sex hormones, the bile acids, oral contraceptives, and many drugs.

Stigmasterol: derived from soya beans to produce progesterone (similar to diosgenin in yams).

Synapse: the membrane-to-membrane contact of one nerve cell with another.

Synarel: a gonadotropin-releasing hormone analog in the form of a nasal spray, used to put women into chemical menopause. Like Lupron, Synarel is often used to treat endometriosis. It is also used to treat severe PMS to see if hysterectomy would be likely to bring relief.

Synthroid (brand name for L-thyroxine, T4): main form of synthetic thyroid. Usually prescribed for hypothyroidism and preferred by physicians and pharmacists because of its dose-reliability and many available dosages. A good match for human thyroid.

Systemic lupus erythematosus: a chronic generalized collagen (connective tissue) autoimmune disease that attacks multiple organs. Symptoms include skin eruptions, joint pains, arthritis, and anemia.

Tamoxifen: a drug that acts as an antiestrogen in the breast tissue. Used in the treatment and prevention of breast cancer. Has some estrogen effects in other parts of the body, including the uterus. Linked with increased incidence of endometrial cancer.

Testes, testicles: male gonads or reproductive glands that produce spermatozoa and male sex hormones. Located in the scrotum, the sac behind the penis.

Thrombosis: the formation or presence of a blood clot.

Thymus: gland-like lymphoid tissue located near the base of the neck. Believed to play a role in the body's immunological responses. Large in infants, but gradually gets smaller as its cells migrate to the rest of the body becoming T-cells.

Thyroid: endocrine gland located at the neck just below the larynx, extending around the front and to either side of the trachea (windpipe) and secreting the hormones thyroxine (T4), and triiodothyronine (T3), both vital to growth and metabolism.

TRH: thyroid-releasing hormone, produced in the hypothalamus.

TSH: thyroid-stimulating hormone, also called thyrotropin, produced in the pituitary gland. It travels to the thyroid gland and stimulates the production of the thyroid hormones.

Tubal ligation: also called tubal sterilization. Involves the tying of the Fallopian tubes as a means of birth-control. There are different methods. Early methods involved cutting, tying, and burning the tubes, and women who had this done typically experienced hormone disturbances. More recent methods, including microsurgery and clipping the tubes, are less likely to cause problems.

Urethritis: inflammation of the urethra, the tube that carries urine out of the body.

Vaginitis: inflammation of the vaginal tissues, due to bacterial infection.

Vitiligo: autoimmune disease wherein depigmented white patches of skin occur.

Westhroid: animal thyroid preparation from New Zealand.

Xanax: a tranquilizer often used to treat premenstrual syndrome and panic attacks.

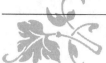

Progesterone and Premenstrual Syndrome

Carpenter, Moira, *Curing PMT the Drug-Free Way.* Arrow Books, 1986. Not available in the U.S. The British address is Arrow Books Limited, 62–65 Chandos Place, London WC2N 4NW, England. It offers her-bal and home-opathic remedies and information about diet and acupressure.

Dalton, Katherina, M.D., *Once a Month,* 5th ed. Hunter House, 1994.

Dalton, Katherina, M.D., *Premenstrual Syndrome and Progesterone Therapy.* Year-Book Publications, 1984.

Harrison, Michelle, M.D., *Self-Help for Premenstrual Syndrome.* Random House, NY, 1982.

Lark, Susan, M.D., *PMS: Premenstrual Syndrome Self-Help Book.* Celestial Arts, Berkeley, 1984.

Lauersen, Nils M.D., and Eileen Stukane, *PMS: Premenstrual Syndrome and You.* Simon & Schuster, 1983.

Lee, John, M.D., with Virginia Hopkins, *Hormone Balance and Natural Progesterone: What your doctor may not tell you about menopause,* Warner Books, 1995.

Lee, John, M.D., *Natural Progesterone: The multiple roles of a remarkable hormone.* BLL Publishing, 1994. P. O. Box 2068, Sebastopol, CA 95473 ($9.95, plus $2.00 postage).

Norris, Ronald, M.D., with Colleen Sullivan, *PMS: Premenstrual Syndrome.* Rawson Associates, Berkeley Edition, 1984.

Menopause, Hysterectomy, and Women's Health

Barbach, Lonnie, Ph.D., *Positive Approaches to Menopause—The Pause.* Penguin Books, 1994.

Cabot, Sandra, M.D., *Smart Medicine for Menopause.* Avery Press, New York, 1995.

Cobb, Janine O'Leary, ed. *A Friend Indeed* (a newsletter for women going through menopause), available from P. O. Box 1710, Champlain, New York 12919-1710. Price $30.00; ten issues a year.

Cone, Faye Kitchener, *Making Sense of Menopause.* Simon & Schuster, New York, 1993.

Cutler, Winnifred B., Ph.D., *Hysterectomy, Before and After.* Harper & Row, New York, 1988.

Cutler, Winnifred B., Ph.D., and Celso-Ramón Garcia, *Menopause: A Guide for Women and the Men Who Love Them* (Revised Edition). W. W. Norton & Co., Inc., New York and London, 1992.

Gaby, Alan, M.D., *Preventing and Reversing Osteoporosis.* Prima Publishing, California, 1994.

Gladstar, Rosemary, *Herbal Healing for Women.* Simon & Schuster, 1993.

Greenwood, Sadja, M.D., *Menopause Naturally*, Volcano Press, 1989.

Ito, Dee, *Without Estrogen: Natural Remedies for Menopause and Beyond.* Carol Southern Books, New York, 1994.

Jacobowitz, RS, *150 Most-Asked Questions About Menopause.* Hearst Books, New York, 1993.

Jacobowitz, RS, *150 Most-Asked Questions About Osteoporosis.* Hearst Books, New York, 1994.

Lark, Susan, M.D., *Menopause Self-Help Book.* Celestial Arts, Berkeley, 1990.

Lark, Susan, M.D., *The Estrogen Decision.* Westchester Publishing Co., Los Altos, California, 1994.

Nachtigall, Lila, M.D., and Joan Rattner Heilman, *Estrogen.* The Body Press, 1986.

Sevener, C. Alan, M.D., *It's Okay to Take Estrogen: In fact, estrogen may be your best friend for life!* Eclectic Publishing, Inc., P. O. Box 28340, Fresno, California 93729-8340. (209) 434-3549.

Sheehy, Gail, *The Silent Passage— Menopause.* Random House, 1992.

Teaff, Nancy Lee, M.D., *Perimenopause: Preparing for the Change.* Prima Publishing, California, 1995.

Vliet, Elizabeth Lee, M.D., *Screaming to Be Heard: Hormonal Connections Women Suspect and Doctors Ignore.* M. Evans & Co., New York, 1995.

Postpartum Depression

Bolton, Wendy (daughter of Katherina Dalton), *Guide to Progesterone for Postnatal Depression.* Available from PMS Help, P. O. Box 100, St. Albans, Hertfordshire, AL1 4UQ, England.

Dalton, Katherina, M.D., *Depression After Childbirth*, Oxford University Press, 1988.

Hamilton, James Alexander, M.D., and Patricia Neal Harberger, eds., *Postpartum Psychiatric Illness: A Picture Puzzle*, University of Pennsylvania Press, Philadelphia, 1992.

Hypothyroidism

Barnes, Broda M.D., and Lawrence Galton, *Hypothyroidism: The Unsuspected Disease.* Harper & Row, 1976.

Langer, Stephen, M.D., *Solved: The Problem of Illness.* Keats Publishing, Inc., Connecticut, 1984.

Rosenthal, M. Sara. *The Thyroid Sourcebook: Everything you need to know.* Lowell House, Los Angeles, 1993.

The Viropause

Hill, A.M. *Viropause/Andropause: The Male Menopause.* New Horizon Press, New Jersey, 1993.

Miscellaneous

Breggin, Peter R., M.D., *Talking Back to Prozac.* St. Martin's Press, 1994.

Reuben, Carolyn, *Antioxidants: Your Complete Guide.* Prima Publishing, Rocklin, CA, 1995.

Waterhouse, Debra, *Outsmarting the Female Fat Cell.* Hyperion, New York, 1993.

Waterhouse, Debra, *Why Women Need Chocolate.* Hyperion, New York, 1995.

NOTES

Introduction
[1] A wedge resection involves removal of a significant wedge-shaped piece of each ovary, and was performed as a treatment for polycystic ovaries.

Chapter One
[1] Mark S. Gold, M.D., *Breakthrough medical treatments that can work for you: The Good News About Depression* (New York: Bantam Books, revised 1995) p. xi.

Chapter Three
[1] Dean Black, M.D., *PMS: When Bodies Lose Their Beat*, available by phone from 1-800-333-4290. See also G Darcourt, Souetre, et al., "Disorders of circadian rhythms in depression," *Encephale*, 18 (Sep 1992), Sec No 4:473–478. The study synthesizes other studies about circadian rhythms in depression and attempts to explain the relationship. They conclude that problems include a drop in melatonin levels, blunted amplitude of each parameter measured, and so on. As possible explanations, they describe problems with oscillators, the decrease in sensitivity to external synthesizers, and problems in rhythm coupling.

Chapter Four
[1] Leon Speroff, M.D., Robert H. Glass, M.D., and Nathan G. Kase, M.D., *Clinical Gynecologic Endocrinology and Infertility* (Baltimore: Williams & Wilkins, 1989), p. 28.

Chapter Five
[1] Rubinow, David R., "The Premenstrual Syndrome: New Views," *JAMA*, October 14, 1992. There were differences in some chemicals in the body, but not in the levels of the main female hormones. Levels of estradiol, progesterone, FSH, LH, sex hormone binding globulin, and ovarian and adrenal androgens were similar among those who had and those who did not have PMS. Some studies showed differences in the pulsatility of the hormones, and other studies showed no difference. The differences Rubinow did note (and these were not cyclical changes, but continual changes) were: the prevalence of abnormal thyroid-stimulating hormone responses

436

to thyrotropin-releasing hormone, decreased slow-wave sleep, phase-advanced temperature minima, offset of melatonin secretion, decreased red blood cell magnesium, blunted growth hormone and cortisol responses to L-tryptophan, and increased cortisol response to corticotropin-releasing hormone infusion. He also mentioned luteal phase decreases in both plasma β-endorphin and platelet serotonin.

[2] Morris K, Ungar S., Natural progesterone surpasses Provera. Available from Hormone Balancing for Women, 5905 Soquel Drive #300, Soquel, CA 95073.

[3] Rubinow, *op. cit.*

[4] Niels Lauersen, M.D., *Listen to Your Body,* (Fireside Books: 1982), p. 354.

[5] Norman Beals, Jr., M.D., personal conversation.

[6] Published in Australia. See book list at back. Dr. Cabot also has a recent book on the U.S. market called *Smart Medicine for Menopause,* (Avery, 1995.)

[7] R.F. Casper, M.T. Hearn, "The effect of hysterectomy and bilateral oophorectomy in women with severe prementrual syndrome," *Am J Obstet Gynecol,* January 1990, 162(1):105–109.

[8] *Consumer Reports,* September 1990, p. 605.

[9] Vicki Hufnagel, M.D., *No More Hysterectomies,* (New York: Penguin, 1989), p. 228.

[10] J. Hargrove and G. E. Abraham, "The ubiquitousness of premenstrual tension in gynecologic practice," *Journ of Reprod Med,* July 1983, 28(7), 435–437. In 137 patients with PMS complaining of pain as a prime symptom, laparoscopy showed 66 as having endometriosis.

[11] See C. deSwaan and N. H. Lauersen, *The Endometriosis Answer Book* (New York: Fawcett Columbine), p. 143. Also see N. H. Lauersen and Z. R. Graves, "A new approach to premenstrual syndrome," *The Female Patient,* April 1983, 8:41–55. "PMS and endometriosis often occur simultaneously."

[12] *The Endometriosis Answer Book,* pp. 197, 198.

[13] Winnifred Cutler, Ph.D., *Hysterectomy: Before and After,* 163.

[14] John Lee, M.D., *Natural Progesterone: The Multiple Roles of a Remarkable Hormone* (BLL Publishing, Sebastopol, 1994), pp. 46–47. Christiane Northrup, M.D., *Women's Bodies, Women's Wisdom* ,(New York: Bantam Books, 1994), p. 165.

[15] E. Othmer, S.C. Othmer, *Life on a Roller Coaster,* (The PIA Press: 1989).

[16] G.E. Abraham, "Nutrition and the premenstrual tension syndrome," *J Appl Nutr,* 1984, 36:103.

[17] K. Dalton, "Premenstrual syndrome and postnatal depression," *Health and Hygiene,* 1990, 11:200.

[18] G.E. Abraham, J.T. Hargrove. "Effect of vitamin B_6 on premenstrual symptomatology in women with premenstrual tension syndrome: a double blind crossover study," *Infertility,* 1980, 3:155–165.

[19] K. Dalton, M.J. Dalton, "Characteristics of pyridoxine overdose neuropathy syndrome," *Acta Neurol Scand,* July 1987, 76(1):8–11.

[20] R.S. London, G.S. Sundaramm, et al., "The effect of alpha-tocopheral on premenstrual symptomatology: A double blind study," *J Am Coll Nutr,* 1983, 2:115. And the second part of the study, *J Am Coll Nutr,* 1984, 3:351.

[21] S. Thys-Jacobs, M.J. Alvir, "Calcium-regulating hormones across the menstrual cycle; evidence of a secondary hyperparathyroidism in women with PMS," *J Clin Endocrinol Metab,* July 1995, 80(7):2227-32. S. Thys-Jacobs, "Vitamin D and calcium in menstrual migraine," *Headache,* October 1994, 34(9)544–546.

[22] R.A. Buist, "The therapeutic predictability of tryptophan and tyrosine in the treatment of depression," *Int Clin Nutr Rev,* 1983 3:1.

[23] Alan Gaby, M.D. describes the sequence of events involved in the banning of L-Tryptophan and the resulting Great B-vitamin bust in the office of Dr. Jonathan Wright, in his book *Preventing and Reversing Osteoporosis,* (Rocklin, California: Prima Publishing, 1994) p. 254.

[24] A.J. Gelenberg, J.D. Wojcik, et al., "Tyrosine treatment of depression," *Am J Psychiatry,* 1980, 137:622. I.K.Goldberg, "L-Tyrosine in depression," *Lancet,* 1980, 2:364.

[25] D.F. Horrobin, "The role of essential fatty acids and prostaglandins in the premenstrual syndrome," *J Reprod Med,* 1983, 28:465. B. Larsson, A. Jonasson, S. Fianu, "Evening primrose oil in the treatment of premenstrual syndrome: a pilot study," *Curr Ther Res,* 1989, 46:58–63.

[26] Debra Waterhouse, *Why Women Need Chocolate,* (New York: Hyperion, 1995).

[27] K. Dalton, M. Dalton, *The Premenstrual Syndrome,* (London: William Heinemann Medical Books), page 115. See also K. Morris, S. Ungar, Natural progesterone surpasses Provera.

[28] Natural Progesterone: Usage and Instructions. Packet insert for Pro-Gest [reg trademark], p. 4, 5.

[29] *Depression After Childbirth,* (Oxford University Press: 1988), pp. 117–118.

[30] See the chapter on Estrogen and Depression.

Chapter Six
[1] Paul Vaughan, *The Pill on Trial* (Penguin Books: 1974) pp. 1–61.

[2] Carl Djerassi, *The Pill, Pygmy Chimps, and Degas' Horse* (BasicBooks, a division of Harper Collins Publishers, Inc.: 1992).

Chapter Seven
[1] James A. Hamilton, M.D. and D. A. Sichel, "Prophylactic Measures," in Hamilton, J. A. and Harberger, P. N., eds., *Postpartum Psychiatric Illness: A Picture Puzzle* (University of Pennsylvania Press: 1992), p. 219.

[2] R. B. Filer, quoting Tulchinsky et al, 1972. "Endocrinology and the Postpartum Period," *Ibid,* 155.

[3] Victor Reus, "Behavioral Aspects of Thyroid Disease in Women," *Psychiatric Clinics of North America*, Vol. 12, No. 1 (March 1989). Reus, who is head of the Psychiatry Department at the University of California at San Francisco, says, "One additional risk factor observed by investigators in this area [the study of thyroiditis] is onset in the postpartum period. This may be related to the risk associated with subclinical hypothyroidism as postpartum thyroid dysfunction is an increasingly recognized phenomena."

[3a] N. Amino and K. Miyai, "Postpartum autoimmune endocrine syndromes," in Davies T (ed), *Autoimmune Endocrine Disease* (New York, John Wiley & Son: 1983).

[3b] H. G. Fein, J. M. Goldman, and B. D. Weintraub, "Postpartum lymphocytic thyroiditis in American women: A spectrum of thyroid dysfunction," *Am J Obstet Gynecol* 138:504, 1980.

[3c] R. Freeman, H. Rosen, and B. Thysen, "Incidence of thyroid dysfunction in an unselected postpartum population," *Arch Intern Med* 146:1361, 1986.

[3d] H-H. Lervang, O. Pryds, and H. P. Kristensen, "Thyroid dysfunction after delivery: Incidence and clinical course," *Acta Med Scand* 222:369, 1987. T. F. Nikolai, S. L. Turney, and R. C. Roberts, "Postpartum lymphocytic thyroiditis," *Arch Intern Med*, 147:221, 1987.

[4] J. C. Davis and M. T. Abou-Saleh, "Manifestations of Postpartum Hypopituitarism," in *Postpartum Psychiatric Illness*, op cit., p. 193.

[5] Dalton K. "Postnatal depression and prophylactic progesterone," *Health and Hygiene*, 1990, 11:199–201.

[6] Harris B, Lovett L, Newcombe RG, Read GF, Walker R, Riad-Fahmy D. Maternity blues and major endocrine changes: Cardiff puerperal mood and hormone study II. *Brit Med Journ*, Apr 9, 1994, 308(6934): 949–53. Women with blues had significantly higher antenatal progesterone concentrations and lower postnatal concentrations than women without blues. Conclusion was that maternal mood in the days immediately after delivery is related to withdrawal of naturally occurring progesterone.

[7] *The Picture Puzzle of Psychiatric Illness After Childbirth*, written for The York Hospital Conference, in York, Pennsylvania, April 6, 1988, and expanded in his book written with Patricia Neal Harberger, *Postpartum Psychiatric Illness: A Picture Puzzle*, University of Pennsylvania Press, Philadelphia, 1992.

Chapter Eight

[1] L. Hegedus, S. Karstrup, and N. Rasmussen, "Evidence of cyclic alterations of thyroid size during the menstrual cycle in healthy women," *Am J Obstet Gynecol*, 1986, 155:142.

[2] Pat Puglio, "Hypothyroidism: the relation to common menstrual disorders," *Women's Health Connection*, complimentary issue II.of Puglio, of the Broda Barnes Foundation in Trumble, Connecticut, says: "In researching the milder forms of hypothyroidism and describing the profound effects it can have on the body, Dr. Eugene Hertoghe, a distinguished Belgian

endocrinologist and a member of the Royal Academy of Medicine, presented a paper in 1914 to the New York Polyclinic Medical School and Hospital. [He] . . . states, 'The thyroid has a great influence on menstruation, pregnancy, lactation, and even uterine involution after childbirth. When the thyroid is normally active the menses are normal; when weak, menorrhagia sets in. The weaker the thyroid, the greater the loss of blood. . . . If we can put aside such causes as fibroids and cancer, we will always think of thyroid deficiency.'"

[3a] V. N. Prilepskaia and T. A. Lobova, "Hypothalamo-hypophyseal-thyroid system in patients with dysfunctional uterine bleeding," *Akush Ginekol* (Mosk) (Sept., 1991), (9):51–54;

[3b] D. L. Wilansky and B. Greisman, "Early hypothyroidism in patients with menorrhagia," *Am J Obstet Gynecol* (Aug., 1990), 163(2):697;

[3c] J. M. Higham and R. W. Shaw, "The effect of thyroxine replacement on menstrual blood loss in a hypothyroid patient," *Br J Obstet Gynaecol* (Aug., 1992), 99(8):695–696;

[3d] P. P. Roy-Byrne, D. R. Rubinow, and M. C. Hoban, et al., "TSH and prolactin responses to TRH in patients with premenstrual syndrome," *Am J Psychiatry*, 1987, 144:480;

[3e] T. Maruo, K. Katayama, E. R. Barnea and M. Mochizuki, "A role for thyroid hormone in the induction of ovulation and corpus luteum function," *Horm Res*, 1992, 37 Suppl 1:12–18;

[3f] E. Kind, T. Steck, and W. Wurfel, "Incidence of functional disorders of the thyroid in a sample of infertile patients with cycle irregularities," *Gynakol Beburtshifliche Rundsch*, 1933, 33 Suppl 1:325;

[3g] V. N. Prilepskaia, T. A. Lobova and I. P. Laricheva, "Secondary amenorrhea caused by hypothyroidism," *Akush Ginekol* (Mosk), (Apr., 1990), (4):35–38;

[3h] L. Bispink, W. Brandle, C. Lindner, and G. Bettendorf, "Preclinical hypothyroidism and disorders of ovarian function," *Geburtshilfe Frauenheilkd*, (Oct, 1989), 49(10):881–888. This study concludes that mild hypothyroidism may cause ovarian insufficiency. Assessment of thyroid function should be mandatory in infertile patients with elevated prolactin levels or chronic anovulation;

[3i] E. Kind, T. Steck, and W. Wurfel, "Incidence of functional disorders of the thyroid in a sample of infertile patients with cycle irregularities," *Gynakol Geburtshilfliche Rundsch*, 1993, 33 Suppl, 1:325;

[3j] T. Maruo, K. Katayama, E. R. Barnea, and M. Mochizuki, "A role for thyroid hormone in the induction of ovulation and corpus luteum function," *Horm Res*, 1992, 37 Suppl 1:12–18;

[3k] G. R. Sridhar and G. Nagamini, "Hypothyroidism presenting with polycystic ovary syndrome," *J Assoc Physicians India*, (Feb, 1993), 41(2):88–90.

Notes two women with hypothyroidism who also had polycystic ovaries. Suggests that correction of hypothyroidism when present would form an important aspect of the management of infertility associated with PCO;

[31] S. K. Singh, "Subclinical hypothyroidism and polycystic ovary syndrome[letter]," *Horm Res*, 1993, 39(1–2):61–66;

[3m] B. J. Van Boorhis, T. W. Neff, et al., "Primary hypothyroidism associated with multicystic ovaries and ovarian torsion in an adult," *Obstet Gynecol*, May 1994, 83(5 Pt 2):885–887. This study reports that profound hypothyroidism can cause multicystic ovaries in an adult. In the absence of ovarian torsion, surgery can be avoided, as thyroid hormone replacement leads to clinical resolution of the cysts within three months;

[3n] S. Ghosh, S. N. Kabir, A. Pakrashi, et al., "Subclinical hypothyroidism: a determinant of polycystic ovary syndrome," *Horm Res*, 1994, 41(1):43–44;

[3o] R. Goi, M. Matsuda, et al., "Two cases of Hashimoto's thyroiditis with transient hypothyroidism," *Intern Med*, Jan 1992, 31(1):64–68. This study reports a woman with polycystic ovary syndrome who had transient hypothyroidism inferred to have been caused by Hashimoto's disease;

[3p] A. J. Shelton and J. H. Harger, "Association between familial autoimmune diseases and recurrent spontaneous abortions," *Am J Reprod Immunol*, Sep 1994, 32(2):82–87;

[3q] M. Bolz and H. Nagal, "The course of pregnancy in congenital thyroid gland aplasia," *Zentralbl Gynakol*, 1994, 116(9):515–521. In this study of a 28-year-old woman, her first pregnancy was complicated by gestational hypertension and pre-eclampsia. Delivery was by forceps. She had repeated bleeding in the first trimester of her second pregnancy. She had no signs of obvious hypothyroidism, but her thyroid dose was increased. The bleeding stopped. It mentions that dysfunction of thyroid gland is associated with reduced fertility. Hypothyroidism in pregnancy is associated with an adverse outcome in fetal health as well as an increase in obstetric complications. Thyroid plays a vital role in fetal development and maturation of the fetal brain. Women with hypothyroidism have a lower rate of pregnancy and a higher rate of spontaneous miscarriages compared to a normal population;

[3r] B. Lejeune, J. P. Grun, P. de Nayer P, et al., "Antithyroid antibodies underlying thyroid abnormalities and miscarriage or pregnancy-induced hypertension," *Br J Obstet Gynecol*, Jul 1993, 100(7):669–672. This study concludes that the presence of thyroid autoantibodies during pregnancy constitutes a marker of increased risk of miscarriages and poor obstetric prognosis;

[3s] L. K. Millar, D. A. Wing, et al., "Low birth weight and pre-eclampsia in pregnancies complicated by hyperthyroidism," *Obstet Gynecol*, Dec 1994, 84(6):946–949. This study reports that lack of control of hyperthyroidism significantly increases the risk of low birth weight infants and severe pre-eclampsia;

[31] L. Vojvodic, V. Sulovic, et al., "The effect of pre-eclampsia on thyroid gland function," *Srp Arh Celok Lek,* Jan–Feb 1993, 121(1–2):4–7. This prospective study looked at 183 women. 15 were normal thyroid, 20 were healthy. The rest had a mixture of thyroid diseases. They found a statistically higher incidence of pre-eclampsia in pregnant women with hyperthyroidism (26.0%) and hypothyroidism (26.8%);

[3u] J. V. Joshi, S. D. Bhandarkar, et al., "Menstrual irregularities and lactation failure may precede thyroid dysfunction or goiter ," *J Postgard Med,* Jul–Sep 1993, 39(3):118–119. "Reproductive function may therefore be considered as one of the presenting symptoms of thyroid disorders in women, keeping in mind both menstrual irregularities and lactation failure may also arise from other common or idiopathic origins. Especially in women with menstrual irregularities in the perimenopausal age if thyroid dysfunction is detected, pharmacotherapy may be a superior alternative to surgical interventions like hysterectomy."

[4] N. D. Brayshaw and D. D. Brayshaw, "Thyroid hypofunction in premenstrual syndrome [letter]," *N Engl J Med,* Dec 1986, 315(23): 1486–87.

[5] B. Catz, "Hypothyroidism," in Falk, S. A., ed., *Thyroid Disease: Endocrinology, Surgery, Nuclear Medicine, and Radiotherapy.* New York: Raven Press, Ltd.: 1990, p. 279–288. Catz says that most patients with hypothyroidism have or have had a goiter or swelling of the thyroid, and that it is an inherited condition. The main causes of the swelling are heredity, defects in enzymes that produce thyroid hormones, or Hashimoto's thyroiditis, an autoimmune disease that leads to tissue alteration and swelling of the thyroid. These factors may be interrelated and it is difficult to separate their coexistence. These thyroid antibodies are passed through the placenta from mother to baby at birth, and may be triggered later in life by trauma, shock, pregnancy, or virus. Catz continues that members of the same family may suffer from hypothyroidism (low thyroid), hyperthyroidism (high thyroid), thyroid cancer, goiter, nodular goiter, chronic lymphocytic thyroiditis (Hashimoto's thyroiditis), or thyroid antibodies. Thus, says Catz, family history becomes extremely important in understanding the chain of events.

[6] Broda Barnes, M.D., *Hypothyroidism: The Undiagnosed Disease* (Harper & Row, 1976). Dr. Barnes says that the ideal test for thyroid function is not even possible because the amount of thyroid hormone needs to be measured on the inside of each cell in the body, an impossible task because there are billions of cells in the body, and analyses could not even be done with computers (pp. 36, 37). Dr. Barnes also says that all the tests done by measuring the amount of thyroid in the gland itself or in the bloodstream don't do what counts: measure what is available and working in the cells. These attempts are something like trying to work out what a thrifty man's spending habits are by looking at what he has in his bank account. How much thyroid there is in the thyroid gland or bloodstream tells us little about how much thyroid is spent in the cells. *Ibid.,* pp. 41–42.

Note also Victor I. Reus, M.D., "How to detect hypothyroidism when screening tests are normal: use of the TRH stimulation test," *Postgraduate Medicine*, Vol 74, No. 2, August, 1983, and "Behavioral Aspects of Thyroid Disease in Women," in Women's Disorders *Psychiatric Clinics of North America*, March, 1989, 12(1):153–165. Dr. Reus is Medical Director of the Department of Psychiatry, Langley Porter Neuropsychiatric Institute, University of California School of Medicine, San Francisco, California.

[7] B. Stone, *American Medical News*, May 23, 1980, cited in Stephen Langer, *Solved: the Problem of Illness* (Keats Publishing, 1984) p. 11.

[8] N. Lauersen, *PMS: Premenstrual Syndrome and You* (Simon & Schuster, 1982), p. 164.

[9] C. M. Intenzo, C. H. Park, S. M. Kim, D. M. Capuzzi, S. N. Cohen, and P. Green, "Clinical, laboratory, and scintigraphic manifestations of subacute and chronic thyroiditis," *Clin Nucl Med*, Apr 1993, 18(4):302–6. The term "thyroiditis" refers to several syndromes with different causes. Chronic or Hashimoto's thyroiditis (HT) is an autoimmune disorder manifested by swelling of the thyroid or a nodule on the thyroid and low thyroid function. It is by far the most common of these syndromes.

Subacute thyroiditis (SAT) includes two different syndromes: subacute granulomatous thyroiditis (SAGT) and subacute lymphocytic thyroiditis (SLT).

SAGT is viral in origin and usually presents with neck tenderness and hyperthyroid symptoms.

SLT is more likely autoimmune in origin and results in goiter and transient hyperthyroidism. SLT is often seen in the postpartum period and is referred to as postpartum thyroiditis (PPT).

Less common forms of thyroiditis include Riedel's struma, characterized by extensive fibrosis of the thyroid gland and acute suppurative thyroiditis, caused by a bacterial infection.

In this study, out of 20 patients studied, 14 had Hashimoto's, 3 had subacute granulomatous thyroiditis, 1 had subacute lymphocytic thyroiditis, and 2 had postpartum thyroiditis.

[10] Some think this is the most frequent thyroid disorder in our population. See D. A. Fisher, T. H. Oddie, D. E. Johnson, et al., "The diagnosis of Hashimoto's thyroiditis," *J Clin Endocrinol Metab*, 1975, 40:795–801.

[11] Irl Extein says that thyroiditis is prevalent in up to 12 percent of the population. Irl Extein quoted in Jeri Miller, "Thyroid dysfunction often found in depressed patients," *Psychiatric Times*, Medicine and Behavior, May 1992, 30–31.

[12] Figures are taken from Dr. Richard Bronson's presentation on the association of premature menopause and autoimmune diseases, called "Immunology of hypergonadotropic ovarian dysfunction: etiology and diagnosis." It was given at the 4th Annual North American Menopause Society meeting in San Diego, California, September 2–4, 1993.

[13] The greater incidence of subclinical thyroid problems in women versus men is well known."The disease is from eight to ten times more common in women than men. Its incidence is highest between age 30 and 50, but it may occur during any period of life." Hall et al, *op cit*, 338.

[14a] Hall and others list a number of sources as saying that there has been a dramatic increase in the incidence of Hashimoto's thyroiditis, and the types of studies indicate that these are real increases not just better detection. R. C. Hall, M. K. Popkin, R. DeVaul, A. K. Hall, et al, "Psychiatric manifestations of Hashimoto's thyroiditis," *Psychosomatics,* Apr 1982, 23(4):337–342. Some of the footnotes to support his theory are as follows:

[14b] J. Furszyfer, L. T. Kurland, L. B. Woolner, et al., "Hashimoto's thyroiditis in Olmsted County, Minnesota, 1935 through 1967," *Mayo Clin Proc,* 1970, 45:586–596;

[14c] E. F. Fowler, "The changing incidence and treatment of thyroid disease," *Arch Surg,* 1960, 81:733–740;

[14d] W. Macksood, R. L. Rapport, and F. Hodges, "The increasing incidence of Hashimoto's disease," *Arch Surg,* 1961, 83:384–387;

[14e] F. J. Kinney and R. E. Hermann, "Increasing occurrence of thyroiditis in the Rocky Mountain area," *Rocky Mt Med J,* 1962, 59:35–37,72–73;

[14f] R. Volpé, "The pathophysiology of autoimmune disease," *Endocr Regul,* Dec 1991, 25(4):187–192;

[14g] R. Volpé and M. Iitaka, "Evidence for an antigen-specific defect in suppressor T-lymphocytes in autoimmune thyroid disease," *Exp Clin Endocrinol,* May 1991, 97(2–3):133–138;

[14h] Y. Hidaka, N. Amino, T. Kaneda, et al., "Increase in peripheral natural killer cell activity in patients with autoimmune thyroid diseases," *Autoimmunity,* 1992, 11(4):239–246;

[14i] Y. Tomer and T. F. Davies, "Infection, thyroid disease, and autoimmunity," *Endocr Rev,* Feb 1993, 14(1):107–120.

[15] B. Catz, *op cit,* p. 279. "Thyroid conditions begin insidiously and may remain undiagnosed for years." He continues, "The condition begins gradually and may remain unnoticed for months or years. The patient may show a goiter, but thyroid laboratory values are normal, except for some patients with evidence of thyroid antibodies. . . . The presence of a palpable thyroid gland is an indication of the presence of a goiter. This in turn is evidence of pathology, such as enzymatic defects and/or lymphocytic thyroiditis (p. 281).

[16] See note 12.

[17] Phyllis Saifer, M.D., and Nathan Becker, M.D., "Allergy and Autoimmune Endocrinopathy: APICH Syndrome," was published overseas in *Food Allergy and Its Intolerance,* Brostoff & Challocombe, eds., (Baillière Tindall, 1991), pp. 781–788.

Chapter Nine

[1] Hypothyroidism was first presented as a cause of psychosis by the Committee on Myxedema (the nonpitting edema or swelling characteristic of severe low thyroid function) of the Clinical Society of London in 1888.

[2] V. Reus, "Behavioral aspects of thyroid disease in women," "Women's Disorders," *Psychiatric Clinics of North America*, Vol 1, No. 1, Mar 1989, 153.

[3] Victor Reus says that women have four to five times as many thyroid problems as men, *ibid*, 153.

[4] B. Nowotny, J. Teuer, W. an der Heiden, B. Scholote, et al., "The role of TSH, psychological, and somatic changes in thyroid dysfunctions," *Klin Wochenschr*, Oct 1990, 68(19):964–970.

[5] Sources that link thyroid problems with particular emotional disorders include:

Depression:
F. Tallis, "Primary hypothyroidism: A case for vigilance in the psychological treatment of depression," *Br J Clin Psych*, Sep 1993, 32(3): 261–270. This study says that primary hypothyroidism is a relatively common endocrine disorder that develops insidiously and can mimic depression. Between 8 and 14 percent of patients diagnosed as depressed may have some degree of hypothyroidism.

M. Fava, J. F. Rosenbaum, R. Birnbaum, K. Kelly, et al., "The thyrotropin response to thyrotropin-releasing hormone as a predictor of response to treatment in depressed patients," *Acta Psychiatr Scand*, July 1992, 86(1):42:5.

D. A. Wilson, R. T. Mulder, and P. R. Joyce, "Diurnal profiles of thyroid hormones are altered in depression," *J Affect Disord*, Jan 1992, 24(1):11–16.

A. J. Prange, P. T. Loosen, I. C. Wilson, et al., "The therapeutic use of hormones of the thyroid axis in depression," in J. C. Ballenger and R. M. Post, eds., *The Neurobiology of Mood Disorders* (Baltimore: Williams & Wilkins, 1983).

R. T. Joffe, R. M. Bagby, and A. J. Levitt, "The thyroid and melancholia," *Psychiatry Res*, Apr 1992, 42(1):73–80.

R. Bunevicius, G. Kazanavicius, et al., "Thyrotropin response to TRH stimulation in depressed patients with autoimmune thyroiditis," *Biol Psychiatry*, Oct 1994, 36(8):543–7.

A. Baumgartner, "Thyroid hormones and depressive disorders—clinical overview perspectives. Part 1: Clinical aspects," *Nervenarzt*, Jan 1993, 64(1):11–20.

A. Baumgartner and A. Campos-Barros, "Thyroid hormones and depressive disorders—clinical overview perspectives. Part 2: Thyroid hormones and the central nervous system—basic research," *Nervenarzt*, Jan 1993, 64(1):11–20. R. H. Howland, "Thyroid dysfunction in refractory depression: implications for pathophysiology and treatment," *J Clin Psychiatry*, Feb 1993, 54(2):47–54. J. J. Haggerty, Jr., R. A. Stern, et al., "Subclinical hypothyroidism: recognition, significance, management," *Clin Neuropharmacol,* 1992, 15 Suppl 1 Pt A:386A.

J. J. Haggerty, Jr., R. A. Stern, et al., "Subclinical hypothyroidism: a modifiable risk factor for depression?" *Am J Psychiatry,* Mar 1994, 151(3):453–454.

R. T. Joffe and A. J. Levitt, "Major depression and subclinical (grade 2) hypothyroidism," *Psychoneuroendocrinology,* May–Jul 1992, 17(2–3): 215–221.

Panic attacks, suicide, and agitation:

M. H. Corrigan, G. M. Gillette, D. Quade and J. C. Garbutt, "Panic, suicide, and agitation: independent correlates of the TSH response to TRH in depression," *Biol Psychiatry,* Oct 1993, 34(7):503–504.

P. Linkowski, J-P Van Wetter, M. Kerhofs, et al., "Violent suicidal behavior and the thyrotropin-releasing hormone-thyroid-stimulating hormone test; a clinical outcome," *Neuropsychobiology,* 1984, 12:19.

M. P. Rogers, K. White, et al., "Prevalence of medical illness in patients with anxiety disorders," *Int J Psychiatry Med,* 1994, 24(1):83–96.

Rapid cycling bipolar affective disorder:

M. S. Bauer, P. C. Whybrow, and A. Winokur, "Rapid cycling bipolar affective disorder. I. Association with grade 1 hypothyroidism," *Arch Gen Psychiatry,* May 1990, 47(5):427–432.

P. Linkowski, H. Brauman, and J. Mendlewicz, "Thyrotropin response to thyrotrophin-releasing hormone in unipolar and bipolar affective illness," *J Affect Dis,* 1981, 3:9.

Schizophrenia:

L. K. Smirnova and T. I. Zorenko, "Thyroid functional activity in schizophrenic patients with aggressive sexual behavior," *Zh Nevropatol Psikhiatr Im SS Korsakova,* 1993, 93(4):68–70.

I. M. Turianitsa, I. I. Lavkai, et al., "Status of the thyroid gland in patients with schizophrenia," *Zh Nevropatol Psikhiatr Im SS Korsakova,* 1991, 91(1):122–123.

P. T. Loosen, A. J. Prange, I. Wilson, et al., "Thyroid stimulating hormone response after thyrotropin-releasing hormone in depressed, schizophrenic and normal women," *Psychneuroendocrinology,* 1977, 2:137.

E. M. Haberfellner, H. Rittmannsberger, and E. Windhager, "Psychotic manifestation of hypothyroidism. A case report," *Nervenarzt,* May 1993, 64(5):336–339.

T. J. Walch, "Enhancing compliance in schizophrenic patients by weekly dosing with levothyroxine sodium [letter]," *J Clin Psychiatry,* Dec 1994, 55(12):543.

S. S. Othman, K. Abdul Kadir, et al., "High prevalence of thyroid function test abnormalities in chronic schizophrenia," *Aust NZ J Psych,* Dec 1994, 28(4):620–624.

Dementia:

E. Hobik, R. Ihl, et al., "Dementia and disorders of the thyroid gland," *Fortscr Neurol Psychiatr,* Sep 1994, 62(9):330–336.

M. Haupt and A. Kurz, "Reversibility of dementia in hypothyroidism," *Z Gesamte Inn Med,* Dec 1993, 48(12):609–613.

C. L. Smith and C. V. Granger, "Hypothyroidism producing reversible dementia. A challenge for medical rehabilitation," *Am J Phys Med Rehabili,* Feb 1992, 71(1):28–30.

Alzheimer's Disease:

G. Pico-Santiago, "Alzheimer's disease: the untold story," *P R Health Sci J,* Jun 1993, 12(2):85–87.

Autism:

T. Hashimoto and R. Aihara, "Reduced thyroid-stimulating hormone response to thyrotropin-releasing hormone in autistic boys," *Dev Med Child Neurol,* Apr 1991, 33(4):313–319.

I. C. Gillberg, C. Gillberg, and S. Kopp, "Hypothyroidism and autism spectrum disorders," *J Child Psychol Psychiatry,* Mar 1992, 33(3): 531–542.

Down's Syndrome:

S. Dinani and S. Carpenter, "Down's sydrome and thyroid disorder," *J Men Defic Res,* Apr 1990, 34(2):187–193.

M. E. Percy, A. J. Dalton, et al., "Autoimmune thyroiditis associated with mild subclinical hypothyroidism in adults with Down syndrome: a comparison of patients with and without manifestations of Alzheimer's disease," *Am J Med Genet,* Jun 1990, 36(2):148–154.

Attention deficit disorder:

P. Hauser, A. J. Zametkin, et al., "Attention deficit disorder in people with generalized resistance to thyroid hormone," *N Engl J Med,* Apr 1993, 328(14):1038–1039.

Obsessive-compulsive disorders:

D. Aizenberg, H. Hermesh, I. Gil-ad, et al., "TRH stimulation test in obsessive-compulsive patients," *Psychiatry Res,* July 1991, 38(1):21–26.

Seasonal Affective Disorder (SAD):

V. Coiro, R. Volpi, C. Marchesi, et al., "Lack of seasonal variation in abnormal TSH secretion in patients with seasonal affective disorder," *Biol Psychiatry,* Jan 1994, 35(1):36–41. This study shows that the secretion of TSH is impaired, regardless of the phase of the psychiatric disease. The low TSH response to TRH in the presence of normal serum thyroid hormone levels and the lack of the TSH nocturnal surge suggest that patients with SAD might be affected by mild central hypothyroidism.

M. N. Raitiere, "Clinical evidence for thyroid dysfunction in patients with seasonal affective disorder," *Psychoneuroendocrinology,* May–Jul 1992,

17(2–3):231–241. The author suggests that SAD may, in part, represent a reformulation in modern neuropsychiatric terms of a previously noted fall-winter decrement, both biochemical and clinical, among hypothyroid patients.

[6] M. M. Fichter, K. M. Pirke, J. Pollinger, G. Wolfram, and E. Brunner, "Disturbances in the hypothalamo-pituitary-adrean and other neuroendocrine axes in bulimia," *Biol Psychiatry,* May 19909, 27(9):1021–1037.

[7] R. C. Hall, M. K. Popkin, R. deVaul, A. K. Hall, E. R. Gardner, and T. P. Beresford, "Psychiatric manifestations of Hashimoto's thyroiditis," *Psychosomatics,* April 1982, 23(4):337–342.

[8] Hall, et al, *op cit,* 339.

[9] *Ibid.*

[10] Victor Reus, "Behavioral aspects of thyroid disease in women," Women's Disorders, *Psychiatric Clinics of North America,* Vol 12, No. 1, Mar 1989, 153. A. J. Prange et al., "Enhancement of imipramine by triiodothyronine in unselected depressed patients," *Excerpta Med Int Cong Serv,* 1968, 180:532–535.

[11] I. Extein I, quoted in Jeri Miller, "Thyroid dysfunction often found in depressed patients," *The Psychiatric Times: Medicine and Behavior,* May 1992, 30–31.

[12] Letter to Gillian Ford, 23rd January, 1995.

[13] T. L. Paul et al., "Long-term L-thyroxine therapy is associated with decreased hip bone density in premenopausal women. *JAMA* 1988, 259:3137–3141. J. M. Coindre et al., "Bone loss in hypothyroidism with hormone replacement. A histomorphometric study," *Arch Intern Med,* 1986, 146:48–53. Quoted in Alan Gaby, *Preventing and Reversing Osteoporosis* (Rocklin, California: Prima Publishing, 1994) pp. 228–232.

[14] J. A. Franklyn et al., "Long-term thyroxine treatment and bone mineral density," *Lancet,* 1992, 340:9–13.

[15] J. Miller, *op cit.* But note the following: M. Maes, H. Y. Meltzer, P. Cosyns, et al., "An evaluation of basal hypothalamic-pituitary-thyroid axis function in depression: results of a large-scaled and controlled study," *Psychoneuroendocrinology,* 1993, 18(8):607–620. This study says that almost all of the unipolar depressed patients were euthyroid (normal); none of the major depressed subjects showed subclinical hypothyroidism. 8.8 percent of the melancholic subjects exhibited some degree of subclinical hyperthyroidism. Basic ultrasensitive TSH was lower in melancholic patients than in healthy ones. Free T4 levels were higher in melancholic patients that in all others. Basal TSH and free T4 levels were significantly correlated with severity of illness. The study argues for using ultrasensitive TSH instead of TRH hormone tests.

[16] Reus, *op. cit.,* page 155.

[17] *Ibid.* Reus quotes D. S. Cooper, R. Halpern, L. C. Wood, et al., "L-thyroxine therapy in subclinical hypothyroidism," *An Intern Med,* 101:18, 1984.

[18] Letter from Dr. Robert Volpé, 27th Feb, 1995. See R. Bunevicius, G. Kazanavicius, and A. Telksnys, "Thyrotropin response to TRH stimulation

in depressed patients with autoimmune thyroiditis," *Biol Psychiatry,* Oct 1994, 15:36(8):543–547. They found that a group with normal thyroid and a group with autoimmune thyroiditis, blunted TSH responses occur as often in one group as the other.

[19] K. Morris, *Hormone Balancing for Women: Medical Protocol for Physicians Assistants,* Oct 1994, 12–13. Dr. Morris's office phone number is (408) 464–7777.

[20] John Lee, M.D., *Natural Progesterone: The Multiple Roles of a Remarkable Hormone* (Sebastopol, California: BLL publishing), pp. 81–82.

[21] Dermoid cysts are one of the more bizarre types of ovarian cysts. They are filled with an oily fluid and can contain hair, teeth, bits of bone, and cartilage. They can also produce hormones. They are the most common ovarian cyst found in women under age 20.

[22] Gary Null, "Prozac, Eli Lilly and the FDA," *Townsend Letter for Doctors,* Feb/Mar 1993, 115/116, pp. 178–187.

[23] G. Csako, D. M. Corso, et al., "Evaluation of two over-the-counter natural thyroid hormone preparations in human volunteers," *Ann Pharmacother,* Apr 1992, 26(4):492–492. They found increased T3 activity, but no definite clinical or laboratory evidence of thyroid hormone excess. However, they felt health professionals should advise against using these over-the-counter medications.

[24] John Lee, M.D., *Natural Progesterone: The Multiple Roles of a Remarkable Hormone* (Sebastopol, California: BLL Publishing), pp. 81–82.

[25] "Should we allow children and adults showing the presence of an enlarged thyroid gland and antibodies to go untreated because the thyroid chemistries are normal? I think not." B. Catz, "Hypothyroidism," *Thyroid Disease: Endocrinology, Surgery, Nuclear Medicine, and Radiotherapy* (New York:, Raven Press, Ltd. 1990) p. 281.

[26] P. Puglio, "Hypothyroidism: the relation to common menstrual disorders," *Women's Health Connection,* complimentary issue II from Women's International Pharmacy.

[27a] Thyroid function in patients receiving long-term levothyroxine treatment should be closely monitored and bone densitometry should be performed in patients at risk for osteoporosis, according to A. W. Kung and K. K. Pun, "Bone mineral density in premenopausal women receiving long-term physiological doses of levothyroxine," *JAMA,* May 1991, 265(20):2688–2691.

[27b] G. Radetti, C. Castellan, L. Tato, et al., "Bone mineral density in children and adolescent females treated with high doses of L-thyroxine," *Horm Res,* 1993, 39(3–4):127–131.

[28] Alan Gaby says that the first study published in 1988 to suggest thyroid medication increased bone loss was flawed. He questions the conclusions because the women were given 175 to 300 mcg of thyroid, which is a large amount (usual dose is between 50 and 150 mcg). A dozen of the women had previous conditions which could cause osteoporosis (6 had Graves' disease; 6 had

Hashimoto's and, in the latter, hyperthyroidism is a common early symptom. The rest were receiving thyroid medication to suppress thyroid cancer and other nodules—these women weren't hypothyroid to begin with, so what they received was extra). Therefore Dr. Gaby believes this study does not prove that taking low or moderate thyroid doses for an underactive thyroid increases osteoporosis. He also states that people who are hypothyroid have abnormal bone modeling as part of the disease—resulting in thicker bones with more old bone. Taking thyroid can take some time to bring the abnormal density back to normal. He feels there is no need for concern if there is an increased rate of bone loss in the first six months, and suggests that there will probably not be continued loss after the initial catch-up period. *Preventing and Reversing Osteoporosis: every women's essential guide*, (Rocklin, CA: Prima Publishing, 1994), pp. 229–232. He adds that a study published last year in the *Lancet* demonstrates that thyroid hormone doesn't cause osteoporosis. The results showed that patients who received thyroid medication had no evidence of lower bone mineral density than the controls at any site. J. A. Franklin et al., "Long-term thyroxine treatment and bone mineral density *Lancet*, 1992,340:9–13.

[29a] J. Dommisse, "T3 is at least as important as T4 in all hypothyroid patients [letter]," *J Clin Psychiatry*, Jul 1993, 54(7):277–279.

[29b] R. G. Cooke, R. T. Joffe, et al., "T3 augmentation of antidepressant treatment in T4-replaced thyroid patients," *J Clin Psychiatry*, Jul 1993, 54(7):277–279.

[30a] T. Csaszar and A. Patakfalvi, "Polyglandular autoimmune syndrome type II," *Orv Hetil*, Jul 1993, 134(29):1591–1593. This study mentions the total remission of illness in a woman with different endocrine disorders who used cyclosporin treatment.

[30b] T. Csaszar and A. Patakfalvi, "Treatment of polyglandular autoimmune syndrome with cyclosporin-A," *Acta Med Hung*, 1992–1993, 49(3–4):187–193.

[30c] A. Antonelli, C. Gambuzza, B. Alberti, A. Saracino, A. Melosi, et al., "Autoimmune polyendocrine syndrome. Treatment with intravenous immunoglobulins," *Clin Ter*, Sep 1992, 141(9 Pt 2):43–38.

[30d] Some studies describe successful use of intravenous methylprednisolone for autoimmune endocrine problems. For example: Y. Hiromatsu, K. Tanaka, et al., "Intravenous methylprednisolone pulse therapy for Graves' ophthalmopathy," *Endocrin J*, Feb 1993, 40(1):63–72.

[30e] Y. Hiromatsu, M. Sato, et al., "Anti-eye muscle antibodies and hypothyroid Graves' disease: a case report," *Endocrinol*, Japan, Dec 1992, 39(6):593–600.

[30f] A. Leovey, G. Bako, et al., "Combined cyclosporin-A and methylprednisolone treatment of Graves' ophthalmopathy," *Acta Med Hung*, 1992–93, 49(3–4):179–185.

[31] M. T. Yilmaz, A. S. Devrim, et al., "Immunoprotection in spontaneous remission of type I diabetes: long-term follow-up results," *Diabetes Res Clin Res Pract*, Feb 1993, 19(2):151–162.

Chapter Ten

[1] R.L. Byyny, L. Speroff, *"A Clinical Guide for the Care of Older Women, op cit,* 76.

[2] Experts saying that about one percent of women go through natural premature menopause before 40 include the following: W. Cutler and C.R. Garcia: "Fortunately, less than 1 percent of women are prematurely menopausal naturally—that is, their menopause is not a result of hysterectomy and oophorectomy." In: *Menopause: A guide for women and the men who love them,* (London: W. W. Norton, 1993), 70. They are quoting S.L. Rabinowe, V.A. Ravnikar, et al., "Premature menopause: monoclonal antibody defined T lymphocyte abnormalities and antiovarian antibodies," *Fertil Steril,* 51(3):450–454. Christine Northrop. "If the age of forty is the cutoff, naturally occurring premature menopause occurs in about one woman in one hundred." In: *Women's Bodies, Women's Wisdom,* (New York: Bantam Books, 1994), 441. She quotes C.B. Coulam, S.C. Adamson, et al., "Incidence of premature ovarian failure," *Amer Journ Obstet and Gynecol,* 1986, 67(4). R.L. Bynny, L. Speroff. "About 1 percent of women will experience menopause before the age of 40." In: *A Clinical Guide for the Care of Older Women,* (Baltimore: Williams and Wilkins, 1990), 75.

[3] Experts saying that about 8 percent of women go through premature nonsurgical menopause include: L. Nachtigall, "If you are among the 8 percent of women who have spontaneous (that is, nonsurgical) menopause before the age of 40, it's probably because you come from a family that tends to run out of eggs very early." In: *Estrogen: The facts can change your life,* (Los Angeles: The Body Press, 1986), 51. Also see R. Bronson (uses the figure of 7–11 percent). "Immunology of hypergonadotropic ovarian dysfunction: etiology and diagnosis," presentation given at the 4th Annual North American Menopause Society meeting in San Diego, California, September 2–4, 1993.

[4] See separate chapter on tubal ligations.

[5] Northrop quotes L.L. Doyle and others. Human Luteal Function following hysterectomy as assessed by plasma progestin," *Am J Obstet and Gynecol,* 1971, 110. Also N. Siddle, P. Sarrel, M. Whitehead, "The effect of hysterectomy on the age of ovarian failure: identificaiton of a subgroup of women with premature ovarian failure and literature review," *Fertility and Sterility,* 1981, 47, no. 1.

[6] W.B. Cutler, *Hysterectomy: Before and After,* 2.

[7] W.B. Cutler, *Hysterectomy: Before and After, op cit.,* 319.

8 The writing group for the PEPI trial. Effects of estrogens or estrogen/progestin regimens on heart disease risk factors in postmenopausal women. *JAMA,* Jan 1995, 273(3):199–208.

[9] Ellen Grant is a British physician who worked as a pathologist with early researchers on the birth control pill. Her book is available in Canada and the U.K., but not in the U.S.

[10] M. Nachtigall, S.W. Smilen, R.D. Nachtigall, R.H. Nachtigall, L.E. Nachtigall, "Incidence of breast chancer in a 22-year-study of women

receiving estrogen-progestin replacement therapy," *Obstet Gynecol,* Nov 1992, 80(5):827–830.

[11] R.D. Gambrell, Jr., *Hormone Replacement and Breast Cancer,* p. 17. Available from R. Don Gambrell, M.D., Dept. of Physiology and Endocrinology, Dept. of Obstetrics and Gynecology, Medical College of Georgia, Augusta, GA 30912.

[12] Gail Sheehey, *The Silent Passage,* p. 20. She quotes Marc Deitch, medical director of Wyeth-Ayerst, which produces Premarin.

[13] John Lee suggests progesterone increases the sex drive; others suggest it dampens the sex drive.

[14a] D. Zava, "Estrogenic and cell growth-inhibitory properties of genestein and other flavonoids in human breast cancer cells" Submitted for publication April, 1995.

[14b] S. Barnes, "Effect of genestein on in vitro and in vivo models of cancer." *J Nutr,* Mar 1995, 125(3 Suppl):777S-783S. V. Persky, L. Van Horn "Epidemiology of soy and cancer: perspectives and directions." J Nutr, Mar 1995, 125(3 Suppl):709S–712S.

[14c] E.J. Hawrylewicz, J.J. Zapata, W.H. Balir, "Soy and experimental cancer: animal studies," *J Nutr,* Mar 1995, 125 (3 Suppl):689S–708S.

[15] A. Vermeulen, "Adrenal androgens and aging." In: A.R. Gemazzini, J.H.H. Thijssen, P.K. Siiteri, et al (eds)., *Adrenal Androgens,* (New York: Raven Press, 1980), 207.

[16] Don Gambrell, "Progestin and Postmenopausal Women," *The Female Patient,* vol 17, April 1992, p. 52.

[17] Natural progesterone: usage and instructions. Package insert with Pro-Gest Cream, is available from Professional and Technical Services with the product at 1-800-648-8211. Local calls to (503) 226-1010.

[18] L. Speroff, "Hormone Replacement Therapy and the Risk of Breast Cancer."

[19] "Update on Estrogen-Progestin Replacement Therapy," by Dr. Leon Speroff quoting D.W. Kaufman, D.R. Miller, L. Rosenberg, S.P. Helmrich, P. Stolley, D. Schootenfeld, S. Shapiro, "Noncontraceptive Estrogen Use and the Risk of Breast Cancer," *JAMA,* 252:63, 1984.

[20] E. L. Vliet, M.D., "New Perspectives on the Relationship of Hormone Changes to Depression and Anxiety in the Menopause," presentation at the North American Menopause Society meeting, September 1992. Dr. Vliet is a clinical assistant professor at Eastern Virginia Medical School, Norfolk, VA. "Estrogen and Memory in Postmenopausal Women," Barbara B. Sherwin, Ph.D., McGill University, Montreal, Canada. "Estrogens Regulate Brain Structure and Chemistry," Bruce S. McEwen, Ph.D., Laboratory of Neuroendocrinology, New York.

[21] W. Cutler, *Hysterectomy: Before and After,* (Harper and Row: 1988), 222–224. L. Nachtigall, J.R. Heilman, *Estrogen: the Facts Can Change Your Life,* (Los Angeles: The Body Press, 1986), 33–34.

[22] P.O. Warner, Use of oral or subcutaneous (pellet) estradiol 17-β with natural progesterone in 200 patients followed for ten years. This is available from the Menopause Institute of Los Gatos, 700 W. Parr Ave., Suite D, Los Gatos, CA 95030. Or call, (408) 379-8640.

[23] Dr. Katherine O' Hanlan, professor of medicine and associate director of the Gynecologic Cancer Service at Stanford University in Palo Alto, California, says she prescribes Estrace for most of her patients beause "it is pure estradiol." *M-News,* Vol. 2, Issue 2. Dr. Antonio Scommegna, a reproductive endocrinologist at the Menopause Clinic at the University of Illinois Hospital, prefers Estrace because it's more physiologic and it's estradiol. When women become sick on Estrace, he puts women on Premarin then Ogen. *M-News,* Vol 2, Issue 5, September/October, 1992. Telephone 1-(800)-241-MENO for subscription information.

[24] Don Gamrell, "Progestins and Postmenopausal Women," *The Famale Patient,* Vol 17, April 1992, p. 52.

[25] According to Maria Danuta Gray, a British Surgeon

[26] Leon Speroff, Women can have regular periods and estrogen decline.

[27] The writing group for the PEPI trial. Effects of estrogens or estrogen/progestin regimens on heart disease risk factors in postmenopausal women. *JAMA,* Jan 1995, 273(3):199–208.

[27a] *Ibid.*

[28] Dr. Winnifred Cutler mentions Drs. Lorraine Dennerstein and Graham Burrows, Australian researchers, who have found that natural progesterone has a hypnotic effect, more pleasant than the tension and irritability incurred by some women on progestins. *Hysterectomy: Before and After,* p. 166. "L. Dennerstein, G. Burrows, (1986), "Psychological Effects of Progestins in the Post-Menopausal Years," *Maturitas,* 8: 101–106.

[29] J.T. Hargrove, W. S. Maxson, et al. "Menopausal hormone replacement therapy with continuous daily oral micronized estradiol and progesterone," *Obstet & Gynecol,* 1989, 73(4), 606–611. J.T. Hargrove, W.S. Maxson, A.C. Wentz, "Absorption of oral progesterone is influenced by vehicle and particle size," *Am Journ Obstet & Gynecol,* 1989, 161(4), 948–951. This article reports that progesterone taken orally is physiologically active, producing a significant increase in tissue progesterone concentrations in breast, endometrium,and myometrium. Orally administered progesterone also induces histologic and biochemical changes in the endometrium after 10 days of administration in estrogen-primed postmenopausal women. Concommitant oral administration of estradiol and progesterone for 1 year did not cause abnormal proliferation or hyperplasia of the endometrium.

[30] According to Dr. Winnifred Cutler, (*Hysterectomy: Before and After,* pp. 168–69), Dr. Malcolm Whitehead and his colleagues concluded that natural progesterone does not harmfully alter blood lipids and might be useful with estrogen for menopause. See article listed under note 4. See also L. Fahraeus, U. Larsson-Cohn, L. Wallentin, (1983), "L-norgestrol and progesterone have different influences on plasma lipoproteins," *Eur. J. Clin. Invest.,* 13:447. See also U.B. Ottoson, B. G. Johansson, B. von Schoultz, (1985), "Subfractions of highly density lipoprotein cholesterol during estrogen replacement therapy: comparison between progestins and natural progesterone." *Am. J. Obstet. Gynecol.* 1151:746.

[31] Kathryn Morris and Sue Ungar. Natural Pogesterone Surpasses Provera. Available from Hormone Balancing for Women, (408) 464-7777.

[32] Personal communication between Dr. Phillip Warner and the author.

[33] J.C. Prior, Y.M. Vigna, et al., "Spinal bone loss and ovulatory disturbances," *New Engl Journ Med,* Nov 1990, 323(18):1221–1227.

Chapter Eleven

[1] Mark S. Gold, M.D., *The Good News About Depression: Breakthrough medical treatments that can work for you,* (New York: Bantam Books, 1995), p. 327.

[2] Judith Bardwick, *The Psychology of Women,* (Harper & Row, 1971).

[3] T. M. Itil, "Rebirth of Hormones in Psychiatry," *Psychiatric Journ of the Univ of Ottawa,* 1976, 1(3):105–112, p. 107.

[4] *Ibid.,* p. 105.

[5a] Edward Klaiber, M.D., Donald Broverman, M.D., and William Vogel, M.D., "Estrogen Therapy for Severe Persistent Depressions in Women," *The Archives of General Psychiatry* (Vol. 6, May, 1979).

[5b] Edward Klaiber, M.D., Donald Broverman, M.D., and William Vogel, M.D., "Estrogens and Central Nervous System Function: Electroencephalography, Cognition, and Depression," in Richard C. Friedman, ed., *Behavior and the Menstrual Cycle* (Marcel Dekker, Inc.: 1982).

[6] Personal communication with Edward Klaiber, M.D., April 18, 1995. Wilkinson, et al., editors, *Brain Research,* 1979, 168:652–655.

[7] D. Keefe and F. Naftolin, "Brain Neurochemistry and Mood," Samuel Smith and Isaac Schiff, *Modern Management of Premenstrual Syndrome,* 1992, pp. 55–70.

[8] *Ibid.,* p. 56.

[9] For example, J. W. Studd and R. N. Smith, "Estrogens and Depression in Women," in Rogerio A. Lobo, *Treatment of the Postmenopausal Woman,* Raven Press, New York, 1994) pp. 129–136.

[10] C. B. Ballinger, "Psychiatric aspects of the menopause," *Br J Psychiatry,* 1990, 1256:773–878.

[11a] J. Studd, S. Chakravarti, and D. Oram, "The climacteric," in R. B. Greenblatt and J. W. Studd, eds., *Clinics in obstetrics and gynaecology, vol 4(1): The Menopause*, (Philadelphia: Saunders, 1977).

[11b] G. T. Bungay, M. P. Vessy, and C. K. McPherson, "Study of symptoms in middle life with special reference to the menopause," *Br Med J*, 1980, 2:181–183.

[12] J. C. Montgomery, L. Appleby, M. Brincat, E. Versi, A. Tapp, P. B. C. Fenwick, and J. W. W. Studd, "Effect of oestrogen and testosterone implants on psychological disorders in the climacteric," *Lancet*, 1987, 1:297–299.

[13] E. C. Ditkoff, W. G. Crary, M. Cristo, and R. A. Lobo, "Estrogen improves psychological function in asymptomatic postmenopause women," *Obstet Gynecol*, 1991, 78:991–995.

[14] B. B. Sherwin, and M. M. Gelfand, "Sex steroids and affect in the surgical menopause; a double blind cross over study," *Psychoneuroendocrinology*, 1985, 10:325–335, pp. 57 and 58.

[15] "New Perspectives on the Hormonal Relationships to Affective Disorders in the Perimenopause," *NAACOG's Clinical Issues* book on mid-life women's health, Oct/Dec 1991, 2(4):453–471.

[16] E. L. Vliet, "New perspectives on the relationship of hormone changes to depression and anxiety in the menopause," Poster presentation at the Scientific Program of the North American Menopause Society, Sept 17–20, 1993.

[17] B. B. Sherwin, "The effect of sex steroids on brain mechanisms relating to mood and sexuality." In Jacques Lorrain, et al, eds., *Comprehensive Management of Menopause* (New York: Springer-Verlag, 1994), pp. 327–333.

[18] Among Dr. Arpel's articles are: "Ovarian hormones and the female brain: from PMS to menopause," *San Francisco Medicine*, Dec. 1993, 19–37, and "The female brain estrogen continuum: from PMS to menopause: a review of supporting data" (manuscript under submission).

Chapter Twelve

[1] However this is an area of contention. For the position saying that there are few side effects with tubal ligations, see "Posttubal sterilization syndrome: does it exist?" *The Contraception Report*, Baylor College of Medicine, 1993 4(4):4–10.

[2] Dr. Nils Lauersen and Eileen Stukane, *Listen to Your Body*, (Berkley Books, pp. 353–355.

[3] Sandra Cabot, *Don't Let Your Hormones Run Your Life*. See chapter on tubal sterilization. Dr. Cabot's books are all worth purchasing. She has several including a general book on gynecology and a book on menopause. They are available from Women's Health Advisory Service, PO. Box 217, Paddington, 2021, NSW, Australia. Their FAX number is 0116123607247 and includes the country and city codes for Sydney, Australia. Remember the time

difference; Australia is 16 to 17 hours ahead of California, so call after 2:00 P.M.). Dr. Cabot has a new book called *Smart Medicine for Menopause* published in the U.S., by Avery Publishing in 1995.

[4a] De Stefano, *et al*, "Long term risk of menstrual disturbance after tubal sterilization," *Am. J. Obstet, and Gynaecol.*, Aug. 1, 1985, Vol 152., No. 7, pt. 1, pp. 835–841.

[4b] "Factors seen as links to posttubal ligation syndrome," *Contraception Tech. Update*, Feb. 1986, Vol. 7, No. 2, pp. 13–15.

[4c] J. Cattanach, "Oestrogen deficiency after tubal ligation," *Lancet*, April 13, 1985, pp. 847–849.

[4d] R.J. Stock, "Sequelae of tubal ligation: An analysis of 75 consecutive hysterectomies," *South. Med. J.*, Oct. 1984, Vol. 77, No. 10, 1255–1260.

[4e] J. Cattanach, "Post-tubal sterilization problems correlated with ovarian steroidogenesis," *Contraception*, Nov. 1988, Vol. 38.

[4f] A. A. Templeton, "Hysterectomy following sterilization," *British Journal Obstetrics & Gynaecology;* Oct. 1982, Vol. 89, No. 10, 845–888.

[5] Sandra Cabot, *Hormones, Ibid.*, p. 85.

[6] But note that Dr. Joel Hargrove and Guy Abrahams say that progesterone is low and serum estradiol is high. See their study on 29 women with posttubal ligation syndrome,"Endocrine Profile of Patients with Post-Tubal-Ligation Syndrome," *Journal of Reproductive Medicine*, July 1981, p. 362. I think that, in most cases, Dr. Cabot is correct in saying that estrogen levels drop.

[7] Vicki Hufnagel, *No More Hysterectomies*, pp. 228–229. Dr. Hufnagel is a surgeon who advocates myomectomies (surgical removal of uterine fibroids) instead of hysterectomies.

[8] Fistulas are abnormal openings that allow substances to travel to the wrong places—in this case, a gap in the fallopian tube that allows endometrial tissue to pass out of the tube and attach to the wrong places as endometriosis.

[9] Dr. Winnifred Cutler believes that if you have a hysterectomy you should try to retain the ovaries. Many doctors will routinely remove them if a women is over 40 or 45, for two inappropriate reasons: 1. they presume that the ovaries are useless and produce no hormones; 2. they believe that retained ovaries may become cancerous. In answer to the first point, Cutler says that while the ovaries stop cycling in 50 percent of hysterectomized women, they may keep cycling for years in the other 50 percent, and the hormones they produce are important.

The second point was based on published research that was reported incorrectly. There is no increased risk for ovarian cancer after a hysterectomy. *Hysterectomy: Before and After,* Harper and Row, New York, 1988. Note that a surgeon may need to go back in to remove the ovaries 7 out of 100 times.

[10] J. Rausch, "Psychobiological aspects of the menopause," in Jacques Lorrain, ed., et al, *Comprehensive Management of Menopause*, (Springer-Verlag, 1994), p. 322. He quotes: C. B. Ballinger, "Psychiatric morbidity and the menopause: survey of a gynaecological outpatient clinic," *Br J Psychiatry*, 1977, 131:83–89. M. Bernardi, M. Sandrini, A. V. Vergoni, et al., "Influence of gonadotropin-induced 'depression' in mice: a behavioral and binding study," *Eur J Pharmacol*, 1990, 187:501–506. S. Chakravarti, W. P. Collins, et al., "Endocrine changes and symptomatology after oophorectomy in premenopausal women," *Br J Obstet Gynaecol*, 1977, 84:769–775.

[11] D. Poad and E. P. Arnold, "Sexual function after pelvic surgery in women," *Aust NZ J Obstet Gynaecol*, Aug 1994, 34(4):471–474. This study of 200 women reports that pain on intercourse developed in 10 women who had never had it before. Of those who had it preoperatively, it stopped in 12 out of 23. Reduced libido was noticed in 16 of 54 (29%), reduced lubrication in 21 (38%), reduced genital sensation in 10 (18%). Lack of information on the potential effects of surgery on sexuality was identified as a major deficit and of considerable concern to 35 of the 66 women. Dr. Christiane Northrup reports that in studies in the United Kingdom, 33 to 46 percent report a decreased sexual response after a hysterectomy-oophorectomy (removal of the uterus and ovaries). *Women's Bodies, Women's Wisdom* (New York: Bantam Books, p. 179, quoting Zussmann, et al., "Sexual Response after Hysterectomy: Recent studies and Reconsideration of psychogenesis," *Amer Journ Obstet and Gynecol*, Aug 1981, 140(7):725–729. Northrop continues, "Even if the ovaries are left intact, some women experience orgasm differently after hysterectomy, probably because the cervix and uterus act as a trigger-point for orgasm."

Chapter Thirteen

[1] *Wellness Letter*, University of California at Berkeley, Vol. 8, Issue 10, July, 1992.

[2] Read Kristin White, *Diet and Cancer*, who says that throughout the Western industrialized world, colon, breast, and prostate cancers are major killers. By comparison, breast cancer among Japanese women was rare for most of this century. She says, "Americans consume about forty percent of their calories in the form of fat, while the Japanese fat consumption accounts for only about 15 to 20 percent of their calories." (Quoted from a section of her book reprinted in *Vegetarian Times*, September, 1984.) White says that breast cancer takes several generations to develop, and that diet in childhood is critical.

[3] ". . . some biomedical experts believe that the simple act of detecting cancer accounts for a longer survival time without enhancing the quality of life. They conclude that while the cancer is discovered sooner and at an earlier stage, this does not actually promote any greater longevity. Women still die of the disease at the same age, but now live with the fear and certain

knowledge of their disease. Because the disease is detected earlier, they have the awareness of it but no guarantee of cure." Winnifred Cutler, *Hysterectomy: Before and After,* (Harper and Row, New York, 1988).

"There is no convincing evidence, as yet, of net health benefits, in terms of reduced mortality or morbidity, accruing to women of any age who practice BSE [breast self-examination] . . . Whether unequivocal evidence of BSE effectiveness can actually be produced in the social climate of widespread BSE promotion is very doubtful. In the meantime, there are substantial risks, as well as many personal costs, for the overwhelming majority of young women who present with breast masses found by BSE, only to have unpleasant subsequent investigations reveal no pathology of significance." J. W. Frank and V. Mai, "Breast self-examination in young women: more harm than good?" *Lancet* 1985 2:654–7.

[4a] D. M. Eddy, V. Hasselblad, W. McGivney, and W. Hendee, "The Value of mammography screening in women under age 50 years. *JAMA* (1988) 259L10:1512–1519.

[4b] J. C. Bailar, "Mammography before age 50 years?" *JAMA* (1988) 259:10: 1548–1549.

[5a] P. Skrabanek, "False premises and false promises of breast cancer screening." *Lancet* 1985; 2:316–20.

[5b] C. R. Lowe, "Breast cancer," *Screening in Medical Care. Reviewing the Evidence* (Nuffield Provincial Hospitals Trust, London: Oxford University Press, 1968) p. 33.

[5c] Both quoted in Tony Dixon, "Breast Cancer: The Debates Continue," *Canadian Family Physician,* Vol 33: April, 1987, pp. 817–818.

[6] Haydn Bush, *Science,* September 1984, p. 34.

[7] Leon Speroff, M.D., "Tamoxifen: Special Considerations for Clinicians," Dr. Speroff has also written many other articles, including "Hormone replacement therapy and the risk of breast cancer."

[8] P. Siiteri, "Hormones, growth and function of the breast," Presentation at the North American Menopause Society, Sep. 1994.

[9] C. W. Lovell, "Breast cancer incidence with parenteral estradiol and testosterone replacement therapy," Presentation at the North American Menopause Society, Sep. 1994.

[10] You can get Don Gambrell, Jr., M.D.'s booklet *Hormone Replacement Therapy and Breast Cancer,* Revised 1992, by writing to R. Don Gambrell, Jr., M.D., Clinical Professor, Department of Physiology and Endocrinology, Department of Obstetrics and Gynecology, Medical College of Georgia, Atlanta, GA 30912.

[11a] For example, J. A. Eden, B. G. Wren, S. Nand, "A study of the effect of hormone replacement therapy on all-cause mortality and recurrence rate in women with breast carcinoma," Fourth Annual Meeting of the North American Menopause Society, San Diego, California, Sep 24, 1995. Dr. Don

Gambrell quotes three prominent gynecologic oncologists who advocate estrogen use in women successfully treated for breast cancer. "In view of the lack of evidence relating estrogen to exacerbations of existing breast cancer, it may be in the best interest of our patients to liberalize our attitude to renewed hormonal exposure in patients with successfully managed breast cancer."

[11b] A. G. Wile and P. J. DiSaia, "Hormones and breast cancer," *Am J Surg*, 1989, 157:438.

"It is no longer justifiable to deprive a woman with a history of breast cancer treatment of a hormonal therapy capable of safely relieving symptoms which are making her life intolerable." B. A. Stoll, "Hormone replacement therapy in women treated for breast cancer," *Eur J Cancer Clin Oncol*, 1989, 25:1989.

"Although there is little or no experience with estrogen use in the woman treated previously for breast cancer, circumstantial evidence suggests that it is not contraindicated in all such cases." W. T. Creasman, "Estrogen replacement therapy: is previously treated cancer a contraindication?" *Obstet Gynecol*, 1991, 77:308.

[12] R. D. Gambrell, Jr., (see ref 10) *op. cit.*, pp. 17, 18. "A good prognostic indicator for survival from breast cancer is the presence of estrogen and progesterone receptors in cancerous tissue." Dr. Gambrell quotes about six studies supporting his thesis.

[13] Answer by George E. Block, M.D., "Questions and Answers," *JAMA*, October 4, 1985—Vol. 254, No. 13, p. 1817.

Chapter Fourteen
[1] For information on Dr. Barnes' work, contact the Broda Barnes Foundation at (203) 261–2101, or write to them at P. O. Box 98, Trumble, CT 06611.

Chapter Fifteen
[1] A. C. Guyton, *Basic Human Physiology: Normal function and mechanisms of disease* (Philadelphia: W.B. Saunders Co., 1971), p. 667.

[2a] W. Krause, "Hormonal changes in the elderly from the viewpoint of the andrologist," *Fortschr Med*, Jun 1990, 108(19):371–374. Although the aging male experiences a decrease in genital function, it is not as pronounced or as complete as in the female ovary, so that this process is only remotely similar to the climacteric. The most important sign is a decrease in erection frequency and other sexual functions. This is, however, not due simply to a decrease in testosterone levels. Numerous studies have clearly shown that the number of sexual performances is independent of current testosterone levels. A qualitative change in Leydig cell function can, however, be concluded from the latent androgen deficit, reduced stimulability of the Leydig cells, and the frequent anomalies of the levels of such other hormones as FSH and LH in patients with impotence. Thus, the treatment of impotence with oral or depot testosterone is indicated in proven manifest or latent androgen deficiency.

[2b] J. Noldus and H. Huland, "Erectile dysfunction and hypogonadism. Is routine endocrine screening necessary?" *Urologe A,* Jan 1994, 33(1):73–75.

[2c] K. Lehmann, W. Schopke, et al., "Which hormone determinations are necessary in the initial assessment of erectile dysfunction?" *Schweiz Rundsch Med Prax,* Sep 1994, 83(37):1030–1033. They suggest that one measurement of testosterone is inadequate. If testosterone levels are low, repeated measurements, combined with LH, FSH, and prolactin will identify erection disorders due to endocrine disease.

[2d] W. Krause, "The male climacteric. A responsibility for dermatologic andrology?" *Hautarzt,* Sep 1994, 45(9):593–598. This study says that there are no adequate institutions for the treatment of the corresponding male complaints. Like ovarian secretion of estrogens, which declines and thus causes the female climacteric syndrome, the endocrine metabolism of the testes decreases with increasing age. The period of this decrease is far more extended than that of estrogen secretion in women. Several recent studies have shown evidence that any disease (irrespective of its kind) influences the decrease of testosterone levels more markedly than a man's age. This particular study finds that sexual dysfunction often occurs because of drug interactions. It indicates that the endocrine changes predate the sexual dysfunction (decrease in healthy men in total testosterone of 1 percent per year; decrease of free testosterone 1.2% per year).

[3a] H. Gall, W. Bahren, et al., "Results of multidisciplinary assessment of patients with erectile dysfunction," *Hautarzt,* Jul 1990, 41(7):353–359. 74.5 percent of the 326 patients studies had erectile problems because of vascular disorders.

[3b] J. E. Morley and F. E. Kaiser, "Sexual function with advancing age," *Med Clin North Am,* Nov 1989, 73(6):1483–1495. Impotence occurs commonly with advancing age. Approximately one half of impotent males over 50 years of age have a vascular cause of their impotence. Vascular impotence is often the harbinger of vascular disease in other organs of the body. Hypogonadism occurs in up to one fourth of older men.

[4] In Gail Sheehy's article "The Unspeakable Passage: Is there a male menopause?" *Vanity Fair,* April 1993, p. 164–227, Sheehy quotes Dr. Spark. "Smoking is absolutely devastating—it's probably the major cause of male sexual dysfunction. Smoking damages the tiny blood vessels in the penis that must enlarge to accept the substantial onrush of blood during the course of an erection." (page 224)

[5] " 'Vasectomy may be another factor that brings on viropause,' according to Dr. Carruthers. Twenty percent of his patients have had a vasectomy [though this is the proportion of men in general society who have had it done]. 'With a complex organ like the testis, I don't think you can shut down one half of the factory without influencing production in the other.' Dr. Lue affirms that a vasectomy can impair blood circulation to the testes." *Ibid,* 224.

[6a] W. Pierpaoli, "The pineal gland as ontogenetic scanner of reproduction, immunity and aging. The aging clock," *Ann N Y Acad Sci,* Nov 1994, 741:46–49. H. A. Schmid, P. J. Requintina, et al., "Calcium, calcification, and melatonin biosynthesis in the human pineal gland: a postmortem study into age-related factors," *J Pineal Res,* May 1994, 16(4):178–183.

[6b] R. Reiter, "Pineal function during aging: attenuation of the melatonin rhythm and its neurological consequences," *Acta Neurobiol Exp (Warsz),* 1994, 54 Suppl:31–39.

[6c] B. Poeggeler, P. J. Reiter, D. X. Tan, et al., "Melatonin, hydroxyl radical-mediated oxidative damage, and aging: a hypothesis," *J Pineal Res,* May 1993, 14(4):151–168.

[6d] P. E. Kloeden, R. Rossler, and O. E. Rossler, "Artificial life extension. The epigenic approach," *Ann N Y Acad Sci,* May 1994, 719:474–482. V. A. Leskinov and Pierpaoli, "Pineal cross-transplantation (old-to-young and vice versa) as evidence for an endogenous aging clock," *Ann N Y Acad Sci,* May 1994, 719:456–460.

[6e] W. Humbert and P. Pevet, "The decrease of pineal melatonin production with age. Causes and consequences," *Ann N Y Acad Sci,* May 1994, 719:43–63. R. J. Reiter, D. X. Tan, et al., "Melatonin as a free radical scavenger: implications for aging and age-related diseases," *An N Y Acad Sci,* May 1994, 719:1–12.

[6f] D. Slowinska-Klencka and A. Lewinski, "Role of melatonin in human physiology and pathology. II. Involvement of melatonin in pathogenesis of affective and chronobiological disorders. Melatonin and the aging process. Melatonin and neoplasms," *Postepy Hig Med Dosw,* 1993, 47(4):267–276.

[7] A. J. Morales, J. J. Nolan, J. C. Nelson, and S. S. Yen, "Effects of replacement dose of dehydroepiandrosterone [DHEA] in men and women of advancing age," *J Clin Endocrinol Metab,* Jun 1994, 78(6):1360–1367. This study reports that aging in humans is accompanied by a progressive decline in the secretion of the adrenal androgens DHEA and DHEAS, paralleling that of the GH-insulin-like growth factor (GH-IGF-1) system. They studied the effect of a replacement dose of DHEA in 13 men and 17 women, 40–70 years of age. The study showed a remarkable increase in perceived physical and psychological well-being for both men (67 percent) and women (84 percent). The study concludes that giving DHEA increased the bioavailability of IGF-1, a growth factor also involved in the aging process.

[8a] C. J. Rosen, "Growth hormone, insulin-growth factors, and the senescent skeleton: Ponce de Leon's Fountain revisited?" *J Cell Biochem,* Nov 1994, 56(3):348–356.

[8b] R. J. Hodes, "Frailty and disability: can growth hormone or other trophic agents make a difference?" *J Am Geriatr Soc,* Nov 1994, 42:11:1208–1211.

[8c] S. E. Borst, W. J. Millard, and D. T. Lowenthal, "Growth hormone, exercise, and aging; the future of therapy for the frail elderly," *J Am Geriatr Soc,* May 1994, 42(5):528–535.

[9a] T. Rosen, T. Hansson, et al., "Reduced bone mineral content in adult patients with growth hormone deficiency, *Acta Endocrinol* (Copenh), Sep 1993, 129(3):188–194.

[9b] There were at least 30 cases of Creutzfeldt-Jakob disease (CJD) after treatment with growth hormone from animal cadavers. These patients developed neurological problems which evolved in a few months to severe neurological deterioration, insanity, and death. V. de Billette and T. Prader, "Iatrogenic Creutzfeldt-Jakob disease. Lessons from cases secondary to extracted growth hormone in France," *Transfus Clin Biol*, 1994, 1(5):333–337. J. Goujard, "Growth hormone and Creutzfeldt-Jakob disease," *Rev Epidemiol Sante Publique*, 1993, 41(6):513–514.

[9c] R. H. Knauer, "Creutzfeldt-Jakob epidemic startles France. The cause is apparently a contaminated growth hormone—parallels to bovine psychosis," *Fortsch Med*, Jun 1993, 111(17):59–60. But, usually, as mentioned in the main text, growth hormone is made in the laboratory.

[10a] See, "A Shot at Youth," *Health*, Nov–Dec, 1993, pp. 39–47.

[10b] Samuel Yen, "Neuroendocrinology of menopause," Keynote speaker, Scientific Program, North American Menopause Society's 4th Annual meeting, held in San Diego, California, Sep 2, 1993.

[11] Particular thanks are extended to Richard S. Wilkinson, M.D., for his generous help with this chapter. See his lecture notes on testosterone, presented at the AAEM national convention, October 1994.

[12] R. L. Byyny and L. Speroff, *A Clinical Guide to the Care of Older Women*, (Baltimore: Williams and Wilkins, 1990), p. 111.

[13] *Ibid.*, p. 111.

[14] Georges Debled, unpublished English translation of his book, *Beyond This Limit, Your Ticket Is Always Valid*, chapter 7.

[15] The Kegel exercise involves contracting the band of muscles that encircle the vagina or the prostate. To strengthen the muscle, both sexes can practice contracting it regularly. Dr. Christiane Northrup tells women how to do it: When you urinate, stop the flow of urination two or three times. As the pubococcygeous muscle (called PC) strengthens, you become able to distinguish it from other muscles. Northrup suggests to begin contracting the PC muscle three times a day, counting to three each time you do it. You can build up to counting to ten each time and doing ten repetitions of ten counts three times a day. *Women's Bodies, Women's Wisdom*, (New York: Bantam Books, 1995, p. 236.

[16] R. L. Young, "Androgens in postmenopausal therapy," *Menopause Management*, May 1993, 22.

[17] *Ibid.*

[18] A. Vermeulen, "Adrenal adrogens and aging," in A. R. Gemazzini, J. H. H. Thijssen, P. K. Siiteri, et al (eds), *Adrenal Androgens* (New York: Raven Press, 1980), p. 207.

[19a] B. B. Sherwin and M. M. Gelfand, "The role of androgen in the maintenance of sexual functioning in oophorectomized women."

[19b] B. B. Sherwin, "A comparative analysis of the role of androgen in human male and female sexual behavior: Behavioral specificity, critical thresholds, and sensitivity," *Psychobiology,* 1988, 16:416–425.

[19c] *Psychosom Med,* 1987, 49:397–409.

[19d] A. D. Mooradian, J. E. Morley, et al., "Biological actions of androgens," *Endocrine Rev,* 1987, 8:1–28.

[20a] J. Møller, *Testosterone Treatment of Cardiovascular Diseases:* Principles and Clinical Experiences (Berlin: Springer-Verlag, 1984).

[20b] J. Møller, *Cholesterol:* Interactions with Testosterone and Cortisol in Cardiovascular Diseases (Berlin: Springer-Verlag, 1987). These books are out of print, but can be obtained from the Broda Barnes Foundation (see Chapter 15 for address).

[21] A. Phillips, *Arteriosclerosis and Thrombosis* (Internal Medicine World Report, 1994), 14:701–716.

[22] R. Wilkinson, Lecture on testosterone, presentation held at the American Academy of Environmental Medicine.

[23] M. Tsushima, et al., "Primary prevention of atheroschlerotic vascular disease with ethylnandrol—an interim report of four year observations," *Japanese Circulation Journal,* Mar 1975, 39:285ff.

[24] M. A. Lesser, "Testosterone propionate therapy in one hundred cases of angina pectoris," *Journ Clin Endocr,* 1946, 6:549–557.

[25a] According to Michael Hansen, M.D., who follows the work of Jens Møller, M.D., of Copenhagen, 60–80 per cent of men with clotting disorders may need testosterone.

See also G. R. Fearnley, "Increase of blood fibronolytic activity by testosterone," *Lancet,* July 21, 1962:128–132.

[25b] J. F. Davidson, et al., "Fibronolytic enhancement by stanozolol: a double blind trial," *Brit Journ of Haematol,* 1972, 22, 543.

[26a] M. D. Jaff, "Effect of testosterone cyprionate on post exercise ST segment depression," *Brit Heart Journ,* 1977, 39, 1217–1222.

[26b] R. Driscoll and C. Thompson, "Salivary testosterone levels and major depressive illness in men," [letter] *Br J Psychiatry,* Jul 1993, 163:122–123.

[27a] R. S. Swerdloff and C. Wang, "Androgen deficiency and aging in men," *West J Med,* Nov 1993, 159(5):579–585.

[27b] A. M. Matsumoto, "Andropause—are reduced androgen levels in aging men physiologically important?" *Ibid,* 618–620.

[28a] A. R. Gaby, "Natural treatment for benign prostatic hyperplasia," *Medical Nutrition Update for Doctors.*

Note also H. J. Schneider, E. Honold, and T. Masuhr, "Treatment of benign prostatic hyperplasia. Results of a treatment study with the phytogenic combination of Sabal extract WS 1473 and Urtica extract WS 1031 in urologic specialty practices," *Fortschr Med*, Jan 1995, 113(3):37–40.

[28b] G. Champault, J. C. Patel, and A. M. Bonnard, "A double-blind trial of an extract of the plant Serenoa in benign prostatic hyperplasia," *Br J Clin Pharmacol*, 1984, 18:461–462.

[28c] E. Cirillo-Marucco et al., "Extract of Serenoa repens (permixon) in the early treatment of prostatic hypertrophy," *Urologia*, 1983, 50:1269–1277.

[28d] V. Tripodi, M. Giancaspro, M. Pascarella, G. D. Pannella, and F. Attanasio, "Treatment of prostatic hypertrophy with Serenoa repens extract," *Med Praxis*, 1983, 4:41–46.

[28e] P. Bassi, et al., "Standardized Pygeum africanum extract in the treatment of benign prostatic hypertrophy," *Minerva Urol Nefrol*, 1987, 39:45–50.

[29] F. Borhan-Manesh and J. B. Farnum JB, "Methyltestosterone-induced cholestasis. The importance of disproportionately low serum alkaline phosphatase level," *Arch Intern Med*, Sep 1989, 149(9): 2127–2129. This study describes a 64-year-old man who developed cholestatic jaundice after receiving 20–40 mg. of methyltestosterne daily for six months for impotence. A normal or mildly elevated alkaline phosphatase level disproportionate to the level of hyperbilirubinemia is characteristic of this phenomenon. Since patients may be reluctant to admit they take MT, this pattern of liver function might offer a clue to the cause of the problem.

[30] Gail Sheehy, "The Unspeakable Passage: Is there a male menopause?" *Vanity Fair*, April 1993, p. 226.

[31a] B. Urman, S. M. Pride, and I. B. H. Yuen, "Elevated serum testosterone, hirsuitism, and virilism associated with combined androgen-estrogen hormone replacement therapy," *Obstet Gynecol*, Apr 1991, 77(4):595–598.

[31b] Harrison's *Textbook of Medicine*, 12th edition says, "All androgens carry the risk of inducing virilization in women. Among the early manifestations are acne, coarsening of the voice, and development of hirsuitism. Menstrual irregularities are common. If treatment is discontinued as soon as these effects develop, the manifestations may slowly subside." It continues that if treatment is continued, symptoms may be irreversible.

[32] R. L. Young, *Menopause Management*, May 1993, p. 24.

[33] Barbara Sherwin, "The effect of sex steroids on brain mechanisms relating to mood and sexuality," in Jacques Lorrain, et. al., eds., *Comprehensive Management of Menopause* (New York: Springer-Verlag, 1994), p. 327.

Chapter Sixteen

[1a] J. R. Lee, "Osteoporosis reversal: the role of progesterone," *Int Clin Rev*, 1991, 10(3):384–391.

[1b] J. R. Lee, "Osteoporosis reversal with transdermal progesterone. *Lancet*, 1990, 336:1327.

[1c] J. R. Lee, "Is natural progesterone the missing link in osteoporosis prevention and treatment? *Med Hypotheses,* 1991, 35:316–318.

[2a] J. C. Prior, Y. Vigna, and N. Alojado, "Progesterone and the prevention of osteoporosis," *Can J Obstet Gynecol Women's Health Care,* 1991, 3(4):178–184.

[2b] J. C. Prior, "Progesterone as a Bone-Tropic Hormone," *Endocr Rev,* 1990, 11(2):336–398.

[2c] R. Lindsay, D. M. Hart, D. Purdie, et al., "Comparative effects of oestrogen and a progestogen on bone loss in postmenopausal women," *Clinical Science and Molecular Medicine,* 1978, 54:193–195.

[2d] J. C. Gallagher, W. T. Kable, and D. Goldgar, "Effect of progestin therapy on cortical and trabecular bone: comparison with estrogen," *Am J Med,* 1991, 90:171–178.

[3] Other physicians have certainly found side effects with natural progesterone and even with the low-dose transdermal creams.

[4] An interview with John R Lee, M.D., by Neal D. Barnard, M.D., "Natural Progesterone: Is estrogen the wrong hormone?" *Community Endeavor News,* July 1994, p. 17.

[5] E. Baracat, M. Simoes, et al., "Endometrial histomorphometric study after oral and transdermal estrogen therapy in menopause," Poster Presentation at the Scientific Program of the North American Menopause Society, San Diego, Sep 2–4, 1993.

[6a] R. D. Gambrell, Jr., "Progestogens in Postmenopausal Women," *The Female Patient,* April 17, 1992, 33–52.

[6b] "Effects of estrogen or estrogen/progestin regimens on heart disease: Risk factors in postmenopausal women," The PEPI Trial. *JAMA,* Jan 1995, 273(3):199–208.

Chapter Seventeen

[1] D. Zava, "The Phytoestrogen Paradox," *The Soy Connection,* 1994, 3(1):1–4.

[2a] *The China Diet Study,* (920 pp.) was discussed in an article, "Huge Diet Study Indicts Fat and Meat," by Dr. Hans Diehl, in *Lifeline Health Letter,* September–October, 1990. The points I list in the text summarize his outline.

See also J. Chen and J. Gao, "The Chinese total diet study in 1990. Part II. Nutrients," *J AOAC Int,* Nov–Dec 1993, 76(6):1193–1205.

[2b] And J. Chen and J. Gao, "The Chinese total diet study in 1990. Part II. Chemical Contaminents," *J AOAC Int,* Nov–Dec 1993, 76(6):1206–1213.

Appendix Three

[1a] A. Loviselli, F. Velluzzi, R. Pala, A. Marcello A, et al., "Circulating antibodies to DNA-related antigens in patients with autoimmune thyroid disorders," *Autoimmunity,* 1992, 14(1):33–36.

[1b] M. Neufeld, N. Maclaren, and R. Blizzard, "Autoimmune polyglandular syndromes. *Pediatr Ann,* 1980, 9(4):43–53.

[1c] M. Gryczynska, A. Baumann-Antczak, and J. Kosowicz, "Polyendocrine autoimmunity in thyroid disease," *Endokrynol Pol*, 1993, 44(1):5–11. This study indicates that thyroid diseases of autoimmune origin (Graves' disease and autoimmune thyroiditis) can be regarded as manifestation of some more generalized autoimmune process. Forty-five patients (25 with Graves'; 20 with autoimmune thyroiditis) were checked for antiadrenal and antipituitary autoantibodies. In the majority of patients with autoimmune diseases of the thyroid, the presence of both these other autoantibodies were found.

In the 20 with hypothyroidism, 13 had anti-adrenal antibodies; 13 had anti-pituitary antibodies. Among the 25 with Graves', 19 had both types.

In the majority of patients with autoimmune thyroid problems, the titers of both types were high, but none of them were symptomatic.

See also K. Bouchou, M. Andre, P. Cathebras, et al., "Thyroid diseases and multiple autoimmune syndromes. Clinical and immunogenetic aspects apropros of 11 cases," *Rev Med Interne*, 1995, 16(4):283–7. This abstract reports 11 cases of multiple autoimmune syndrome, and a total of 15 different autoimmune diseases. It suggests that Graves' disease and Hashimoto's thyroiditis are a common feature of multiple autoimmune syndromes and antithyroid antibodies are a constant among their patients.

[2] B. Catz, "Hypothyroidism," in S.A. Falk, ed., *Thyroid Disease: Endocrinology, Surgery, Nuclear Medicine, and Radiotherapy* (New York: Raven Press, Ltd., 1990), pp. 279–288. See also C. Patrick, "Organ-specific autoimmune diseases," *Immunol Ser*, 1993, 58:423–436.

[3] M. Neufeld, N. MacLaren, and R. Blizzard, "Autoimmune polyglandular syndromes," *Pediatr Ann* 1980, 9(4), 43–53.

[4] I. M. Roitt, P. R. Hutchings, K. I. Dawe, et al., "The forces driving autoimmune disease," *J Autoimmun*, Apr 1992, 5 Suppl A:11–26.

[5a] **Polyglandular autoimmune syndromes:** F. Chuard, R. Munger, P. Kaeser, and B. Ruedi, "Polyglandular autoimmune syndrome," *Rev Med Suisse Romand*, Nov 1993, 113(11):897–900.

[5b] M. A. Graber and H. A. Freed, "Polyglandular autoimmune syndrome: a cause of multiple and sequential endocrine emergencies," *Am J Emerg Med*, Mar 1992, 10(2):130–132. This study says that the polyglandular autoimmune syndromes are a rare, inherited constellation of disorders characterized by multiple endocrine end-organ failure.

[5c] **Diabetes mellitus:** R. E. Davis, V, J, McCann, and K. G. Stanton, "Type 1 diabetes and latent pernicious anemia," *Med J Aust*, Feb 3, 156(3): 160–162. Links diabetes mellitus, pernicious anemia, and hypothyroidism.

[5d] N. Chikuba, S. Akazawa SY. Yamaguchi, et al., "Type 1 (insulin-dependent) diabetes mellitus with coexisting autoimmune thyroid disease in Japan," *Intern Med*, Sep 1992, 31(9):1076–1080.

[5e] K. Bech, M. Hoier-Madsen, U. Feldt-Rasmussen, B. M. Jensen, L. Molsted-Pedersen, and C. Kuhl, "Thyroid function and autoimmune

manifestations in insulin-dependent diabetes mellitus during and after pregnancy," *Acta Endocrinol* (Copenh), May 1991, 124(5):534–539.

[6a] **Addison's disease:** Note that there is a difference between what is termed idiopathic (of unknown cause) Addison's disease and Schmidt Syndrome. The former is an isolated problem, the second is polyglandular. This is because two different cytochrome enzymes are involved in the different forms of Addison's. See O. Winqvist, J. Gustafsson, F. Rorsman, et al., "Two different cytochrome P450 enzymes are the adrenal antigens in autoimmune polyendocrine syndrome type I and Addison's disease," *J Clin Invest,* Nov 1993, 92(5):2377–2388.

On the link with thyroid, see K. Schmidtt, G. Tulzer, and W. Tulzer, "Polyglandular type I autoimmune syndrome," *Wien Klin Wochenschr,* 1992, 104(11):325–327.

[6b] R. Govindarajan and O. P. Galpin, "Coexistence of Addison's disease, ulcerative colitis, hypothyroidism, and pernicious anemia," [letter] *J Clin Gastroenterol,* Jul 1992, 15(1):82–83. In this study, two identical twin sisters developed PAS I, with hypoparathyroidism and Addison's disease. One of them also developed diabetes mellitus, and low ovarian function.

[6c] S. Okuno, M. Inaba, Y. Nishizawa, and H. Morii, "Isolated ACTH deficiency associated with Hashimoto disease," *Nippon Rinsho,* Oct 1993, 51(10):2721–2725.

[6d] **Schmidt Syndrome:** A. Kasperlik-Zaluska, B. Czarnocka, and W. Czech, "High prevalence of thyroid autoimmunity in idiopathic Addison's disease," *Autoimmunity,* 1994, 18(3):213–216.

[6] **Addison's anemia:** T. Sasinska, M. Izbicka, and Kierat, "Association of primary autoimmune hypothyroidism with Addison's anemia," *Endokrynol Pol,* 1991, 42(3):407–413.

[8a] **Ovarian failure:** S. Savastano, A. P. Tommaselli, et al., "The ovary and the immune function: our experience," *Acta Neurol* (Napoli), Oct 1991, 13(5):442–447.

[8b] E. K. Muechler, K. E. Huang, and E. Schenk, "Autoimmunity in premature ovarian failure," *Int J Fertil,* Mar–Apr 1991, 36(2):99–103.

[8c] C. Betterle, A. Rossi, S. Dalla Pria, A. Artifoni, B. Pedini, S. Gavasso, and A. Caretto, "Premature ovarian failure: autoimmunity and natural history," *Clin Endocrinol* (Oxf), Jul 1993, 39(1):35–43. They studied the association of clinical and latent autoimmune diseases in different groups of women. They looked for the presence of circulating steroid-producing cell autoantibodies (SCA) in the following groups:

- **Group 1:** 50 females (age 16–39) with premature ovarian failure;
- **Group 2:** 3,677 females with autoimmune disease that was organ-specific, but the women did not have premature ovarian failure. This group was divided into subgroups:
- **Group 2a:** 99 women with Addison's disease (low adrenal function), alone or with other endocrine problems, or with hypoparathyroidism (low parathyroid);

• **Group 2b:** 3,578 women with insulin-dependent diabetes mellitus or thyroid autoimmune diseases.

Conclusions of the Study: The results confirmed the strong relationship between premature ovarian failure and other clinical autoimmune diseases, as well as the strong link existing between primary ovarian failure, Addison's disease, and antibodies to steroid-producing cells.

[8d] M. H. Mignot, J. Schoemaker, B. Kleingeld, et al., "Premature ovarian failure I: The association with autoimmunity," *Eur J Obstet Reprod Biol*, 1989, 30(59):461–462. Also see its companion article in *Eur J Obstet Reprod Biol*, 1989, 39(67).

[8e] P. Bannatyne, P. Russell, and R. P. Shearman, "Autoimmune oophoritis: a clinicopathologic assessment of 12 cases," *Int J Gynecol Pathol*, 1990, (9):3):191–207.

[9a] **Hypophysitis (swollen pituitary):** A. Mizuno, H. Wada, C. Hirose, M. Ishikawa, D. Tsujino, and K. Someya, "Case of primary hypothyroidism with pituitary enlargement treated by thyroid-hormone-supplement therapy," *Nippon Naika Gakkai Zasshi*, Jun 1994, 83(6): 988–989.

[9b] C. Adams, H. J. Dean, S. J. Israels, A. Patton, and D. H. Fewer, "Primary hypothyroidism with intracranial hypertension and pituitary hyperplasia," *Pediatr Neurol*, Mar 1994, 10(2):166–168.

[9c] Y. Ozawa and Y. Shishiba, "Recovery from lymphocytic hypophysitis associated with painless thyroiditis: clinical implications of circulating antipituitary antibodies," *Acta Endocrinol* (Copenh), June 1993, 128(6):493–498.

[9d] G. Fulcher, J. Roche, and A. McElduff, "Primary hypothyroidism with pituitary enlargement and a visual field abnormality," *Austras Radiol*, Feb 1992, 36(1):37–39.

[9e] O. P. Tadmor, I. Barr, and Y. Z. Diamant, "Primary hypothyroidism presenting with amenorrhea, galactorrhea, hyperprolactinemia and enlarged pituitary," *Harehuah*, Jan 1992, 122(2):76–78.

[9f] S. Natori, T. Karashima, S. Koga, et al., "A case report of idiopathic myxedema with secondary amenorrhea and hyperprolactinemia: effect of thyroid hormone replacement on reduction of pituitary enlargement and restoration of fertility," *Fukuoka Igaku Zasshi*, Aug 1991, 82(8):461–463.

[9g] R. Miranda-Ruiz, M. Chavez, et al., "Primary hypothyroidism associated with a chiasmatic syndrome simulating a prolactinoma," *Gac Med Mex*, Jan–Feb 1990, 126(1):51–54.

[9h] M. Chadli, L. Chaieb, M. Makhlouf, et al., "Hyperprolactinemia in primary hypothyroidism," *Tunis Med*, Jan 1989, 67(1):17–21.

[9i] J. L. Wemeau, D. Dewailly, et al., "Pseudoprolactinoma caused by subclinical hypothyroidism," *Presse Med*, Jan 1985, Jan 1985, 14(3):167.

[9j] S. Arlot, J. D. Lalau, B. Guerlin, and J. Quichaud, "Postpartum amenorrhea with hyperprolactinemia disclosing a transient hypothyroidism," [letter] *Presse Med*, Jan 1985, 14(1):48.

[9k] C. Christopoulos, "Primary hypothyroidism presenting as amenorrhoea and galactorrhea with hyperprolactinemia and pituitary enlargement," [letter] *Br Med J* (Clin Res Ed), Sept 1986, 293(6547):624–625.

[9l] P. J. Heyburn, O. M. Gibby, et al., "Primary hypothyroidism presenting as amenorrhea and galactorrhoea with hyperprolactinaemia and pituitary enlargement," *Br Med J*, Jun 1986, 292(6536):1660–1661.

[9m] L. H. Fish and C. N. Mariash, "Hyperprolactinemia, infertility, and hypothyroidism. A case report and literature review," *Arch Intern Med*, Mar 1988, 148(3):709–711.

[9n] M. R. Grubb, D. Chakeres, and W. B. Malarkey, "Patients with primary hypothyroidism presenting as prolactinomas," *Am J Med*, Oct 1987, 83(4):765–769.

[9o] L. Poretsky, J. Garber, and J. Kleefield, "Primary amenorrhea and pseudoprolactinoma in a patient with primary hypothyroidism. Reversal of clinical, biochemical, and radiologic abnormalities with levothyroxine," *Am J Med*, Jul 1986, 81(1):180–182.

[9p] L. Chaieb, M. Chadli-Chaieb, A. Chaieb, et al., "Primary amenorrhea-galactorrhea with hyperprolactinemia and huge pituitary enlargement in juvenile primary hypothyroidism," *Eur J Obstet Gynecol Reprod Biol*, Sep 1992, 46(2–3):159–162.

[10a] **Hypoparathyroidism:** Y. Sumida, M. Matsumura, H. Goto, et al., "A case of idiopathic hypoparathyroidism associated with primary hypothyroidism and diabetes mellitus," *Nippon Naibunpi Gakkai Zasshi*, Aug 1994, 70(6):609–614.

[10b] K. Yoshioka, A. Ohsawa, T. Yoshida, and S. Yokoh, "Insulin-dependent diabetes mellitus associated with Graves' disease and idiopathic hypoparathyroidism," *J Endocrinol Invest*, Sep 1993, 16(8):643–646.

[10c] E. R. McRorie, J. Chalmers, and I. W. Campbell, "Riedel's thyroiditis complicated by hypoparathyroidism and hypothyroidism," *Scott Med J*, Feb 1993, 38(1):27–28.

[11] **Graves' disease:** C. Osorio-Salazar, P. Lecomte, P. Madec, A. M. Madec, and J. L. Baulieu, "Basedow disease [a form of hyperthyroidism] following autoimmune primary hypothyroidism," *Ann Endocrinol* (Paris), 1994, 55(5):185–189.

[12] **Progressive ophthalmopathy:** J. R. Wall, N. Bernard, A. Boucher, et al., "Pathogenesis of thyroid-associated ophthalmopathy; and autoimmune disorder of the eye muscle associated with Graves' hyperthyroidism and Hashimoto's thyroiditis," *Clin Immunol Immunopathol*, Jul 1993, 68(1):1–8.

[13a] **Lupus erythematosus:** E. V. Hess, "Prevalence of antithyroid antibody in patients with systemic lupus erythematosus," [letter; comment] *J Rheumatol,* Aug 1991, 18(8):1193–1195.

[13b] M. Magaro, A. Zoli, L. Altomonte, et al., "The association of silent thyroiditis with active systemic lupus erythematosus," *Clin Exp Rheumatol,* Jan–Feb 1992, 10(1):67–70. This study says that autoimmune thyroid disorders have been shown to occur in patients with connective tissue diseases. Hypothyroidism and thyrotoxicosis have been recognized in system lupus erythematosus (SLE). Moreover a high prevalence of antithyroid antibodies has been found in patients with SLE. It concludes that there exists a mild hypothyroidism in SLE that is clinically silent. The altered thyroid function appears to be dependent on the activity of the systemic autoimmune process.

[13c] M. L. Boey, P. H. Fong, J. S. Lee, W. Y. Ng, and A. C. Thai, "Autoimmune thyroid disorders in SLE in Singapore," *Lupus,* Feb 1993, 2(1):51–54. This study states that there was a high prevalence in this group of antimicrosomal and antithyroglobulin antibodies (32.2%). Aberrations in thyroid function tests are common in SLE, but the incidence of thyroid failure is low.

[13d] M. M. Konstadoulakis, G. Kroubouzos, A. Tosca, et al., "Thyroid autoantibodies in the subsets of lupus erythematosus: correlation with other autoantibodies and thyroid function," *Thyroidol Clin Exp,* Apr 1993, 5(1):1–7.

[13e] M. Hashizuma, R. Okiyama, S. Orimo, et al., "Oculopharyngeal myopathy with autoimmune disease," *Rinsho Shinkeigaku,* Mar 1993, 33(3):334–337. This study links SLE, Hashimoto's disease, and other problems, and ascribes this to an autoimmune cause.

[13f] R. T. Tsai, T. C. Chang, C. R. Wang, et al., "Thyroid disorders in Chinese patients with systemic lupus erythematosus," *Rheumatol Int,* 1993, 13(1):9–13.

[14] **Multiple sclerosis:** P. Klapps, S. Seyfert, T. Fischer, and W. A. Scherbaum, "Endocrine function in multiple sclerosis," *Acta Neurol Scand,* May 1992, 85(5):353–357. Noted preclinical endocrine insufficiency including impairment of thyroid-stimulating hormone.

[15a] **Myasthenia gravis:** Y. L. Yu, B. R. Hawkins, M. S. Ip, et al., "Myasthenia gravis in Hong Kong Chinese. 1. Epidemiology and adult disease," *Acta Neurol Scand,* Aug 1992, 86(2):113–119. This study says that autoimmune thyroid disease was the most commonly associated disease in people with MG, along with diseases of the thymus.

[15b] S. Ichiki, C. Komatsu, H. Ogata, et al., "A case of myasthenia gravis complicated with hyperthyroidism and thymic hyperplasia in childhood," *Brain Dev,* May–Jun 1993, 15(3):246.

[15c] H. Y. Chu, S. G. Shu, S. C. Mak, and C. S. Chi, "Graves' disease associated with myasthenia gravis: report of one case," *Acta Paediatr Sin,* Nov–Dec 1992, 33(6):457–461.

[16a] **Rheumatoid arthritis:** V. Taneja, R. R. Singh, A. N. Malaviya, et al., "Occurrence of autoimmune diseases and relationship of autoantibody ex-

pression with HLA phenotypes in multicase rheumatoid arthritis families," *Scand J Rheumatol*, 1933, 22(4):152–157.

[16b] G. Bianchi, G. Marchesini, et al., "Thyroid involvement in chronic inflammatory rheumatological disorders," *Clin Rheumatol*, Dec 1993, 12(4):479–484.

[16c] P. Caron, S. Lassoued, C. Dromer, et al., "Prevalence of thyroid abnormalities in patients with rheumatoid arthritis," *Thyroid Clin Exp*, Dec 1992, 4(3):99–102.

[16d] J. B. Shiroky, M. Cohen, M. L. Ballachey, and C. Neville, "Thyroid dysfunction in rheumatoid arthritis: a controlled prospective survey," *An Rheum Dis*, Jun 1993, 52(6):454–456. Concludes that thyroid dysfunction is seen at least three times more often in women with RA than in women with similar demographic features with noninflammatory rheumatic diseases such as osteoarthritis and fibromyalgia.

[16e] S. Sakata, K. NagaiK, T. Shibata, et al., "A case of rheumatoid arthritis associated with silent thyroiditis," *J Endocrinol Invest*, May 1992, 15(5):377–380.

[16f] C. M. Deighton, A. Fay, D. J. Walker, "Rheumatoid arthitis in thyroid disease positive and negative same-sexed sibships," *Br J Rheumatol*, Jan 1992, 31(1):13–17.

[16g] Y. Yamada, K. Kuroe, "A case of rheumatoid arthritis complicated with idiopathic thrombocytopenic purpura and Hashimoto's disease," *Ryumachi*, Aug 1991, 31(4):413–419.

[16h] M. P. Spina, A. Cerri, V. Piacentini, et al., "Seronegative hashitoxicosis in patient with rheumatoid arthritis," *Minerva Endocrinol*, Jul–Sep 1980, 15(3):173–176. This study states that Hashimoto's thyroiditis is known to occur in conjunction with other autoimmune disorders including rheumatoid arthritis. The occurrence of these autoimmune diseases in individual patients suggests an imbalance in immune function which affects more than one organ system. The predisposition to this spectrum of autoimmune diseases may be genetically determined, with specific HLA haplotypes associated with a variety of autoimmune diseases. However there can be an association of the diseases without there being a systemic autoimmune problem.

[16i] V. G. Sereriakov, Z. S. Alekberova, et al., "The characteristics of the course of rheumatoid arthritis combined with thyroid pathology," *Ter Arkh*, 1990, 62(5):48–51.

[16j] F. Herrmann, K. Hambsch, et al., "Incidence of goiter and thyroiditis in chronic inflammatory rheumatism," *Z Gesamte Inn Med*, Jn 1990, 45(2):52–55. This study found a clearly higher prevalence of goiter in women with RA, but not among men.

[17a] **Sjøgren's Syndrome:** B. U. Hansen, U. B. Ericsson, V. Henricsson, et al., "Autoimmune thyroiditis and primary Sjøgren's syndrome: clinical and laboratory evidence of the coexistence of the two diseases," *Clin Exp Rheumatol*, Mar–Apr 1991, 9(2):137–141.

[17b] G. T. Ko, C. C. Chow, V. T. Yeung, H. Chan, and C. S. Cockram, "Hashimoto's thyroiditis, Sjøgren's syndrome and orbital lymphoma," *Postgrad Med J*, Jun 1994, 70(822):448–451.

[17c] B. Gudbjornsson, A. Karlsson-Parra, et al., "Clinical and laboratory features of Sjøgren's syndrome in young women with previous postpartum thyroiditis," *J Rheumatol*, Feb 1994, 21(2):215–219.

[17d] E. A. Sycheva and T. S. Khein, "A case of Sjøgren's disease associated with autoimmune thyroiditis," *Probl Endokrinol* (Mosk), Jan–Feb 1994, 40(1):30–31.

[17e] S. Yamazaki, I. Katayama, et al., "Acral ichthosiform mucinosis in association with Sjøgren's syndrome: a peculiar form of pretibial myxedema?" *J Dermatol*, Nov 1993, 20(11):715–718.

[17f] H. Foster, A. Fay, C. Kelly, P. Charles, D. Walker, and I. Griffiths "Thyroid disease and other autoimmune phenomena in a family study of primary Sjøgren's syndrome," *Br J Rheumatol*, Jan 1993, 32(1):36–40.

[17g] G. Warfvinge, A. Larsson, V. Henricsson, et al., "Salivary gland involvement in autoimmune thyroiditis, with special reference to the degree of association with Sjøgren's syndrome," *Oral Surg Oral Med Oral Patho*, Sep 1992, 74(3):288–293. It concludes that significant involvement of salivary glands may occur in cases of autoimmune thyroiditis, which indicates that common mechanisms may frequently be operative in the development of thyroid and salivary gland immune disease.

[17h] M. Bouanani, R. Bataille, et al., "Autoimmunity to human thyroglobulin. Respective epitopic specificity patterns of anti-human thyroglobulin autoantibodies in patients with Sjøgren's syndrome and patients with Hashimoto's thyroiditis," *Arthritis Rheum*, Dec 1991, 34(12):1585–1593.

[18a] **Pernicious anemia:** S. J. Wang, T. Shohat, C. Vadheim, W. Shellow, J. Edwards, and J. I. Rotter, "Increased risk for type I (insulin-dependent) diabetes in relatives of patients with alopecia areata (AA)," *Am J Med Genet*, Jul 1994, 51(3):234–239. This study links thyroid disease, vitiligo, Addison's disease, and pernicious anemia.

[18b] N. J. Sheehan and K. Stanton-King, "Polyautoimmunity in a young woman," *Br J Rheumatol*, Mar 1993, 32(3):254–256. This study presents a young woman with rheumatoid arthritis, pernicious anemia, Hashimoto's thyroiditis, systemic sclerosis, insulin-dependent diabetes mellitus, and other autoimmune problems. A family study showed rheumatoid arthritis, pernicious anemia, and diabetes mellitus among her close relatives. The study shows the clinical and immunological links between the different autoimmune diseases.

[18c] N. Suzuki, R. Mitamura, H. Ohmi, Y. Itoh, et al., "Hashimoto thyroiditis, distal renal tubular acidosis, pernicious anaemia and encephalopathy: a rare combination of autoimmune disorders in a 12-year-old girl," *Eur J Pediatr*, Feb 1994, 153(2):78–79.

[19a] **Atrophic Gastritis:** M. Certo, A. Mancini, C. Fiumara, et al., "Gastroenterologic pathology and replacement organotherapy in thyroidectomized patients," *Minerva Clin*, Nov 1993, 48((21–22):1319–1323. This study underlines the frequent association of gastroenteric disease and hypothyroidism.

[19b] P. Burman, O. Kampe, W. Kraaz, et al., "A study of autoimmune gastritis in the postpartum period and at a 5-year follow-up," *Gastroenterology*, Sep 1992, 103(3):934–942.

[20a] **Chronic Active Hepatitis:** A. Tran, J. F. Quaranta, C. Beusnel, V. Thiers, et al. Hepatitis C virus and Hashimoto's thyroiditis. *Eur J Med*, May 1992, 1(2):116–118. They report two cases of Hashimoto's thyroiditis associated with chronic active hepatitis (HCV). Their data suggest that HCV infection might be involved in this autoimmune disease.

[20b] D. Pateron, D. J. Hartmann, J. C. Cuclos-Vallee, et al., "Latent autoimmune thyroid disease in patients with chronic HCV hepatitis," [letter] *J Hepatol*, Mar 1993, 17(3):417–419, and *J Hepatol*, Sep 1992, 16(1)–2):244–245.

[20c] M. Tomsic, V. Ferlan-Marolt, T. Kveder, et al., "Mixed connective tissue disease associated with autoimmune hepatitis and thyroiditis," *An Rheum Dis* Apr 1992, 51(4):544–546.

[20d] T. M. Michele, J. Fleckenstein, et al., "Chronic active hepatitis in the type I polyglandular autoimmune syndrome," *Postgrad Med J*, Feb 1994, 70(820):128–131.

[20e] A. Tran, J. F. Quaranta, et al., "High prevalence of thyroid autoantibodies in a prospective series of patients with chronic hepatitis C before interferon therapy."

[21] **Primary Biliary Cirrhosis:** M. Horita, N. Takahashi, M. Seike, S. Nasu, R. Takaki, "A case of primary biliary cirrhosis associated with Hashimoto's thyroiditis, scleroderma, and Sjøgren's syndrome," *Intern Med*, Mar 1992, 31(3):418–421.

[21a] F. Gaches, P. Sauvage, E. Vidal, et al., "Multiple autoimmune syndrome," *Rev Med Interne*, Mar 1993, 14(3):177–178. Reports a case of multiple autoimmune syndrome with autoimmune thyroiditis, Sjøgren's syndrome, and primary biliary cirrhosis.

[21b] M. Horita, N. Takahashi, et al., "A case of primary biliary cirrhosis associated with Hashimoto's thyroiditis, scleroderma and Sjøgren's syndrome," *Intern Med*, Mar 1992, 31(3):418–421.

[22a] C. E. Counsell, A. Taha, et al., "Coeliac disease and autoimmune thyroid disease," *Gut* Jun 1994, 35(6):844–846. This study reports that 14 percent of their coeliac patients had thyroid disorders. This is a clinically important association.

[22b] P. Collin, T. Reunala, et al., "Coeliac disease—associated disorders and survival," *Gut*, Sep 1994, 35(9):1215–1218.

[22c] R. Lazzari, A. Collina, et al., "Celiac disease and autoimmune thyroiditis. Description of a case," *Pediatr Med Chir,* May–Jun 1992, 14(3):339–340. This study reports that there is more than a fortuitous association between coeliac disease and a whole range of autoimmune conditions, and mentions a young girl with both coeliac disease and autoimmune thyroiditis.

[23a] **Vitiligo:** L. Hegedus, M. Heidenheim, M. Gervil, et al., "High frequency of thyroid dysfunction in patients with vitiligo," *Acta Derm Venereol,* (Stockh), Mar 1994, 74(2):120–123.

[23b] L. G. Curti, M. Siccardi, et al., "Full-blown hypothyroidism associated with vitiligo and acropachy," *Thyroidol Clin Exp,* Dec 1992, 4(3):111–114.

[23c] Y. K. Shong and J. A. Kim, "Vitiligo in autoimmune thyroid disease," *Thyroidol Clin Exp,* May 1991, 3(2):89–91.

[23d] A. Torrelo, A. Espana, J. Balsa, and A. Ledo, "Vitiligo and polyglandular autoimmune syndrome with selective IgA," *Int J Dermatol,* May 1992, 31(5):343–344.

[24a] **Alopecia:** H. Pasaoglu, U. Soyuer, M. Astaal, "Thyroid antibodies in alopecia totalis," *Cent Afr J Med,* Oct 1991, 37(10):337–339.

[24b] S. J. Wang, T. Shohat, C. Vadheim, et al., "Increased risk for type I (insulin-dependent) diabetes in relatives of patients with alopecia areata (AA)," *Am J Med Genet,* Jul 1994, 51(3):234–239. States the commonality of thyroid disease, vitiligo, Addison's disease, pernicious anemia, and alopecia areata. States that AA protects these women from diabetes mellitus (there is a strong incidence of it in other relatives with no alopecia).98

[24c] **Chronic Mucocutaneous Candidiasis:** T. Appleboom and F. Flowers, "Ketoconazole in the treatment of chronic mucocutaneous candidiasis secondary to autoimmune polyendocrinopathy-candidiasis syndrome," *Cutis,* 1982, 30:71–72.

[25a] K. Arulanantham, J. M. Dwyer, and M. Genel, "Evidence for defective immunoregulation in the syndrome of familial candidiasis endocrinopathy," *N Engl J Med,* 1978, 300(4):164–168.

[25b] F. Segawa, H. Yamada, H. Tomi, et al., "A case of autoimmune polyglandular deficiency associated with progressive myopathy," *Rinsho Shinkeigaku,* May 1992, 32(5):501–505. This studies a 29-year-old woman with autoimmune polyglandular deficiency with progressive myopathy (muscle disease). She had mucocutaneous candidiasis at age 3, primary hypothyroidism at age 12, insulin-dependent diabetes at age 27, and adrenal insufficiency at age 29 years.

[25c] G. Proto, S. Leoni, I. Torossi, et al., "Autoimmune polyendocrinopathy and chronic mucocutaneous candidiasis," *Minerva Med,* Jul–Aug 1992, 83(7–8):475–478. This study states that a chronic mucocutaneous infection due to candida yeasts can be part of the autoimmune polyglandular syndrome. The authors describe a young patient with mucocutaneous candidiasis, hypoparathyroidism, and adrenal insufficiency. Candidiasis was first

diagnosed in early childhood, followed by hypoparathyroidism at age 4, and adrenal insufficiency at age 5.

[26a] **There are many other unusual linkages of other autoimmune problems.** For example, N. J. Sheehan and K. Stanton-King, "Polyautoimmunity in a young woman," *Ibid.*, (see footnote 18).

[26b] O. Fain, M. Rainfray, P. Callard, et al., "Dermatopolymyositis, Gourgerot-Sjøgren's syndrome, Hashimoto's thyroiditis, and glomerulopathy," *Nephrologie*, 1990, 11(4):223–225.

[26c] P. Collin, J. Salmi, O. Hallstrom, T. Reunala, and A. Pasternack, "Autoimmune thyroid disorders and coeliac disease," *Eur J Endocrinol*, Feb 1994, 130(2):137–140.

[26d] N. Kojima, S. Sakata, S. Nakamura, K. Nagai, et al., "Serum concentrations of osteocalcin in patients with hyperthyroidism, hypothyroidism, and subacute thyroiditis," *J Endocrinol Invest*, Jul–Aug 1992, 15(7):491–496.

[26e] K. I. Papadopoulos and B. Hallengren, "Polyglandular autoimmune type III associated with coeliac disease and sarcoidosis," *J Intern Med*, Dec 1994, 236(6):661–663.

[26f] G. Leibowitz, G. Amir, I. S. Losses, R. Eliakim, "Autoimmune polyglandular failure associated with malabsorption and gastric carcinoid tumour."

[26g] F. Segawa, H. Yamada, H. Tomi, et al., "A case of autoimmune polyglandular deficiency associated with progressive myopathy," *Ibid.*, (see footnote 25).

[27] Note P. Bosze, "Autoimmune ovarian inflammation," *Orv Hetil*, Jun 1994, 135(26):1403–1410. This article says that autoimmune oophoritis, which is frequently associated with other autoimmune diseases, including other endocrine glands (autoimmune polyglandular syndrome), may precede the associated disease by several years. The clinical significance of this association has increasingly been emphasized. The report urges early diagnosis since early initiation of replacement therapy can be life-saving. The article says this subject should be of interest not only for gynecologists but for internists, general practitioners, and others.

[28] Dr. Richard Bronson, "Immunology of hypergonadotropic ovarian dysfunction: etiology and diagnosis," presented at the Fourth Annual North American Menopause Society meeting in San Diego, California, September 2–4, 1993.

[29] C. Betterle, A. Rossi, S. Dalla Pria, A. Artifoni, B. Pedini, S. Gavasso, A. Caretto, "Premature ovarian failure: autoimmunity and natural history," *Clin endocrinol* (Oxf), Jul 1993, 39(1):35–43. They studied the association of clinical and latent autoimmune diseases in different groups of women. They looked for the presence of circulating steroid-producing cell autoantibodies (SCA) in the following groups:

- **Group 1**: 50 females (age 16–39) with premature ovarian failure.
- **Group 2**: 3,677 females with autoimmune disease that was organ-specific, but the women did not have premature ovarian failure. This group was divided into number of subgroups:

- **Group 2a**: 99 women with Addison's disease (low adrenal function) alone or with other endocrine problems, or with hypoparathyroidism (low parathyroid);

- **Group 2b**: 3,578 women with insulin-dependent diabetes mellitus or thyroid autoimmune diseases.

Conclusions of the study: The results confirmed the strong relationship between premature ovarian failure and other clinical autoimmune diseases, as well as the strong link existing between primary ovarian failure, Addison's disease and antibodies to steroid-producing cells.

[30] M.H. Mignot, J. Schoemaker, B. Kleingeld, et al., "Premature ovarian failure I: The association with autoimmunity," *Eur J Obstet Reprod Biol,* 1989, 30(59):461–462. See also companion article in *Eur J Obstet Reprod Biol,* 1989, 39(67).

INDEX

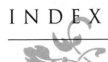